RADIOLOGY

FOR THE

DENTAL PROFESSIONAL

RADIOLOGY

FOR THE

DENTAL PROFESSIONAL

NINTH EDITION

Herbert H. Frommer BA, DDS, FACD
Diplomat of the American Board of Oral and Maxillofacial Radiology
Professor Emeritus of Radiology
New York University
College of Dentistry
New York, New York

Jeanine J. Stabulas-Savage RDH, BS, MPH
Assistant Clinical Professor of Radiology
New York University
College of Dentistry
New York, New York

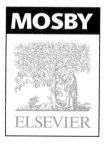

MOSBY

ELSEVIER

MOSBY
ELSEVIER

3251 Riverport Lane
St. Louis, Missouri 63043

RADIOLOGY FOR THE DENTAL PROFESSIONAL,
NINTH EDITION

ISBN: 978-0-323-06401-9

Notice

Neither the Publisher nor the Authors assume any responsibility for any loss or injury and/or damage to persons or property arising out of or related to any use of the material contained in this book. It is the responsibility of the treating practitioner, relying on independent expertise and knowledge of the patient, to determine the best treatment and method of application for the patient.

The Publisher

Library of Congress Cataloging-in-Publication Data
Frommer, Herbert H., 1933-
    Radiology for the dental professional. – 9th ed. / Herbert H. Frommer, Jeanine J. Stabulas-Savage.
        p. ; cm.
    Includes bibliographical references and index.
    ISBN 978-0-323-06401-9 (pbk. : alk. paper) 1. Teeth–Radiography. I. Stabulas-Savage, Jeanine J.
II. Title.
    [DNLM: 1. Radiography, Dental. 2. Technology, Radiologic. WN 230 F932r 2011]
    RK309.F76 2011
    617.6'07572–dc22

                                                                                    2010001726

Vice President and Publisher: Linda Duncan
Executive Editor: John Dolan
Developmental Editor: Joslyn Dumas
Publishing Services Manager: Julie Eddy
Project Manager: Marquita Parker
Designer: Paula Catalano

Printed in United States

Last digit is the print number: 9   8   7   6   5   4   3   2   1

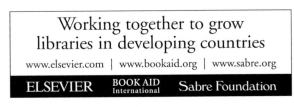

Working together to grow
libraries in developing countries

www.elsevier.com | www.bookaid.org | www.sabre.org

ELSEVIER   BOOK AID International   Sabre Foundation

For my grandchildren,
EVAN, ADAM, and ARIELLA FROMMER.

For my darling daughters,
VALERIE JUDITH and VANESSA THERESE SAVAGE,
whose inspiration lights up my world.

Preface

As we sit here planning the ninth edition of this textbook we are overwhelmed by the changes in dental radiology since the first edition was published. We have grown from a textbook consisting of nine chapters and 160 pages to our present textbook of 25 Chapters and over 500 pages with an accompanying Study Guide and Instructor's Resource Manual. In addition, this text is currently augmented by a related computer resource. One has to be impressed with the changes that have taken place both in the fields of Radiology and specifically in Dental Radiology. The ninth edition now includes increased mention of utilization of faster speed film, rectangular collimation, Cone Beam Tomography, automatic processing, digital radiography, recognition by the American Dental Association of Dental Radiology as a specialty, the advent of established Dental Radiology private practice, implant placement, concern with radiation protection and the universal use of the Paralleling technique. We feel that we are a part of these monumental advancements and hope to reflect this in the current edition of our textbook.

Once again, we have some words of thanks for our families and colleagues who have encouraged and helped us in preparing the ninth edition. We could not have completed the manuscript without the help of our colleagues here at NYU, Drs. Rajinder Jain, Alan Friedman, Debra Ferraiolo, Shailesh Kottal, Lewis Lampert, Milton Palet and our chairperson Dr. Joan Phelan. A special recognition goes to the President of New York University, Dr. John Sexton; the former Dean of the College of Dentistry and present Executive Vice President of the University, Michael C. Alfano; the Dean of New York University's College of Dentistry, Charles N. Bertolami; and the Vice Dean of New York University's College of Dentistry, Richard Vogel, for creating an academic environment that encourages and supports faculty scholarship.

Finally, to our spouses Eleanor Frommer and John Paul Savage, without whose encouragement, patience, and support this project could not have been completed.

Herbert H. Frommer
Jeanine J. Stabulas-Savage

Contents

CHAPTER 1

Ionizing Radiation and Basic Principles of X-Ray Generation

CHAPTER OUTLINE

EDUCATIONAL OBJECTIVES

1. Understand the nature and production of ionizing radiation.
2. Be able to apply these concepts and principles to clinical radiography.

KEY TERMS

anode
atom
atomic number
binding energy
bremsstrahlung
cathode
cathode ray
duty cycle
duty rating
electromagnetic
    radiation

electromagnetic spectrum
electron
focal spot (area)
ionization
isotope
molecule
neutron
nucleus
photon
proton
radiation

radioactive
radionuclide
shell
target
thermionic emission effect
wavelength
x-rays

RADIATION

Radiation is the emission and propagation of energy through space or a substance in the form of waves or particles. Particulate radiation consists of atoms or subatomic particles that have mass and travel at high speeds to transmit their kinetic energy. Some examples of particulate radiation are electrons (sometimes called beta particles), protons, neutrons, and alpha particles. Particulate radiations most commonly are emitted from radioactive substances called **radionuclides**. *The term radiation should not be confused with radioactive, which is the process whereby certain unstable elements undergo spontaneous degeneration and produce high-energy waves called gamma and particulate radiations. Dental radiology deals with x-radiations. However, patients who are undergoing cancer therapy may receive radiation from radioactive materials.*

X-rays are invisible waves or bundles of energy that possess certain properties that allow practitioners to see differences in densities in opaque objects, among other things. The use of x-rays is an intricate and essential part of dental diagnosis and is applied in many of the diagnostic imaging systems in both dentistry and medicine. The images produced are seen on either film or a digital display device and *should be* referred to as radiographs or images but not as "x-rays." X-rays are energy waves with no mass and are part of a grouping called electromagnetic radiation.

ELECTROMAGNETIC SPECTRUM

The electromagnetic spectrum is a grouping of energy waves that has in common the weightlessness of the waves and the speed at which they travel (186,000 miles per second). The individual radiations of the spectrum differ in their wavelengths and frequencies and thus in many of their properties. Those with shorter wavelengths and higher frequencies have more photon energy. Looking at Figure 1-1, the reader can immediately recognize energy waves that are encountered every day.

It is not known whether these electromagnetic radiations are actually waves of energy or the individual units of energy called photons. Some phenomena can be best explained using the wave theory and others by considering the theory of discrete units of energy. If the radiation is considered a wave, its length is measured in angstrom units. If it is considered a bundle of photon energy, it can be measured in ergs. This text uses both forms, sometimes referring to waves of energy and at other times to photons of energy.

An energy wave travels in the same way that a ripple crosses a body of still water. The height of the wave is called the crest, and the depth of the wave is called the trough. The distance from one crest to another is called the wavelength and is usually abbreviated with the Greek letter lambda (λ). The frequency of a wave is the number of oscillations per unit of time (Figure 1-2). The wavelength of x-rays is very short and is measured in angstrom units, which are 1/100,000,000 of a centimeter and can be expressed as 10–8 cm.

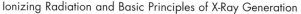

Measured in angstrom units

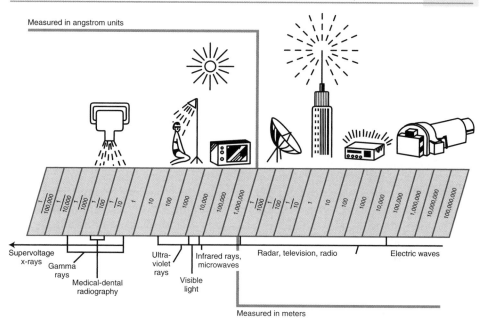

Measured in meters

Figure 1-1. Electromagnetic spectrum. The shorter, more energized waves to the left are measured in angstrom units; the longer waves are measured in meters.

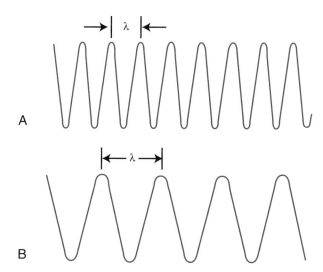

A

B

Figure 1-2. X-ray energy wave. The distance between the two crests is the wavelength lambda (λ) and the number of oscillations is the frequency. Wave A has a shorter wavelength and a higher frequency than does B.

The difference in the electromagnetic spectrum between visible light and x-rays is their wavelengths; x-rays have shorter wavelengths. The shorter the wavelength and the greater the frequency, the more energy it bears. This energy gives the x-ray the ability to penetrate matter—specifically, the teeth, bones, and gingiva of the dental patient—as well as cause ionization in tissue. Light waves cannot penetrate teeth and bone because the wavelength is too long and does not have sufficient energy.

The effect of electromagnetic radiation on living organisms varies depending on the wavelength. Television and radio waves, which are ever-present in the atmosphere, have no effect on human tissue. Microwaves, which are low-energy radiations, can produce heat within organic tissues and are so employed in microwave ovens. Microwaves do not have enough energy to be ionizing and therefore do not have the same effects on living tissue as x-rays, gamma rays, or particulate radiations. Electromagnetic radiations that are too low in energy to cause ionization are employed in magnetic resonance imaging (MRI) for diagnostic purposes. These radiations are located in Figure 1-1 near the radio waves.

Figure 1-1 also shows that there is an overlap between gamma rays and the x-rays used for diagnostic purposes in medicine and dentistry because the two have identical wavelengths. Gamma rays and x-rays have identical properties if their wavelengths are the same; they differ only in their source. X-rays are the result of electron and atomic interactions within an x-ray tube, whereas gamma rays originate in the nuclei of radioactive materials.

Ultrasonic radiation, which is not part of the electromagnetic spectrum, is another type of radiation used in medicine, and dental patients often question dentists about its use and relationship to dental x-rays. Ultrasound is a nonelectromagnetic, nonionizing radiation, with no effect on tissue, that can be used to image internal structures. Because it is nonionizing, its use is acceptable in cases in which ionizing radiation might prove harmful (e.g., fetal imaging in pregnant women).

To explain the energy aspect of radiation, take the example of throwing a ball. Energy is imparted to the ball, which is expressed by the speed with which the ball travels. As this energy is lost, the ball falls, hits the ground, and rolls to a stop. The total energy is lost when the ball stops. This is also true of radiation. As x-rays travel over a distance, they lose their energy. For this reason, in the dental office the operator stands a safe distance (6 ft) away from the patient being exposed to x-rays to avoid any exposure. If the ball is caught in midair, the energy can be felt by the impact on the hand catching the moving ball. The impact of the ball is in part a product of the weight of the ball and the speed with which it was thrown. X-rays and other radiations have no weight; they have only speed and energy, but their effect is as tangible as the sting of the ball on the hand. This effect is produced by interaction with the basic unit of matter, the atom, and the resultant ionization, which may adversely affect living tissue.

A preliminary understanding of x-rays and x-ray generation can be acquired simply by visualizing the everyday office procedure of taking a radiograph of a patient. The patient is seated in the dental chair and draped with a lead apron. Following the infection control protocol, which is described in Chapter 9, a film packet or a digital sensor in a holding device is positioned in the patient's mouth. An activating switch already has turned on the dental x-ray machine (Figure 1-3). The open-ended, position-indicating device then is aimed at the film packet or sensor in the patient's mouth. The operator leaves the room or stands 6 ft away. Radiation is produced for the desired length of time, and the film is exposed by pressing a button attached to an electric cord leading to the x-ray machine. The film is then processed and interpreted.

From this description, some important observations can be made on the properties of x-rays. X-rays are produced by a machine whose source of energy is electricity; x-rays are produced by pushing a button that completes an electric circuit. Because no sign of x-ray production is apparent during the interval of exposure, x-rays must be invisible. The x-ray beam is directed at the film packet or sensor, so x-rays must travel in straight lines.

The ability of x-rays to produce an image on a film packet inside a patient's mouth by a machine positioned outside the mouth indicates that x-rays can penetrate an opaque structure such as skin, teeth, or bone.

After penetrating the dense tissue, x-rays can produce an effect on an imaging system, such as the dental film or sensor placed in the patient's mouth. This effect becomes visible by processing the film in the darkroom or computer imaging so that an image of the penetrated structures appears on the film or screen.

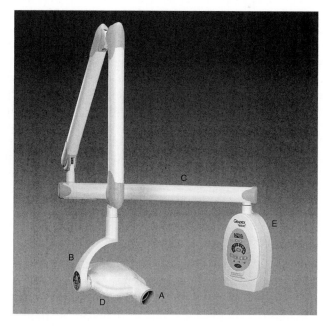

Figure 1-3. Dental x-ray machine. **A,** Position-indicating device. **B,** Yoke. **C,** Arm. **D,** Tube head. **E,** Control panel. *(Courtesy KaVo Dental/GENDEX Imaging, Lake Zurich, IL.)*

Because x-rays produce undesirable effects, the patient is draped with a lead apron and collar for protection, and the operator either leaves the room or stands 6 ft away from the machine or behind a suitable barrier during the exposure.

In summary, the following properties of x-rays have been observed:

1. X-rays are produced by the conversion of electric energy into radiation.
2. X-rays are invisible.
3. X-rays travel in straight lines.
4. X-rays can penetrate opaque tissues and structures.
5. X-rays can affect a photographic emulsion or digital sensors, which, when processed, produce a visible image.
6. X-rays can adversely affect human tissue.

HISTORY OF X-RAYS

It has been more than 110 years since the discovery of x-rays, and radiation can be best appreciated and understood by looking at the history of the discovery and development of x-rays. One can also learn about the hardships and injuries sustained by the early radiation workers and how far science has come in reducing radiation exposure to patients and practitioners alike while improving diagnostic capabilities.

The x-ray was discovered on November 8, 1895, by Wilhelm Conrad Roentgen, a professor of physics at the University of Würzburg in Germany. He was working with a vacuum tube called a *Hittorf-Crookes tube*, through which an electric current from a battery was flowing (Figure 1-4). Roentgen, like many of his colleagues, was interested in the cathode ray and the type of light produced across a vacuum tube when an electric current was applied. Because he was concerned with light, he was working in a darkened room with black cardboard covering the Hittorf-Crookes tube, and there were many fluorescent plates in his laboratory. Thus the stage was set for a discovery that would aid medical and dental science and has been ranked in importance with the discoveries of Pasteur, Lister, and Wells and Morton.

One evening while working in his darkened laboratory, Roentgen noticed that one of the fluorescent plates at the far side of the room was glowing. He quickly realized that something coming from the Hittorf-Crookes tube was striking the fluorescent plate and causing it to glow. Because he did not know what it was, he called the phenomenon x-ray, *x* being the algebraic designation for the unknown. He also noted that when he moved the plate closer to the tube, the glow grew stronger and, conversely, when the distance increased, it weakened. This observation made over 110 years ago is the basis of today's "inverse square law," which is dealt with in later chapters. By placing various objects in the path of the x-ray beam, he could produce images on the screen. He inadvertently placed his hand between the tube and the screen and saw the faint outline of the bones of his hand. Roentgen went on to expose and produce images on photographic plates. Some of the first

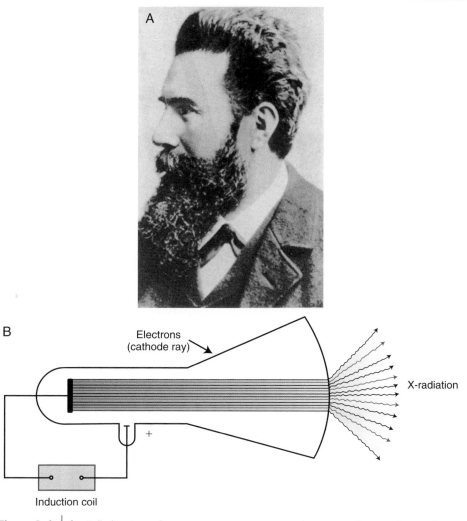

Figure 1-4. | **A,** Wilhelm Conrad Roentgen (1845 to 1923), discoverer of x-rays. **B,** Crookes tube, which Roentgen worked with at the time he discovered x-rays in 1895.

radiographs Roentgen took were of his wife's hand with a 15-minute exposure (Figure 1-5) and his shotgun. Thus the first medical and industrial use of x-radiation was seen. It is interesting to note how closely the essential parts of Roentgen's tube and the modern x-ray tube resemble each other. They both are highly exhausted vacuum tubes with an anode and a cathode through which an electric current passes. Roentgen's tube had a fixed number of electrons available, in contrast to the present variable source (milliamperage), and the potential across his tube was fixed, whereas today it is variable (kilovoltage).

Within a few weeks of his discovery, Roentgen presented a paper titled "On a New Kind of Rays: A Preliminary Communication." In January 1896

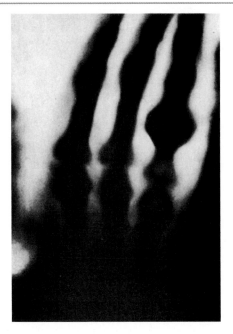

Figure 1-5. | Radiograph taken of the hand of Mrs. Wilhelm Conrad Roentgen in 1895. (*From Goaz PW, White SC: Oral radiology and principles of interpretation, ed 2, St Louis, 1987, Mosby.*)

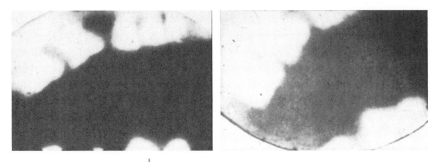

Figure 1-6. | Early radiographs taken by Dr. Walkhoff.

Dr. Otto Walkhoff, a dentist in Braunschweig, Germany, made the first dental use of an x-ray, a radiograph of a lower premolar (Figure 1-6).

He used a small glass photographic plate wrapped in black paper and covered with rubber that he placed in his own mouth while lying on the floor. The exposure time was 25 minutes. Because of the plate's position in his mouth, the image showed parts of the upper and lower teeth and he was actually taking a bitewing radiograph. This was followed in February 1896 by the work of physicist Walter Koenig, who obtained a clearer image using only 9 minutes of exposure. Today, for comparable exposure, about one tenth of a second (six impulses) would be used.

Interestingly Roentgen's work was not greeted with universal acclaim because the potential for diagnosis of disease was overshadowed by the public's concern about "something that could see through people's clothing." His discovery was exploited by many who commercialized the use of x-rays. There were x-ray parlors in the United States in which individuals could have an image made of any part of their body made suitable for framing. These images were often referred to as *skiagraphs* from the Greek word meaning "shadow pictures." At the same time in Victorian England, Roentgen was vilified for inventing a machine that could see through women's dresses.

For many years the science of imaging with the use of x-rays was called *roentgenology*. His name is still used today, expressing the amount of x-ray exposure in roentgens. For his work in the discovery of x-rays, Roentgen was awarded the first Nobel Prize in physics in 1901. Roentgen died in 1923.

The announcement of Roentgen's discovery was reported in the United States in 1896, and within 2 days, Thomas Alva Edison and his staff at Menlo Park, New Jersey, had duplicated Roentgens' work. One of Edison's assistants was the first person to die as a result of repeated radiation experiments on himself and demonstrations on patients. Edison himself noted the development of redness around his eyes. He discontinued his work with radiation and developed a fear of radiation that stayed with him for the rest of his life.

Dr. C. Edmund Kells, a New Orleans dentist, is credited with taking the first intraoral radiographs in the United States in April 1896. He had read about Roentgen's work and the new rays and immediately recognized its potential use in dentistry. Within a year, he set about acquiring the electrical equipment needed to produce the voltage necessary to charge the vacuum tubes available. He assembled all the equipment in Asheville, North Carolina, and gave the first demonstration of the use of x-rays before the Southern Dental Society. He used a variety of glass tubes, depending on the extent of the vacuum, age of the patient, and weather conditions to make his choice. Because the hand-blown tubes were not standardized, the usual way for him to determine which tube was best for any procedure on a given day was to place his hand between the tube and a hand-held fluoroscope and "set the tube" in that manner. This setting of the tube could take a considerable amount of time, and as a consequence Kells developed radiation burns that led to amputation of his fingers, then his hand, and finally his arm. These injuries led to his committing suicide.

Another early worker with intraoral radiographs was William Rollins, who developed the first dental x-ray unit in 1896. Many of the early workers with dental x-rays suffered from effects of their work. Rollins reported burns to the skin on his hands and recommended lead shielding of both the tube and the patient.

It was not until 1913 that film was used instead of glass photographic plates to record dental images. Dr. Frank Van Woert, a New York dentist, was one of the first dentists to use and lecture about the new Kodak dental film.

Dr. Howard Riley was the first to introduce radiology into the dental school curriculum at the University of Indiana. He also invented the dental bitewing.

The next great breakthrough was in 1913 when William D. Coolidge invented the hot-cathode x-ray tube, which is the prototype of x-ray tubes used today. The hot filament provided a variable source of electrons in the tube and eliminated the need for residual gas as a source for ionization in the tube.

Also in 1913 the first American dental x-ray machine was manufactured. In 1923 the Victor X-ray Corporation, which later became General Electric X-ray Corporation and now Gendex Corporation, introduced a dental x-ray machine with a Coolidge tube in the head of the unit cooled by oil immersion.

The x-rays were produced in Roentgen's vacuum tube by the electric current applied to the tube, which caused ionization of the gas molecules in the tube; that is, the neutral molecules were broken into negative and positive ions. Because of the difference in electric potential, the negative particles (electrons) were attracted to the positive side of the tube, where they collided with the tube wall, and x-rays were produced. Modern dental x-ray tubes employ the same principle with some modifications, the most significant being a higher voltage, or difference in potential across the tube, and a variable source of electrons (hot filament). Today's tubes also have radiation safety features and cooling devices.

Atomic Structure

To understand x-ray production and the effect of radiation on tissue, the basic structure of matter (Figure 1-7) must be understood. All matter is made of molecules. A molecule is the smallest particle of a substance that retains the property of the substance. Molecules are composed of atoms (Figure 1-8). An atom contains a relatively heavy inner core, or nucleus, which possesses a positive electric charge, and a number of light negatively charged subatomic particles called *electrons* that orbit around the nucleus. The nucleus of an atom is composed of positively charged subatomic particles, called protons, and particles that have no charge, called *neutrons*. The number of protons in the nucleus of an element is specific for each element, determines its atomic number, and is designated by the symbol Z. The total number of protons and neutrons in the nucleus of an atom is the mass number and is designated by the letter A. An atom of an element that has the required number of protons but a different number of neutrons in the nucleus is said to be an *isotope* of the element. Isotopes of an element have the same atomic number (number of protons) but a different atomic mass number (number of neutrons) of the element (e.g., carbon-14). They may be stable or unstable, and the unstable isotopes may give off gamma rays, which are a component of the electromagnetic spectrum. Many isotopes are used as tracer elements in diagnosis or for management of malignancies.

In the neutral or stable atom, the number of orbiting electrons (−) equals the number of protons (+) in the nucleus; hence the atom is electrically neutral.

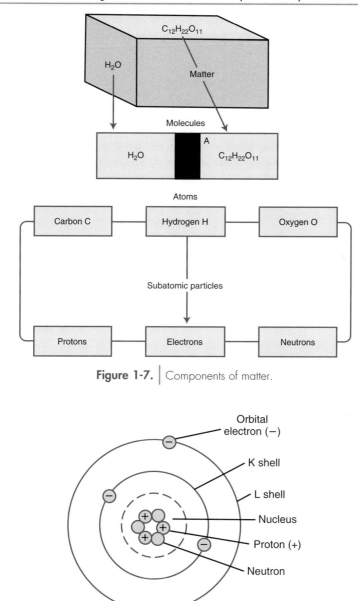

Figure 1-7. Components of matter.

Figure 1-8. An atom. This is a lithium atom, whose atomic number (Z) is 3 and mass number (A) is 6.

Electrons travel around the nucleus in definite orbits called *shells*. There is a maximum of electrons that can occupy each shell and a definite energy level that binds the electrons in each shell to the nucleus. The shells farthest from the nucleus have less binding energy than the inner shells. The shell closest to the nucleus is called the *K shell*, the next outer shell the *L shell*, and then successively the M, N, and O shells. More energy is needed to remove an electron from the K shell than from the outer shells because the binding energy is greater. This factor will come into play during the discussion of characteristic x-ray production.

IONIZATION

When an orbiting electron is ejected from its shell in an electrically stable or neutral atom, the process is called *ionization* (Figure 1-9). The electrically neutral atom is then changed into two ions, one positively charged and one negatively charged. The remainder of the atom has a positive charge, and the ejected electron has a negative charge. Electrons can be removed from atoms by heating or interaction with x-ray photons. In all cases, however, the energy must be greater than the binding energy that holds the electron in orbit around the nucleus of the atom. Thus the inner-shell electrons can be dislodged only by high-energy photons such as x-rays, gamma rays, or particulate radiations, whereas the loosely bound electrons of the outer shell can be dislodged by low-energy photons, such as in ultraviolet light. The new ions do not have all the same properties of the former neutral atom. Because

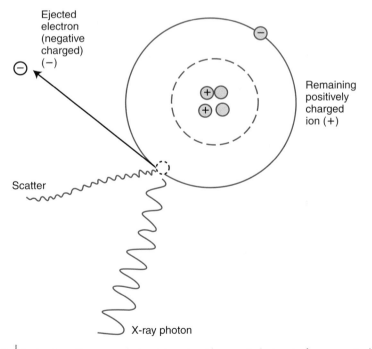

Figure 1-9. | Ionization. The x-ray photon interacts with a neutral atom to form negatively and positively charged ions.

x-rays, gamma rays, and some particulate radiation can cause this type of reaction, they are classified as ionizing radiations. The ionizing potential of certain radiations accounts for their harmful biologic effects. A simple illustration is the water molecule, H_2O. If it is ionized, as it can be by radiation, two hydroxyl ions are formed (free radicals). The two ions may recombine to form water, or in certain instances they may recombine as H_2O_2, which is hydrogen peroxide, a tissue poison (Figure 1-10).

X-Ray Tube

The dental x-ray tube (Figure 1-11), although housed in a large machine, is about 6 in long and $1\frac{1}{2}$ in in diameter. The three basic elements of an x-ray tube needed to produce x-rays are (1) high voltage to accelerate electrons across the tube, (2) a source of electrons within the tube, and (3) a target to stop the electrons.

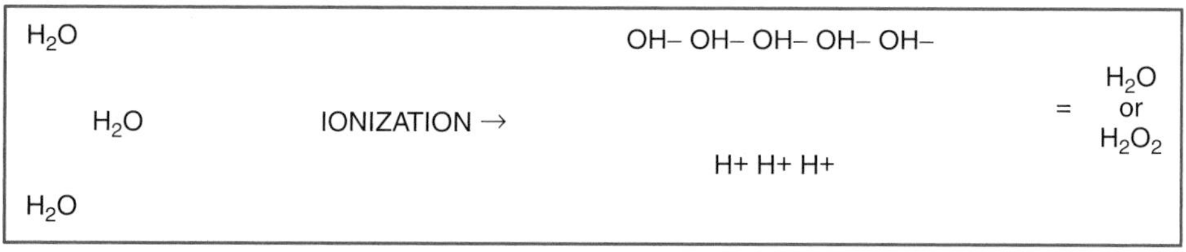

H_2O		OH– OH– OH– OH– OH–		
				H_2O
H_2O	IONIZATION →		=	or
		H+ H+ H+		H_2O_2
H_2O				

Figure 1-10. Ionization of a water molecule.

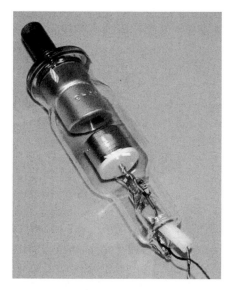

Figure 1-11. Dental x-ray tube. (Courtesy Xintec, Inc., Research Triangle Park, NC.)

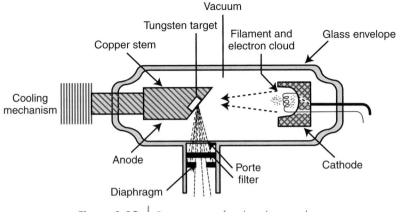

Figure 1-12. Components of a dental x-ray tube.

High Voltage

As shown in Figure 1-12, the x-ray tube has a positive side (pole), called the *anode,* and a negative side, called the *cathode.* Electric current flows from a negative pole to a positive pole. This voltage can be varied by adjusting the kilovoltage dial that controls the autotransformer, which then affects the step-up transformer and thus the kilovoltage across the tube. The greater the kilovoltage or potential across the tube, the faster the electrons will travel and the greater the energy that will be released when the electrons strike the target at the anode and hence the greater the penetration capability.

Source of Electrons

The main source of electrons in the x-ray tube is the tungsten filament found at the cathode. This is a variable source of electrons, unlike Roentgen's tube, in which electrons were produced from the ionization of a fixed volume of gas. The tungsten filament is connected to the step-down transformer circuit. The hotter the resistant filament becomes, the more electrons are produced at the cathode. This production, or "boiling off," of electrons from the heated tungsten filament is called the *thermionic emission effect.* The milliamperage dial controls the amount of current in the filament circuit and hence the number of electrons that boil off. The tungsten filament is surrounded by a focusing cup, which directs electrons toward the anode that contains the target.

Target

The target in the x-ray tube also can be called the *focal spot* or *area.* At the anode side of the tube, and when the circuit is complete, it has a positive (+) charge. It is made of tungsten and measures about 0.8 × 1.8 mm. This is the actual target. The effective target or focal area is smaller because of the tilting of the target that geometrically makes the target smaller when viewed from the opening in the tube. All modern dental x-ray machines have approximately the same size target. Tungsten is used as the target material because it has a high melting point and a low vapor pressure at high temperatures and thus is not affected by the heat produced. The element tungsten also is desirable as a target material because of its high atomic number and thus its density and because when it is bombarded by electrons, x-ray production is more efficient. However, tungsten does not have a high degree of thermal conductivity and must be embedded in a copper stem. The heat is dissipated into the head of the x-ray machine by the copper stem attached to the anode and cooled by air or oil immersion.

Heat Production

The dental x-ray machine is an extremely inefficient machine. Of the total energy produced at the anode by the collision of the electrons with the target, less than 1% is x-ray energy; the remaining 99% is in the form of heat. This is why the highly conductive copper sleeve and oil immersion tube surround the target. Although difficult to do, care must be taken not to overheat the tube.

Heat production at the target is the limiting factor of the milliampere (mA) setting of a dental x-ray machine. With a milliampere setting of more than 15, too many electrons hit the target and too much heat is produced. This overheating soon will destroy the target. Some panoramic and extraoral units have rotating anodes (Figure 1-13) to dissipate the heat and thus can use higher milliampere settings. The standard dental x-ray machine has a fixed anode and a limit to the amount of milliamperage.

Overheating of a dental x-ray machine is not very likely under ordinary use. Each machine has a *duty rating* and a *duty cycle*. The duty rating refers to the number of consecutive seconds a machine can be operated before it overheats, and the duty cycle refers to the portion of every minute that the dental machine can be used without overheating. To damage the x-ray tube, one would have to make about a 17-second exposure or work so fast that four exposures would be made per minute.

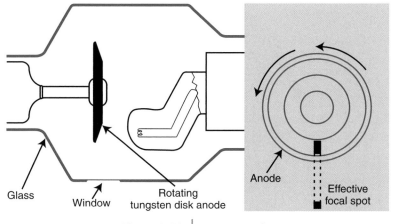

Glass   Window   Rotating tungsten disk anode   Anode   Effective focal spot

Figure 1-13. Rotating anode.

X-RAY PRODUCTION

X-rays used in dentistry are produced in an x-ray tube, and, as previously mentioned, with modifications the modern tube resembles the cathode ray tube used by Roentgen. The principles of high-speed electrons being attracted to and colliding with a positively charged target to produce x-rays and heat are still valid. Figures 1-14 to 1-16 are schematic drawings of the production of x-rays in the dental x-ray tube.

When a dental x-ray machine is turned on and the indicator light is glowing, it is ready to produce x-rays. Turning on the machine closes the filament circuit and heats the tungsten filament, causing electrons to boil off by the thermionic emission effect. The electrons stay at the filament and are referred to as an *electron cloud* (see Figure 1-14). The electrons are attracted across the tube only when there is a difference in electric potential across the tube or, stated another way, when the high-voltage circuit is closed or completed.

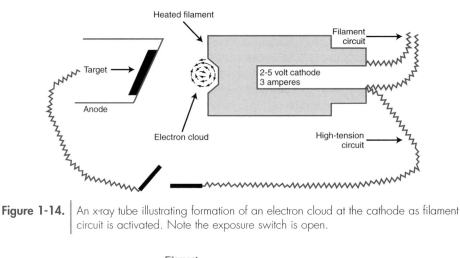

Figure 1-14. An x-ray tube illustrating formation of an electron cloud at the cathode as filament circuit is activated. Note the exposure switch is open.

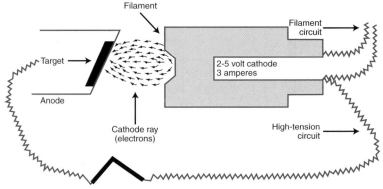

Figure 1-15. An x-ray tube showing electrons traveling across the tube from the cathode to anode (target) as high-tension circuit (exposure switch) is activated.

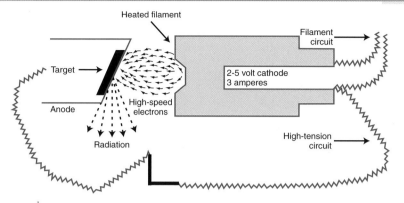

Figure 1-16. An x-ray tube showing production of x-rays as high-speed electrons collide with target.

This high-voltage circuit is activated by the exposure switch and remains active for the length of time for which a timer is set as long as the operator maintains pressure on the switch.

With the high-voltage circuit completed by closing the exposure switch, the electrons produced by the thermionic emission effect at the cathode are attracted to the positively charged anode, which contains a tungsten target (see Figure 1-15). This stream of electrons crossing the tube is called the *cathode ray*.

Federal regulations require that new dental x-ray machines emit an audible signal when an exposure is being made, in addition to the signal lights in the control panel.

X-rays and heat are produced in the tube when the high-speed electrons strike the tungsten target (see Figure 1-16). This is transference of energy. The kinetic energy of the moving electron is converted to the energy-laden x-ray photon and heat energy. The faster the electrons travel across the tube, the more energized and penetrating are the x-rays produced. The speed of the electrons across the tube is determined by the kilovoltage.

As illustrated in Figure 1-13, the tungsten target is angled and the x-rays produced are directed to an exit point (porte) in the tube. The rest of the x-ray tube is lead-lined, and x-rays can leave the tube only through the porte. If x-rays leave the tube in any area other than the porte, the machine is said to have head leakage. This is a safety hazard to both patient and operator and a violation of the radiation safety code.

BREMSSTRAHLUNG AND CHARACTERISTIC X-RAYS

This section examines the formation of x-rays at the level of the atom; that is, what is the atomic mechanism of the formation of x-rays when the high-speed electrons strike the tungsten target?

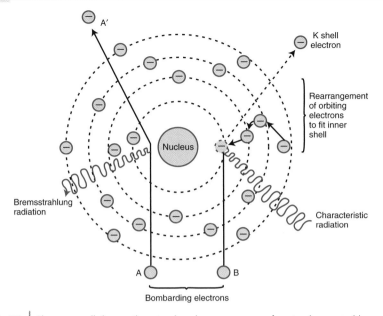

A′

K shell
electron

Rearrangement
of orbiting
electrons
to fit inner
shell

Nucleus

Bremsstrahlung
radiation

Characteristic
radiation

A   B

Bombarding electrons

Figure 1-17. | Electrons colliding with a simulated tungsten atom, forming bremsstrahlung radiation (**A**) and characteristic radiation (**B**).

The phenomenon of x-ray production can be best understood by considering the tungsten atom and the possibilities that arise when a high-speed electron enters its orbit, as it would at the target of a dental x-ray machine (Figure 1-17, *A*). The tungsten target consists of an infinite number of tungsten atoms. Only one surface atom will serve as a representative example for the rest of the atoms in the tungsten target.

The first possibility, which rarely occurs, is that the high-speed electron might hit the nucleus of the tungsten atom and give up all its energy. The second possibility, represented by entering electron A in Figure 1-17, is that the entering high-speed electron might be slowed down and bent off its course by the positive pull of the nucleus. This slowing down represents a loss of energy that is given off as x-rays and heat and is the major source of x-ray production in the dental x-ray tube. The slowing down and veering off course of the entering high-speed electron with its loss of energy expressed in x-rays and heat is called *bremsstrahlung,* the German word for "braking radiation."

Because the tungsten target is not just one atom thick, this bremsstrahlung is repeated an infinite number of times. The exiting electron A′ (see Figure 1-17, *B*) will enter another tungsten atom, and the reaction will be repeated with the production of more x-rays. A′ and the succeeding A″, A‴, and so forth each will have less energy than the original entering electron A; hence the x-rays produced at each succeeding bremsstrahlung will have less energy or longer wavelengths. Because of the multiple bremsstrahlung reactions, all of the x-rays produced do not have the same energy content (wavelength).

A heterogeneous x-ray spectrum is produced. The later bremsstrahlung reactions produce x-rays whose energy is not sufficient to penetrate teeth and bone and, as will be seen, are removed by filtration.

The third possibility, represented by entering electron B, is that the high-speed electron might hit and dislodge one of the orbiting electrons of the tungsten atom. This can happen only when the entering electrons possess more energy than that binding the orbiting electrons to the nucleus. In the dental machine, this means it can happen only at settings of 70 kVp (70,000 V) and above because the binding energy of the K shell of electrons is 69,000 electron volts. If an orbiting electron is dislodged, a rearrangement or cascading of electrons inward fills up the electron vacancies in the inner shells. This rearrangement produces a loss of energy that is expressed in x-ray energy. The x-rays thus produced are called *characteristic x-rays* and account for a very small part of the x-rays produced in the dental machine and only in those machines operating at 70 kVp and above. Bremsstrahlung and characteristic radiation can be produced at the same time and are additive.

SUGGESTED READINGS

American Academy of Dental Radiology Quality Assurance Committee: Recommendations for quality assurance in dental radiology, Oral Surg Oral Med Oral Pathol 55:421-426, 1983.

American Dental Association Council on Scientific Affairs: An update on radiographic practices: information and recommendations, J Am Dent Assoc 132:234-238, 2001.

Code of Federal Regulations 21, subchapter J Radiol Health, part 1000, Washington, D.C., Office of the Federal Register, General Services Administration, 1994.

Frommer HH: History of dental radiology, Texas Dent J 119:417-427, 2002.

Frommer HH, Fortier P: History of the American Academy of Oral and Maxillofacial Radiology, Oral Surg Oral Med Oral Pathol Oral Radiol Endod 80:511-516, 1995.

Langland OE, Langlais RL: Early pioneers of oral and maxillofacial radiology, Oral Surg Oral Med Oral Pathol Oral Radiol Endod 80:496-511, 1995.

National Council on Radiation Protection and Measurements: NCRP Report No. 145, Radiation in dentistry, 2004.

White SC, Pharoah MJ: Oral radiology: principles and interpretation, ed 5, St Louis, Mosby, 2004.

CHAPTER 2

The Dental X-Ray Machine

EDUCATIONAL OBJECTIVES

1. Understand the generation of x-rays in the dental x-ray unit, the variables of the control panel, and the properties of the x-ray beam.
2. Be able to apply these concepts and principles to clinical radiography.

KEY TERMS

alternating current
ampere
central ray
collimation
collimator cutoff
cone
cone cutting
cycle
direct current
electric current

filter
half-value layer
half-wave rectified
impulse
intensity
kilovolt
kilovolt peak
milliampere
position-indicating
   device

rectification
scatter radiation
self-rectified
step-down transformer
step-up transformer
transformer
useful beam
voltage

ELECTRICITY

Because the primary source of energy for the x-ray machine is electricity, it is necessary to learn or review some basic concepts of electricity.

Electric current is the flow of electricity through a circuit; it can be either *alternating current* (AC) or *direct current* (DC). Direct current flows in only one direction in an electric circuit, whereas alternating current flows in one direction and then reverses and flows in the opposite direction in the circuit (Figure 2-1). In the dental x-ray tube, this means that the tungsten filament is only the negative pole half the time because of the reversal of the direction of the current. During this part of current flow, almost no x-rays are produced and still fewer leave the tube. There are usually 60 *cycles* per second in most AC circuits.

Rectification

If the dental x-ray machine is operating on alternating current, in the x-ray tube itself the polarity is reversed 60 times per second. When the direction of the current flow is reversed, the tungsten target becomes the negative pole, or cathode, and the tungsten filament becomes the positive pole, or anode. During the alternating $1/120$ second (half of a cycle) when the current is reversed, few x-rays are produced because there are few electrons available at the filament to travel across the tube and strike the target; thus the current is blocked from traveling across the tube. This blocking of the reversal is called *rectification,* and because the dental x-ray tube is designed to produce this effect, it is said to be *self- or half-wave rectified* (Figure 2-2).

X-rays are not produced in a steady stream but in spurts or *impulses,* and these pulses take place only during one half of the alternating current cycle. Most alternating current is 60 cycles, so the dental x-ray machines express exposure units in pulses or sixtieths of a second instead of the usual ½ second or $3/10$ second. A ½-second exposure is equal to 30 pulses. An exposure time of

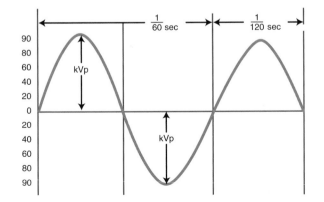

Figure 2-1. | Sine wave of 60-cycle alternating electric current operating at 90,000 V (90 kVp).

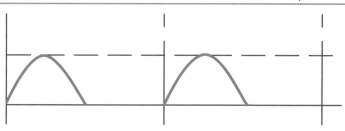

Figure 2-2. | Half-wave rectification.

$1/7$ second, for example, is not possible because it is not divisible into 60, and it is impossible to get a fraction of a cycle of alternating current. Some newer-model dental x-ray machines are designed to supply full-wave rectification (Figure 2-3). In this circuitry, the negative portion of the alternating current cycle is reversed. If currents are then superimposed, there is less of a drop in voltage between cycles. These machines do not produce pulses of x-radiation but rather a constant stream of x-rays. Thus exposure time can be reduced by one-half because x-rays are not being produced half the time, as they are in the self-rectified circuit, but all the time. The radiation exposure to the patient is the same; it just requires half the time. Considering the very short exposure times used today, a reduction in exposure time has no effect on work patterns except in digital radiography (see Chapter 15, in which short exposure times are used).

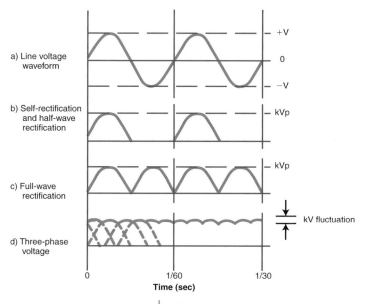

Figure 2-3. | Full-wave rectification.

Voltage is the term used to describe the electric potential or force that drives an electric current through a circuit. The unit of measurement is the volt. The *kilovolt* (kV) is 1000 V. In an alternating current, where the direction of the current is constantly changing, the voltage is also changing, and the term *kilovolt peak* (kVp) is used to denote the maximum or peak voltage that is described by the sine wave that plots the alternation of the current (see Figure 2-1). A dental x-ray machine that is set for a potential of 90 kVp will reach 90 kVp only at the peak of the alternating current during exposure. As seen in the diagram of the exposure's sine wave (see Figure 2-1), other voltage levels also occur during the exposure. This has great clinical significance because these differences in voltage contribute to the heterogeneity of the x-ray beam and the need for filtration.

Ampere is the unit of measurement used to describe the amount of electric current flowing through a circuit. The *milliampere* (mA) is equal to $^1/_{1000}$ of an ampere.

A *transformer* is a device that can either increase or decrease the voltage in an electric circuit. It is composed of two coils of electric wire insulated from one another. The magnetic field from one coil induces an electric current in the second coil. The number of turns in the induction coil in relation to the number of turns in the second coil determines the action of the transformer (Figure 2-4). The dental x-ray machine also has an autotransformer, which uses only one coil and can be used only for making minor changes in voltage. If the transformer increases the voltage, it is referred to as a *"step-up"* trans-former, and if it decreases the voltage, it is referred to as a *"step-down"* trans-former. The dental x-ray machine uses both types in taking ordinary line or house voltage of 110 V and stepping it up to a range of 65,000 to 100,000 V (65 to 100 kVp) in the high-voltage circuit or stepping line voltage down to 3 to 5 V in the filament circuit—these being the two basic circuits in the dental x-ray machine.

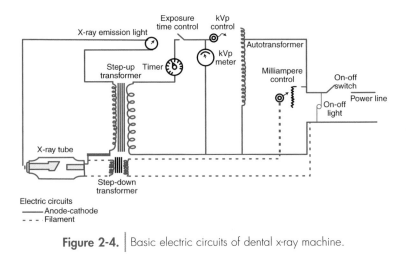

Figure 2-4. | Basic electric circuits of dental x-ray machine.

CIRCUITRY

Dental x-ray machines use 110-V alternating current. The two major circuits in the x-ray machine are the filament circuit and the high-voltage circuit. Each circuit uses a transformer to convert the line voltage and current. The filament circuit uses 3 to 5 V, so the 110-V line current is reduced by means of a step-down transformer (see Figure 2-4). The heating of the cathode filament by the electric current is controlled by a rheostat in this circuit, is a function of the milliamperage selector on the control panel of the machine, and determines the quantity of the x-rays produced. The high-voltage circuit in the dental x-ray machine requires voltage in the range of 65,000 to 100,000 V. This increase in voltage is achieved by the use of a step-up transformer. An auto-transformer also is used in the circuit as a line compensator to control fluctuations in line voltage. The relationship of the input circuit to a variable number of coils is changed in the autotransformer, by the kVp dial on the control panel, to change the quality of the x-rays emitted.

CONTROL PANEL

The control panel of the dental x-ray machine (Figure 2-5) contains an on-off switch and indicator light, an exposure button and indicator light, timer dial, and kVp and mA selectors. The exposure button is on a 6-ft retractable cord or linked to a remote station that is behind a suitable barrier. Some *newer* machines have preset fixed milliamperage choices, usually 7, 10, or 15 mA, or adjustable. The kVp values may be fixed or have a range from 65 to 100. Some units, instead of having numerical choices for kVp, have icons or diagrams of a small, medium, or large patient because kilovolt peak is linked

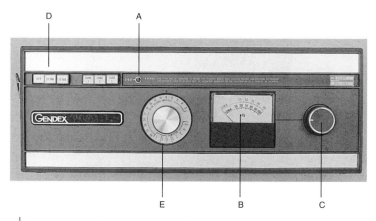

Figure 2-5. Control panel of dental x-ray machine. **A,** Exposure indicator. **B,** kVp meter. **C,** kVp control. **D,** mA control. **E,** Timer control. *(Courtesy KaVo Dental/GENDEX Imaging, Lake Zurich, IL.)*

to the penetration of a large or small patient (Figure 2-6). When the size of the patient icon is changed, the x-ray unit automatically adjusts the milliamperage to maintain the film density.

Timer

As previously discussed, the dental x-ray tube does not emit a continuous stream of radiation but rather a series of impulses of radiation. The number of impulses depends on the number of cycles per second in the electric current being used. In 60-cycle alternating current, there are 60 pulses of x-ray per second (Figure 2-7). Each impulse lasts only $^1/_{120}$ second because no x-rays are emitted in the negative half of the cycle when the polarity of the tube is reversed. The exposure dials on newer-model dental x-ray machines are not calibrated in fractions of seconds but more realistically in impulses. On the timer dial, "24" means 24 impulses per second, which is equivalent to $^2/_5$ or $^{24}/_{60}$ second of exposure. With the advent of more sensitive or faster films or digital sensors calling for decreasing exposure times, all machines should have electronically controlled timers so that these short exposure times can be achieved accurately and repeatedly. The old mechanical timers with increments of ¼ second, which were usually inaccurate by at least $^1/_8$ to ¼ second, are unacceptable for the shorter exposure times in use and in many instances are violations of the radiation code.

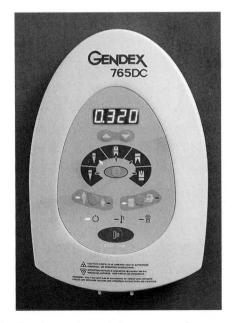

Figure 2-6. Icons on the dental control panel showing size of patient icons. *(Courtesy GENDEX Dental Systems, Lake Zurich, IL.)*

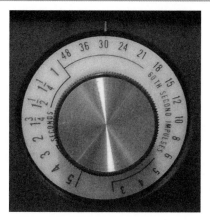

Figure 2-7. | Timer dial. Note the increments in impulses ($\frac{1}{60}$ second). *(From Langlais RP:* Exercises in oral radiology and interpretation, *ed 4, Philadelphia, 2004, Saunders.)*

The x-ray machine should be turned off after use. Warm-up time is almost instantaneous for the x-ray tube, so there is no need to keep the machine on during the work day. Most offices have definite settings for mA and kVp that are used for all patients. As discussed in the next chapter, the kVp is determined by the density of the object and the type of contrast desired, whereas the mA is determined by the speed of the film, the exposure time, and the source-to-patient distance.

The control panel should be checked each day to ensure that the mA and kVp settings have not been changed inadvertently. As seen in Figure 2-6, some control panels have preset values for different types of patients, and the selectors are labeled with such terms as "large patient," for which the kVp is increased, and "child," for which the kVp is decreased. If one understands the principles of radiology, this type of panel is unnecessary and very limiting.

X-RAY BEAM

The x-ray photons produced at the target in the dental x-ray tube emanate from and leave the tube as a divergent beam. The x-ray at the center of the beam is called the *central ray*. The x-rays closest to the central ray are more parallel, and those farthest away are more divergent. The more parallel rays produce less magnification of the image; thus they are most useful (Figure 2-8).

The x-ray beam is positioned or aimed at the film in the patient's mouth by an open-ended device, either a rectangle or a cylinder, called a *position-indicating device* (PID). These PIDs should be lead-lined to prevent the escape of *scatter radiation* and are usually 8, 12, or 16 in long (Figure 2-9). Originally all dental machines had short, 8-in, plastic, pointed cones as position-indicating devices. To this day, people incorrectly refer to open-ended cylinders as *"cones,"* although the proper term is position-indicating device.

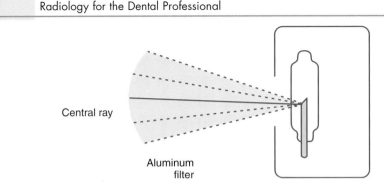

Figure 2-8. The divergent x-ray beam. The aluminum filter removes longer wavelength x-rays from the beam.

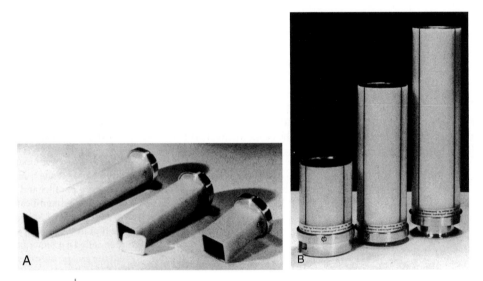

Figure 2-9. Position-indicating devices: open-ended, lead-lined 8, 12, and 16 inch. **A,** Rectangles. **B,** Cylinders. *(Courtesy Margraf Dental Mfg., Jenkintown, PA.)*

The pointed cone was designed as a user-friendly aiming device, with the tip of the cone indicating the position of the central ray. The technique called for aiming the tip of the cone at the center of the film packet placed in the patient's mouth or the extraoral anatomic landmark being used. One of the unfortunate outcomes of this type of instrumentation was that some practitioners came to believe that the x-ray beam was coming out only from the tip of the cone and that the size of the beam was that limited.

The problem with the pointed plastic cone is the secondary radiation that is produced by the interaction of the primary beam of x-ray photons with the plastic cone (Figure 2-10). These secondary x-rays increase the long-wavelength radiation to the patient's face and degrade the diagnostic image

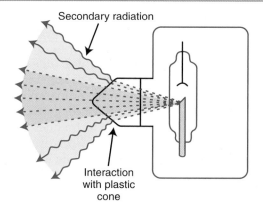

Secondary radiation

Interaction
with plastic
cone

Figure 2-10. | Production of secondary radiation resulting from interaction of the primary beam with the closed-end plastic cone.

on the film. X-rays interact with plastic, even though one might not consider plastic to be very dense material.

X-rays interact and cause secondary radiation with any form of matter, from a piece of tissue paper to a bar of steel. The density of the material and the quality of the x-ray beam determine the type and extent of interaction. When the open-ended PID is used, there is no material at the end of the PID with which to interact. Some practitioners have complained about open-ended PIDs, claiming that they are difficult to aim properly and that *"cone cutting"* results. In reality, the rectangle or the cylinder is not difficult to use, and the change from using the pointed cone is not difficult. Novice students starting instruction in radiology have no more difficulty using open-ended PIDs than their predecessors had with the pointed models. Because all new dental x-ray machines are made with open-ended PIDs, the problem of closed-ended PIDs will eventually disappear.

Radiation protection codes in ALMOST ALL states have required the use of open-ended PIDs. Even in jurisdictions that allow the use of pointed cones, it is strongly recommended that their use be terminated in favor of using open-ended, lead-lined rectangles or cylinders instead. The standard of care in radiation risk prevention calls for open-ended, lead-lined PIDs.

Quality and Quantity of X-Rays: The Difference Between Milliamperage and Kilovoltage

The three parameters of the dental x-ray beam that are adjusted from the control panel by either the dental professional or the dentist are (1) the energy or penetrating power (quality) of the x-ray beam, (2) the number of x-rays produced (quantity), and (3) the length of time for which these x-rays will be produced.

Quality

The quality, or penetrating power, of the x-ray beam is controlled by the kilovoltage. The suitable range for dental radiography is 65 to 100 kVp. Some units can deliver this complete range, whereas others have more limited ranges or even a fixed kVp value. As a rule, the kilovoltage in a dental office remains fixed at one setting for all intraoral radiography. The dentist determines what kilovoltage will produce the most diagnostic radiographs for the particular use of that office. There are some techniques that call for a variable kilovoltage and time with a fixed mA; that is, increased kVp in denser areas and reduced kVp in less dense areas. For every increase of 15 kVp, exposure time is reduced by 50% to maintain the density of the film.

Dental diagnostic radiology is confined to the 65- to 100-kVp range. The density of the structures dealt with in dentistry (teeth, bone, etc.) determines the useful penetration range. Kilovoltage settings below 40 would not give adequate penetration of the object. Kilovoltage from 40 to 65 would penetrate and produce a diagnostic radiograph but not without undue production of secondary x-radiation, and kilovoltage above 100 causes overpenetration. The overall objective of diagnostic radiology is to record differences in densities on the film of the objects being radiographed. A kilovoltage range is chosen that will indicate the difference of penetration and absorption so that the differences in structural densities can be recorded. The choice of kVp setting within the acceptable range is discussed in the section on density and contrast. Thus a kilovoltage is selected that allows complete absorption of some x-rays, partial absorption of others, and passage of other x-rays through the object to reach the film.

Differential absorption of the x-ray beam by the object being radiographed produces the image. That is why less dense structures, such as the dental pulp, appear radiolucent (black) on the dental film and highly calcified denser structures, such as the enamel, appear radiopaque (white or gray). The less dense areas in the object allow greater passage of x-rays than do denser areas, and more x-rays strike the film in these areas to darken it.

Low kilovoltage, in the 45- to 65-kVp range, produces a diagnostic radiograph but should not be used because the radiation produced contains many long, nonpenetrating wavelengths that unnecessarily increase the facial exposure to the patient (see Figure 5-6).

Half-Value Layer

The term *half-value layer* (HVL) is more appropriate than kilovoltage to describe beam quality and penetration. Kilovoltage is a description of the electric energy put into an x-ray tube. HVL represents the quality (penetration) of the x-rays emitted from the tube. Two similar x-ray machines operating at the same kilovoltage may not produce x-rays of the same penetration. The HVL is defined as the thickness of aluminum (measured in millimeters) that will reduce the intensity of the x-ray beam by 50%. For example, a dental x-ray beam could be described as having an HVL of 2 mm. This means that the energy of this particular beam is such that a thickness of 2 mm of aluminum

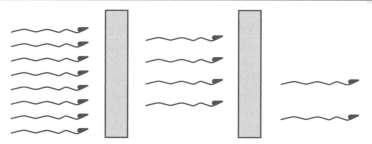

Figure 2-11. Half-value layer of an x-ray beam. Note how the thickness of aluminum used reduces the intensity of x-ray photons by half.

would be necessary to decrease its intensity by half (Figure 2-11). A beam with an HVL of 1 mm would not be as energized, because only 1 mm of aluminum is necessary to decrease its energy by half. The normal HVL for a dental x-ray beam is about 2.75 mm of aluminum.

Quantity

The mA dial determines the number of x-rays produced in a given exposure period by controlling the heating of the tungsten filament to produce electrons at the cathode of the tube. Just as the kilovoltage determines the quality (penetrating power) of the x-rays produced, the milliamperage determines the quantity (amount) of x-rays produced.

It is better to consider the concept of milliampere seconds (mAs) than milliamperage alone. An exposure, at a given kVp, of 1 second using 10 mA is 10 mAs. A 2-second exposure, at the same kVp, using 5 mA would produce an identical film because the mAs are again 10 ($10 \times 1 = 10$; $5 \times 2 = 10$).

The sensitivity of the film and the focal-film distance (FFD) used determine the milliampere seconds required at a given kilovoltage. The more sensitive the film to radiation, the fewer milliampere seconds required. The advantage of higher milliamperage is that a shorter exposure time can be used. This does not represent a decrease in the patient's x-ray exposure, but a decrease in the time necessary to expose the film. This reduces the chance of blurring caused by patient motion.

Ideally, the shortest exposure time with high milliamperage is the best way to achieve the desired milliampere seconds. The range of milliamperage on dental x-ray machines is usually 5 to 15 mA. As mentioned, the limiting factor is the heat produced at the desired small target. Milliamperage higher than 15 produces too many electrons bombarding the target and thus too much heat. As mentioned, some x-ray machines in dentistry are made specifically for extraoral radiography and have rotating anodes. A rotating anode is a spinning disk composed of many tungsten targets instead of one stationary target, as found in the standard intraoral x-ray unit. Because the targets are rotating, they are struck by the electrons through only part of their 360-degree rotation. During the rest of the rotation, the targets can cool. Because the heat is dissipated in this manner, milliamperage of 50 or 100 can be used (see Figure 1-13).

Intensity

The beam intensity is affected by the kVp, mA, exposure time, and FFD. As shown the kVp determines the quality (penetration) of the x-ray beam and the mA determines the quantity of the x-rays produced. Quality and quantity are linked together with FFD and exposure time in the expression of the intensity of the x-ray beam. The intensity of the beam is the product of the quality and quantity of the beam per unit of area per unit of exposure time. (The quality multiplied by the quantity divided by the product of beam area and exposure time equals the intensity of the beam.)

$$\text{Intensity} = \frac{(kVp) \times (mA)}{(area) \times (exposure)}$$

Higher kVp and mA settings increase the intensity of the beam, and an increase in exposure time will also increase the x-ray beam intensity. However, as the FFD increases, the intensity of the beam decreases because the divergence of the beam produces a larger field size. This concept is applied clinically in Chapter 3 in the discussion of the inverse square law.

Filtration

As shown the x-ray beam that originates at the anode is not homogeneous because of the multiple bremsstrahlungs and sine wave variation of alternating current. The beam consists of a spectrum of long and short wavelengths. In fact very few of the x-ray photons produced have energy or penetration power corresponding to the desired kilovoltage called for on the control panel. In other words if one sets the kVp dial for any desired kilovoltage, only a few of the x-ray photons produced will correspond to this setting. Almost all the x-ray photons produced will have wavelengths longer than those corresponding to the desired setting and thus will be less penetrating. This is partially the result of the electrons in the tube bombarding multiple atomic layers of the tungsten target with the resulting bremsstrahlung and characteristic x-ray production and the effect of alternating current with its sine wave voltage buildup. As shown in the graph in Figure 2-12, the x-ray beam is not homogeneous but heterogeneous, having a full range of wavelengths. The longer, lower kVp wavelengths do not penetrate tooth and bone and are absorbed by the skin or produce secondary radiation.

The function of the *filter* is to remove from the primary beam the long, nonpenetrating wavelength x-rays (see Figure 2-8). After the primary beam has been filtered and collimated, it is referred to as the *useful beam*. There is some "inherent filtration" of the x-ray beam as it passes through the glass window and the insulating oil, which is equivalent to about 0.5 to 1 mm of aluminum. "Added filtration" is the thickness of aluminum disks that are added to achieve "total filtration."

Federal regulations specify that for dental x-ray machines operating at kilovoltage up to 70 kVp, 1.5 mm total filtration is required. For those machines operating at 70 kVp and higher, 2.5 mm of total filtration is required.

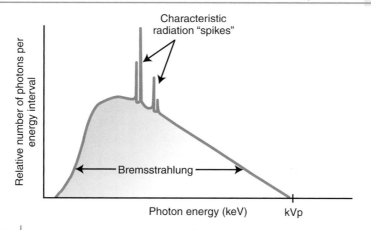

Figure 2-12. Spectrum of x-ray beam from dental x-ray machine operating at 65 kVp. Note number of low-energy photons produced. Note where the characteristic x-rays occur.

Collimation

A collimating device (Figure 2-13) restricts the size and shape of the x-ray beam as it leaves the tube head. In intraoral radiography the beam should be just large enough to cover the film packet or digital sensor. Circular *collimation* allows a margin of error in film beam alignment (Figure 2-14). A beam size any larger than this would expose the patient's face to unnecessary primary radiation. Historically in dentistry the diameter of the x-ray beam measured at the patient's face has been decreasing. From no limitation at all in the early days of dental radiology, the beam diameter has gone to 3½ inches, to 3 in, and presently to 2³/₄ in (7 cm).

The collimating devices most often used are a lead diaphragm with a circular aperture (Figure 2-15) and the metallic PID. The size of this aperture, at a selected FFD, determines the beam size. PIDs, whether open-ended cylinders or rectangles, lead-lined, or made of metal, also can serve as collimating

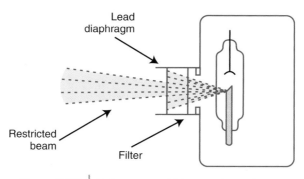

Figure 2-13. Collimation and filtration of x-ray beam.

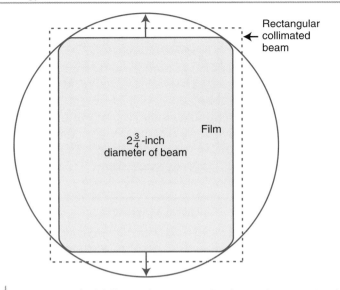

Figure 2-14. Relative size of adult film packet compared with x-ray beam 2³/₄ inches (7 cm) in diameter and rectangularly collimated beam.

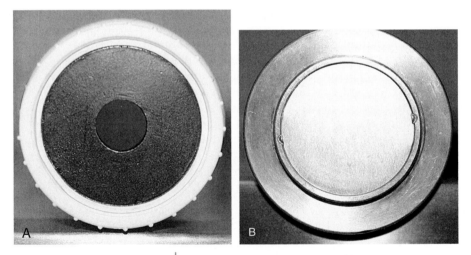

Figure 2-15. **A,** Lead diaphragm. **B,** Aluminum filter.

devices. Federal regulations presently require that the x-ray beam not exceed 2³/₄ inches (7 cm) in diameter when measured at the patient's skin.

Rectangular Collimation

The shape of the dental x-ray beam always has been circular. The question can be asked, "Why is a circular beam used when the film packet is rectangular in shape?" The circular beam covers a greater facial area, and it exposes the

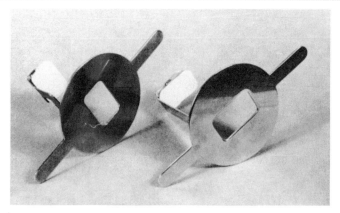

Figure 2-16. Rectangular collimating device. *(Courtesy Precision Instruments, Isaac Masel Co., Philadelphia.)*

patient to more primary radiation than does a tightly collimated rectangular beam. The movement in the dental profession is now toward rectangular collimation. It is taught as the primary technique at most dental schools and is recommended by the American Dental Association and the American Academy of Oral and Maxillofacial Radiology. This change to rectangular collimation can be accomplished without an increase in *collimator cutoff* (cone cutting) with the use of proper equipment. Collimator cutoff occurs when the beam is not centered on the film and thus part of the image is cut off. X-ray beams can be aligned to film easily using the Precision film-holding device (Isaac Masel Co., Philadelphia) (Figure 2-16). The XCP Beam Alignment System (Rinn Corp., Elgin, IL) and the RAPD Positioning System can be used in conjunction with a metal rectangular PID collimator (Figure 2-17). The use of these devices in rectangular collimation is illustrated and described in Chapter 10.

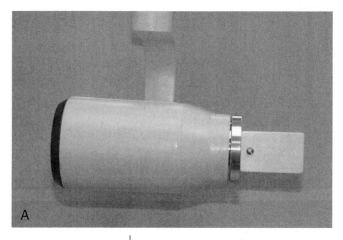

A

Figure 2-17. **A,** Rectangular PID collimator.

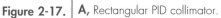

Continued

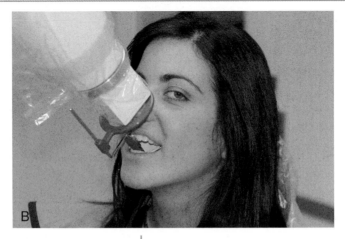

Figure 2-17—cont'd. | **B,** with Paralleling Positioning Device.

SUGGESTED READINGS

American Dental Association Council on Scientific Affairs: An update on radiographic practices: information and recommendations, J Am Dent Assoc 132:234-238, 2001.

Code of Federal Regulations 21, subchapter J Radiol Health, part 1000, Washington, D.C., Office of the Federal Register, General Services Administration, 1994.

National Council on Radiation Protection and Measurements: NCRP Report No. 145, Radiation in dentistry, 2004.

White SC, Pharoah MJ: Oral radiology: principles and interpretation, ed 5, St Louis, Mosby, 2004.

Image Formation

EDUCATIONAL OBJECTIVES

1. Understand the principles of image formation and the factors that influence the image in dental radiography.
2. Be able to apply these principles to the clinical situation in taking proper radiographs with the least amount of radiation exposure to the patient.

KEY TERMS

actual focal area
bisecting-angle technique
blurred image
contrast
density (film or object)
detail
effective focal area
focal-film distance
illuminator

image
intensity
inverse square law
line pairs per millimeter
long-scale contrast
magnification
object-film distance
paralleling technique
penumbra

radiolucent
radiopaque
recessed target
recessed tube
short-scale contrast
umbra

No matter what imaging system is used to produce radiographs of dental and maxillofacial structures, the goal is to create an *image* with the proper degree of density and contrast, detail sharpness, and minimal enlargement and distortion. These factors enable the most diagnostic information for the amount of radiation expended.

FILM DENSITY AND CONTRAST

The two types of related densities that are factors in image formation are the *object density* (teeth, bone, soft tissue), which is determined by the structure of the object being radiographed, and the *film density*, which is the degree of blackness on a film. *Contrast* is the difference in the degrees of blackness on the film between adjacent areas. When comparing a black (dense) area on a film with a white area, a great deal of difference, or high contrast, is seen. When comparing gray with white or gray with black areas or shades of gray, less or low contrast is seen. The density of a film is determined by the relative transmissions of the x-rays through parts of the object and the absorption of the x-rays in the emulsion of the film. These two factors, the object being radiographed (object contrast) and the properties of the film (film contrast), determine the overall density and contrast of the finished radiograph.

Object Contrast

The object contrast is determined by: (1) the thickness of the object, (2) the density of the object, (3) the chemical composition of the object, (4) the quality of the x-ray beam, and (5) scatter radiation. The thickness, density, or atomic number of the structures being radiographed (teeth, bone, etc.) cannot be controlled. However, these parameters determine the range of kVp that is used in dentistry. Therefore a kVp range that produces a differential absorption pattern to portray differences in object density on the film is used. Using a kVp setting greater than 100 in dentistry results in overpenetration, and using a kVp of below 40 results in underpenetration. In both cases the selective penetration desired is not achieved.

This can be demonstrated with the use of an aluminum step wedge (Figure 3-1). As the wedge gets thicker, there is a decrease in x-ray penetration. The only variables of object contrast are the quality or penetration of

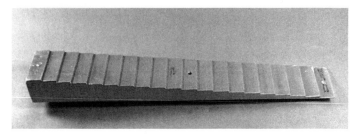

Figure 3-1. | Aluminum step wedge.

the x-rays within the dental diagnostic penetration range of 65 to 100 kVp and the amount of scatter radiation produced.

The image difference between films produced at the different kVp settings in the dental range is the resulting contrast. By varying the kilovoltage, and thus the quality of the radiation, and keeping scatter to a minimum, either high- or low-contrast films can be produced. It should be noted again that kilovoltage in the 45- to 65-kVp range will produce a diagnostic image, but should not be used because of the amount of secondary radiation produced (Figure 3-2).

Short Scale

High-contrast films appear mainly black and white with very few gray tones. They also are referred to as *short-scale contrast* films and are produced by kilovoltage of about 65 kVp. These films are said to be "crisper" and more pleasing to the eye, but they may not reveal early pathologic changes. The short-scale film is a yes-or-no situation: either the x-ray beam penetrates the object or it does not. Areas appear black (*radiolucent*) or white (*radiopaque*), with few gray tones in the middle range (Figures 3-3 and 3-4).

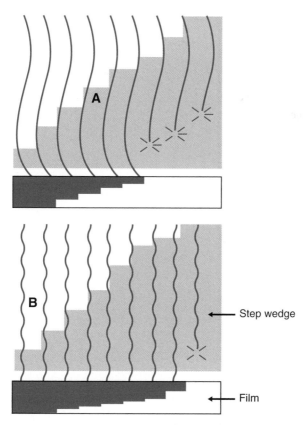

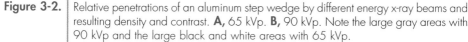

Figure 3-2. Relative penetrations of an aluminum step wedge by different energy x-ray beams and resulting density and contrast. **A,** 65 kVp. **B,** 90 kVp. Note the large gray areas with 90 kVp and the large black and white areas with 65 kVp.

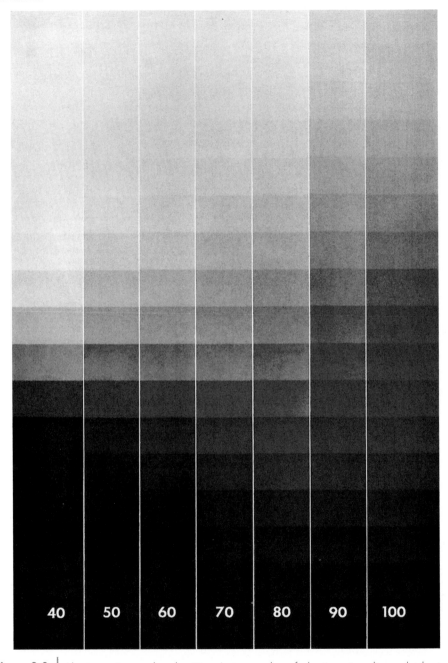

Figure 3-3. Aluminum step wedge densities. A step wedge of aluminum is radiographed using increasing kVp (penetration). The thinner portion of the step wedge shows complete penetration of all kVps. At the thicker portion of the wedge, the lower kVp does not penetrate, whereas the higher kVp penetrates, as shown by the gray tones. *(Courtesy Eastman Kodak Co., Rochester, NY.)*

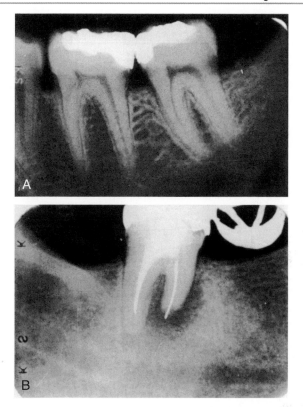

Figure 3-4. **A,** High-contrast radiograph taken at 65 kVp. Note predominance of black and white tones. **B,** Low-contrast radiograph taken at 90 kVp. Note predominance of gray tones.

Furthermore the lower kVp ratings (below 65) are undesirable because they result in increased facial absorption and scatter, which degrades the image, as a result of their less penetrating wavelengths.

Long Scale

The low-contrast films, also referred to as *long-scale contrast*, are produced by the high kilovoltage range of 90 to 100 kVp. In these films there are many tones of gray in addition to the blacks and whites. The long-scale film is not as visually pleasing as the short-scale film, but early changes in object density, such as early bone loss or incipient decay, may be seen in the gradation of the gray tones because of more selective penetration (see Figure 3-3), which is not present in the high-contrast films. Many in the field believe that the human eye can detect changes better in the 70- to 75-kVp range and therefore choose that setting. With this in mind one could question the advantage of purchasing or having an x-ray unit that has a variable kVp range if one is using a fixed-kilovoltage technique.

In addition to its effect on other parts of the patient's body, scattered radiation produces a uniform exposure or darkening over the film and in doing so reduces the contrast. Scatter radiation is one of the causes of "film fog," and it degrades the diagnostic image. Most scatter radiation originates in the object itself; thus the larger the field, the more that object scatter becomes a factor. As noted in Chapter 13 grids are sometimes used to eliminate object scatter in extraoral radiography. In intraoral radiography, scatter radiation is reduced by using as small a beam as possible, open-ended position-indicating devices (PIDs), lead backing in the film packet, and kVp settings of 65 and above.

Film Contrast

Film contrast is determined by (1) the amount of radiation transmitted (object contrast); (2) the properties of the film; (3) intensifying screens, if used; (4) film processing; and (5) viewing conditions. All of these factors are discussed in their respective chapters. It is important to remember that any secondary radiation or light that affects the film decreases the desired contrast, or "fogs" the film and degrades the image. Fogging of the film must be differentiated from the overall grayish appearance of radiographs produced at high kVp settings. Definition can also be judged by the size of the penumbra the image produces.

IMAGE DETAIL AND DEFINITION

Image *detail* is the visual quality of a radiograph that depends on definition or sharpness. It is measured in the number of *line pairs per millimeter* that can be seen on an imaging device. For example, film has 12 line pairs per millimeter. The factors that influence detail are (1) size of the tube focal or target area; (2) *focal-film distance* (FFD); (3) *object-film distance* (OFD); (4) movement of patient, film, or x-ray machine; (5) type of intensifying screen, if used; and (6) image contrast.

The *penumbra* is the unsharpness or blurring that surrounds the edge of a radiographic image, whereas the *umbra* is the sharp area. It is desirable to keep the penumbra as small as possible. This is done by using a small focal spot, angulation of the target, an increased FFD, and a small OFD (Figure 3-5).

Size of Tube Focal (Target) Area

The smaller the focal area (spot) at the anode (see Figure 1-12) of the x-ray, the better the image detail will be. As discussed in Chapter 1, the heat produced limits how small the focal area can be. The focal area in the tube is tilted, usually at an angle of 20 degrees to the cathode (Figure 3-6), and when viewed from below the focal area appears to be smaller than it actually is and

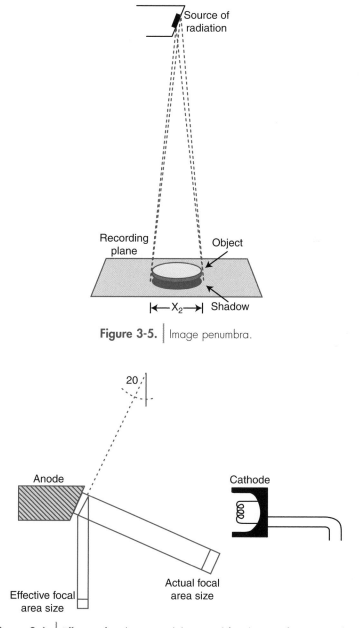

Figure 3-5. | Image penumbra.

Figure 3-6. | Effective focal area and the actual focal area of an x-ray tube.

functions as the desired smaller focal area. This is called the *effective focal area,* in contrast to the *actual focal area.* The effective focal area is always smaller than the actual focal area. Most dental x-ray machines are equipped with the smallest fixed focal area possible, given the heat production restrictions.

Focal-Film Distance and Object-Film Distance

The ideal radiograph of a tooth or other object, in terms of definition, image enlargement, and distortion, can be made by meeting the following criteria:

1. Establish a maximum FFD. This is the distance between the focal spot (target) at the anode and the film in the patient's mouth. The maximal distance allows the more parallel rays from the center of the x-ray beam to strike the object and the film, and not the more divergent x-rays from the periphery of the beam, which would cause image enlargement on the film (Figure 3-7).

2. Determine a minimal OFD. The tooth and the film should be as close together as possible. The closer they are, the less enlarged the image is on the film (Figure 3-8).

3. Position the object and the film parallel to each other in their long axes and the central ray perpendicular to both.

These are the optimal requirements. Because of anatomic constraints in intraoral radiography, it is impossible to meet all of these requirements at the same time. In most periapical projections it is not possible for the tooth and film to be parallel and still be close together.

Focal-Film Distance (Source-Film Distance)

The most common FFDs used in dentistry are 8, 12, and 16 in. An FFD of less than 8 in may cause *magnification* of the image that is larger than the film (see

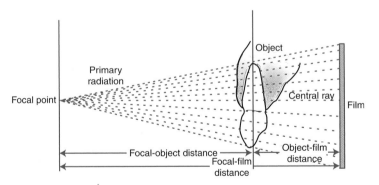

Figure 3-7. Relationships among focal point, object, and film.

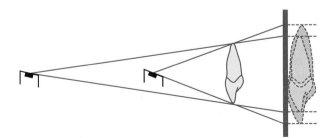

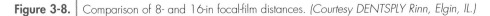

Figure 3-8. Comparison of 8- and 16-in focal-film distances. *(Courtesy DENTSPLY Rinn, Elgin, IL.)*

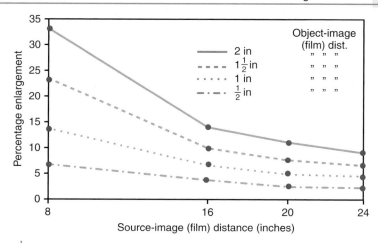

Figure 3-9. Relationship of image magnification to object-film distance and focal-film distance. (Courtesy DENTSPLY Rinn, Elgin, IL.)

Figure 3-8). As the FFD is increased to 12 or 16 in, the magnification of the image decreases because the image is formed by the more parallel x-rays from the center of the beam. However, this decrease in magnification is not linear beyond 16 in. Figure 3-9 shows that as the FFD increases beyond 16 in, the percentage of magnification does not decrease significantly, and the difference cannot be seen by the naked eye. Therefore using a 24-in FFD does not give a significantly better image clinically than a 16-in FFD. The 16-in FFD is the distance of choice. The extended or 16-in FFD also results in exposure of less tissue volume (see Chapter 6, Figure 6-10). The 16-in FFD produces a better image because of the decrease in magnification, with less radiation to the patient. For these reasons its use is strongly recommended.

Tube Position

The x-ray tube is positioned in the anterior part of the head of the machine close to the PID or "cone" (Figure 3-10). The rest of the head of the x-ray machine contains electric circuitry and cooling devices. The open-ended, rectangle or cylinder, PID placed on the head of the machine serves as the aiming device for the x-ray beam, and the length of this PID determines the focal distance to be used.

Some practitioners objected that the longer PIDs (cones) were bulky, cumbersome, and difficult to use in small operatories. Others said the long "cone" tended to unbalance the head of the x-ray machine. With the increasing popularity of the paralleling technique and the need for an extended FFD (16 in), a new design for the tube head was introduced. Figure 3-10 illustrates the operation of the new design. The x-ray tube is placed in the rear part of the machine's head, and the rest of the components are placed on both sides of the beam. This concept is known as a *recessed tube* or *recessed target*. The advantage of this design is

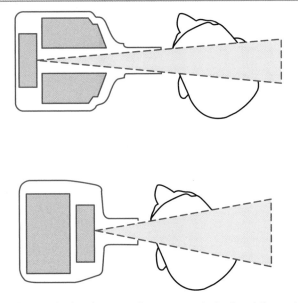

Figure 3-10. | Long-beam tube head (*top*) and conventional tube head (*bottom*). Note different position of x-ray tube that allows increased focal-film distance.

in the extended focal distance and the elimination of the longer PID. The terms *short cone* and *long cone* are no longer appropriate. Cones are now outdated because of radiation hygiene, having been replaced by open-ended, lead-lined cylinders and rectangles. In addition, the machine with the short "cone" really may have a long FFD, depending on the placement of the x-ray tube in the head of the machine.

Inverse Square Law
One factor that must be considered in choosing or changing an FFD is the *inverse square law* (Figure 3-11), which states that "the intensity of radiation varies inversely with the square of the distance." This is attributable to the fact that as the FFD increases, the intensity of the beam decreases because of the divergence of the x-ray beam, which produces a larger field size. More simply stated, if the FFD doubles, the exposure time quadruples. This assumes that the mA and kVp remain the same. The inverse square law is discussed again in Chapter 7 regarding its relationship to radiation protection for the operator.

As seen in Figure 3-11 the intensity of the radiation at 16 in is much less than at 8 in because it is spread out over 16 boxes. To achieve the same intensity of radiation, the exposure time must be increased by a factor of 4. In Figure 3-11 the field size at 16 in would be kept to four boxes by decreasing the aperture of the collimating device.

Before the advent of more sensitive films the inverse square law presented more of a limiting factor than it does today. For instance, if one were using an 8-in FFD at 1-second exposure and then changed to a 16-in FFD, a 4-second exposure time would be necessary to produce a comparable film at

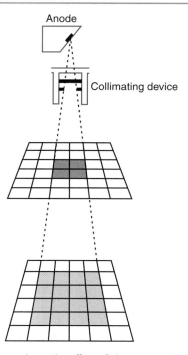

Figure 3-11. | Inverse square law. The effect of distance on the intensity of the radiation.

the same mA and kVp. This 4-second exposure time would be inordinately long, and patient movement could occur. With the use of faster x-ray film and exposure times of ²/₁₀ second at an 8-in FFD, a 16-in FFD would need only ⁸/₁₀-second exposure time. Clinically, ⁸/₁₀-second exposure time, when compared with ²/₁₀-second exposure time, presents no more or less of a problem with patient movement. The same amount of radiation reaches the film in the 8- and 16-in techniques; it just takes more time to achieve the required x-ray intensity with the increased distance.

Another clinical application of the inverse square law is in the correction of an error that can cause underexposed, light (thin) films. The correct position of the PID is almost touching the patient's face when intraoral radiographs are taken. This gives the desired FFD, depending on the length of the PID. If the operator is careless in placement and does not approximate the skin, the result is an increased FFD and decreased intensity of the x-ray beam by a factor of the square of the distance from the patient's face. A small distance, when squared, can result in underexposed film. Most dental offices select an FFD and keep this technique constant.

Object-Film Distance

The closer the object (tooth, bone, etc.) is to the film, the better the detail and the less the enlargement (Figure 3-12). The OFD is determined by the anatomy of the area of the mouth being radiographed and whether the paralleling or

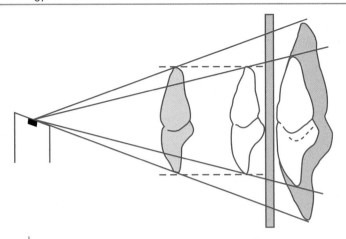

Figure 3-12. │ Comparison of object-film distances and the effect on image magnification.

bisecting-angle technique is used. In the paralleling technique in some areas of the mouth the OFD will have to be increased to have the film parallel to the long axis of the tooth. Compare the OFD needed for parallelism in the mandibular molar area with that needed in the maxillary molar area. In the lower area the film is very close to the tooth and still parallel, whereas in the upper area the film has to be positioned in the midline of the palate to achieve parallelism.

IMAGE DISTORTION AND ENLARGEMENT

Because of the mouth's anatomy it is impossible to satisfy ideal criteria 2 and 3 (p. 44), which refer to OFD and parallelism between the object and the film. If the film is held close to the teeth, then the parallelism is lost; if the teeth and film are to be parallel, then there must be an increased OFD.

This is the basis for the two techniques used in film placement for intraoral radiography: the paralleling technique and the bisecting-angle technique. The clinical methods of performing these techniques, as well as their advantages and disadvantages, are described in Chapters 10 and 11. In the *paralleling technique* the film is held parallel to the long axis of the tooth. This results in an increased OFD in most areas of the mouth; that is, for the film to remain parallel to the tooth, it must be positioned away from the tooth (Figure 3-13). The compensation for enlargement caused by the increased OFD is using an increased FFD (12 or 16 in). The use of the increased FFD is the reason for the misnomer "long-cone technique." It is not the long cone with its increased distance that is of primary importance, but the parallelism between the tooth and the film.

In the *bisecting-angle technique* the film is held as close to the tooth as possible. At this point the long axis of the tooth and the plane of the film cannot be

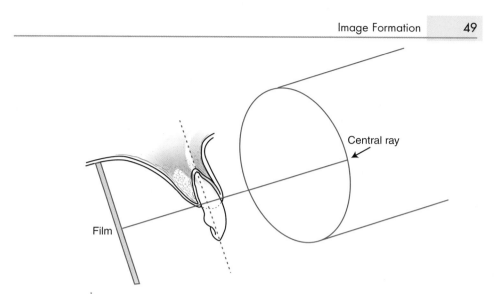

Figure 3-13. | Relationships of central ray, tooth, and film packet in the paralleling technique.

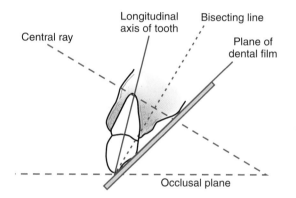

Figure 3-14. | Relationships of central ray, tooth, and film packet in the bisecting-angle technique.

parallel. A geometric trick is then used to project the proper image of the tooth onto the film. An imaginary line is drawn that bisects the angle formed by the long axis of the tooth and the plane of the dental film (Figure 3-14). The central ray of the x-ray beam then is directed perpendicularly at this bisecting line. This projects the proper linear dimensions of the tooth onto the film without elongation or foreshortening.

Movement

Image detail is affected by patient movement, film movement, and x-ray source movement (Figure 3-15). Patient and film movement are controlled by good chairside technique and are discussed later in the book. Source movement, or tube and arm movement, is caused by improper upkeep and quality

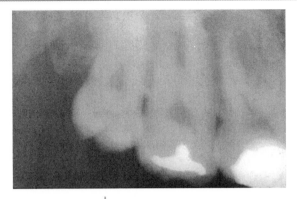

Figure 3-15. | Radiograph showing movement.

control of x-ray equipment. If the arm or head moves or vibrates, image quality is compromised causing a *blurred image*. There is no excuse for this type of error, and an effective quality control program should detect this malfunction. In many jurisdictions, tube or arm movement is a violation of the Radiation Health Code.

Viewing Conditions

Radiographs should always be viewed on an *illuminator* or *viewbox* (Figure 3-16). A magnifying glass can be used to examine fine changes. A darkened room for using an illuminator is the ideal setting for viewing radiographs. The darkened room may not be practical in all dental offices, but certainly viewing radiographs on an illuminator is always feasible. Holding radiographs up to the light on the unit or ceiling or in front of the window is no substitute for an illuminator. Valuable information can be lost or never seen if the proper viewing conditions are not used and maintained.

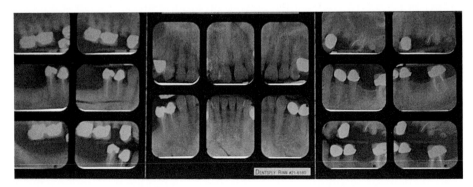

Figure 3-16. | Viewing radiographs on a viewbox (illuminator).

SUGGESTED READINGS

American Dental Association Council on Scientific Affairs: An update on radiographic practices: information and recommendations, J Am Dent Assoc 132:234-238, 2001.

National Council on Radiation Protection and Measurements: NCRP Report No. 145, Radiation in dentistry, 2004.

New York City Health Code, Article 175, Feb 1998.

White SC, Pharoah MJ: Oral radiology: principles and interpretation, ed 5, St Louis, Mosby, 2004.

CHAPTER 4

Image Receptors

EDUCATIONAL OBJECTIVES

1. Know and understand the imaging systems available in dental radiography today.
2. Be able to apply this knowledge to clinical situations that call for the use of intraoral panoramic or extraoral projections, as well as their processing and duplication.

KEY TERMS

American National
 Standards Institute
 (ANSI)
calcium tungstate
double film packet
duplicating film
emulsion
film base

film contrast
film speed (film sensitivity)
fog
fluorescence
group D film
group E film
group F film
image receptor

intensifying screen
packet
phosphor
rare earth elements
silver bromide
silver halide

The *image receptors* used in dentistry today are film, film-screen combinations, the electronic sensors used in digital imaging and computed tomography (CT). All of these use x-rays to generate an image on a receptor. Some medical imaging systems, such as fluoroscopy systems, use x-rays as the energy source without film. Other systems, such as CT, ultrasound (sound waves), and magnetic resonance imaging (MRI) (radio waves) systems, also do not use film to record the image. The "films" seen in CT and MRI are actually print-outs, referred to as hard copies, of the electronic image. Even with the ever-increasing use of digital imaging (see Chapter 15), film remains by far the most commonly used image receptor in dentistry today.

At the present time, three types of dental film are being manufactured: (1) intraoral, including periapical, bitewing, and occlusal; (2) extraoral, including panoramic; (3) and duplicating film.

HISTORY

Dental x-ray film has evolved since the discovery of x-rays in 1895 and the taking of the first dental radiograph in 1896. To appreciate how far dentistry has come in reducing radiation and improving the diagnostic image, review the evolution of dental x-ray film. In the early days from 1896 through 1913, the *x-ray packet* consisted of glass photographic plates or film cut into pieces and hand-wrapped by the dentist in black paper or rubber dam. These packets were prepared by the dentist just before use. The corners of the packets were square, and the packets were thick and rigid, resulting in a great deal of patient discomfort.

In 1913 the Eastman Kodak Company introduced the first commercially available prepackaged dental x-ray film. The film packets were still made by hand and consisted of two pieces of film but with the emulsion coating only one side of each film. In 1921 the first machine-made packet was placed on the market, and the packet began to resemble the one used today in that it was flatter, contained a thin sheet of lead to prevent backscatter, had rounded edges, and was easier to open. All of these factors led to greater patient comfort.

By 1923 Kodak was producing dental film packets in two speeds: regular and extrafast. In 1925 double-coated emulsion film was introduced, which greatly reduced the amount of exposure necessary because of the more efficient use of the radiation. Film speed has increased over the years, the x-ray emulsion has been made less sensitive to darkroom safelighting by a factor of 10, and the packet itself has been made more flexible.

The diagnostic quality of dental x-ray film has improved in spite of the increases in film speed and film contrast, while at the same time the patient's exposure to ionizing radiation has decreased. Exposures in the neighborhood of $1/10$ of a second are being used currently, whereas 50 years ago, exposure times were 6 to 8 seconds and resulted in diagnostic images that were not as good as those seen today.

FILM SIZE

Intraoral film packets come in five basic sizes (Figure 4-1): (1) child size, #0; (2) narrow anterior film, #1; (3) and adult size, #2. (4) Occlusal film packets, #4, and (5) preformed long bitewing films, #3, also are available.

All the film packets must be light-tight and resistant to salivary seepage. These packets must have some degree of flexibility and should be easy to open in the darkroom.

The dental x-ray film packet has an outer, plastic-like wrapper. Inside the wrapper is the x-ray film, covered by black paper, and a lead-foil backing. The lead backing is placed on the side of the film away from the x-ray tube to absorb any unused radiation and backscatter secondary to irradiation and prevent them from affecting the patient or fogging the film (Figure 4-2).

A film packet may contain one or two pieces of film. The so-called *double film packet* requires slightly more exposure time than the single-film packet. Some dental offices prefer the double packets to *duplicating films*.

The film also has a button or dot on it (Figure 4-3). This is a small convex-concave area that indicates which side of the film was closest to the tube and helps to orient the developed film in mounting (see Chapter 19).

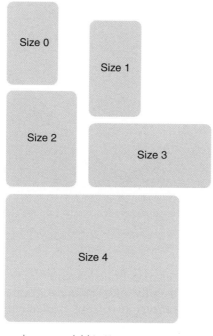

Figure 4-1. Intraoral film packet sizes: child (#0), narrow anterior (#1), adult size (#2), preformed bitewing (#3), and occlusal (#4).

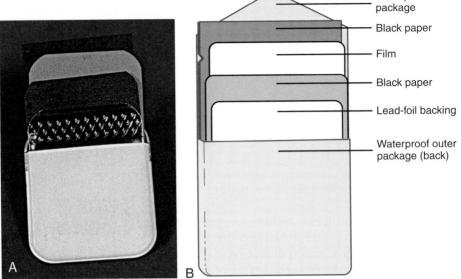

Waterproof outer package

Black paper

Film

Black paper

Lead-foil backing

Waterproof outer package (back)

A

B

Figure 4-2. | **A,** Back of an opened dental film packet. **B,** Diagram of (**A**).

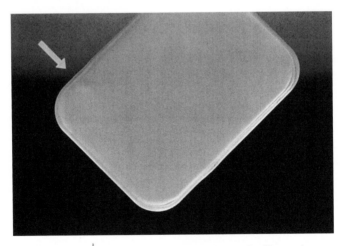

Figure 4-3. | The orientation marker (*dot*) on the film packet.

Composition

X-ray film is composed of a clear cellulose acetate *film base* that is coated with an *emulsion* of *silver halide* (usually *silver bromide*) grains suspended in a layer of gelatin (Figure 4-4). The emulsion with its protective coating is attached to the acetate base by an adhesive. The emulsion is sensitive to x-rays, visible light, and static electricity. The film base is coated on both sides and thus is referred to as a double emulsion. Less radiation is used than with the old,

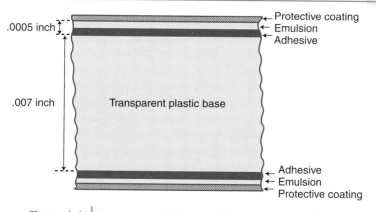

.0005 inch — Protective coating
← Emulsion
← Adhesive

.007 inch   Transparent plastic base

← Adhesive
← Emulsion
Protective coating

Figure 4-4. | Cross-sectional diagram of film base and emulsion.

single-sided emulsion film. Clinically this means that a radiograph can be viewed correctly from either side. Previously with single-emulsion film, the film had to be viewed from the side with the emulsion on it.

Sensitivity (Speed)

The size of the silver halide crystals, the thickness of the emulsion, and the presence of special radiosensitive dyes determine the *film speed*, or *film sensitivity*. Film sensitivity determines how much radiation for what period of time (mAs) is needed to produce an image on the film.

More sensitive films require fewer mAs and are said to have greater film speed; these are the fast films. Films that require more mAs are less sensitive to radiation and are called *slow films*. The size of the silver bromide crystals is the main factor in determining the film speed: the larger the crystals, the faster the film. Film sensitivity is compared or expressed by means of a characteristic curve (H & D curve, Figure 4-5). The curve expresses the relationship between radiation exposure to the film and resulting film density. A fast film requires less exposure to produce a desired density than a slow film.

Different film manufacturers give different brand names to their various film speed types. No slow-speed film is made today. At 65 kVp and 10 mA, slow film would take an average exposure time of about 3 seconds per film. Under the same conditions, the intermediate-speed film takes about 1½ seconds and the fast film about $3/10$ of a second of exposure per film. One manufacturer's "ultra-speed" (Eastman Kodak) may equal another's "lightning" or "very fast" film speed. It is obvious that some standards and nomenclature are necessary. Film speed is designated by group by the *American National Standards Institute* (ANSI) using the letters A through F, *A* for the slowest film and *F* for the fastest. F-speed film is the fastest film available. To obtain comparable film sensitivities when changing from one manufacturer to another, one should consult the ANSI speed group ratings found on the package and not be misled by descriptive names.

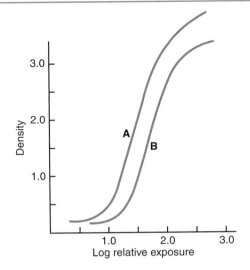

Figure 4-5. Characteristic curve. Note that film (**A**) requires less exposure to achieve a given film density than film (**B**).

Presently, *group D film*, *group E film*, and *group F film* are the only film speed groups that should be used. The American Dental Association (ADA) and the American Academy of Oral and Maxillofacial Radiology recommend that E- or F-speed film be used. The ADA further recommends that films in a speed group slower than group D should not be used. Certain health codes forbid the use of film slower than group D. Group E film is twice as fast as group D; thus, the patient receives half the radiation exposure for a comparable diagnostic film. The new F-speed film reduces radiation exposure 20% and 70% compared with E-speed film and D-speed film, respectively.

Film Contrast

Film contrast is the characteristic of the x-ray film that enables it to portray differences in subject contrast. It is inherent to each type of film and is determined by the manufacturer of the film. Film with inherent high contrast is more desirable for diagnosis. When type E film was first introduced, although the speed of the film was increased by 50%, some practitioners objected to the perceived decrease in film contrast. The manufacturers have increased film contrast in later generations of the E-speed film. Film contrast is usually expressed as the slope of the line in the diagnostically useful part of the characteristic curve (see Figure 4-5).

Film Definition and Detail

The definition or detail on a film also depends on the size of the silver bromide crystals. Theoretically the larger crystals, despite the fact that they allow reduced exposure time, give poorer definition when compared with the smaller, slower crystals.

The present dilemma is whether to reduce the amount of radiation the patient receives by using fast films with large crystals, thereby sacrificing definition, or increase exposure time by using small crystals to give better definition, thereby increasing radiation exposure. The human eye, which must view the finished radiograph, cannot easily distinguish among the definition of D-, E-, or F-speed films. The literature strongly suggests that it is difficult to tell the difference among them and that the decrease in radiation far outweighs the slight possible loss of definition. Eastman Kodak, the major supplier of E-speed film, had improved and changed its group E emulsion; now the film is called Ektaspeed Plus. The new film has better contrast and is not as sensitive to variations in storage and processing conditions as the original Ektaspeed emulsion. Kodak also introduced an F-speed emulsion, called Insight, which is a faster film, and then withdrew all of its E speed film from the market because of sales strategy.

Film Fog

X-ray film *fog* occurs when all or part of the radiograph is darkened by sources other than the primary beam of radiation to which the film was exposed. Fogging degrades the diagnostic image, and use of a good-quality assurance program should minimize its deleterious effects. Sources of fogging may include the following:
1. Chemical fog results from an imbalance or exhaustion of processing solutions (see Chapter 8).
2. Light fog results from unintentional exposure from light leaks and improper safelighting to which the film emulsion is sensitive, either before or during processing (see Chapter 8).
3. Scatter radiation fog results from radiation striking the film from sources other than the intentional exposure of the primary beam. Examples are scatter from the patient or unprotected storage of films before or after exposure (see Chapter 8).

DUPLICATING FILM

In recent years with the increase in dental insurance programs and a more mobile patient population, dental offices and institutions receive many requests to provide radiographs to insurance carriers or to forward films to the patient's new dentist. Coupled with this has been the increase in the number of dental malpractice suits, for which the defendant-dentist's records are of the utmost importance. Radiographs are an essential part, if not the most important part, of these records. The use of radiographic duplicating film can satisfy requests for radiographs and still maintain the integrity of office records. Radiographs should never leave the dental office unless they have been duplicated. There should be no exception to this rule. This is a litigious society, and dentists must protect themselves. Duplication of radiographs is a relatively easy process that requires only a few additions to normal darkroom equipment, namely, duplicating film, appropriate size film hangers, a light source (ultraviolet is preferable), and a photographic printing frame (Figure 4-6). Duplicating devices are also commercially available that can duplicate all film sizes (Figure 4-7).

Radiographic duplicating film is readily available from dental supply firms. It is supplied in 8 × 10- or 5 × 12-in sheets and individually wrapped periapical size duplicating film. The photographic duplicating emulsion is present on only one side of the film, so one must be careful in identifying the emulsion side when positioning the film. Under safelight conditions the emulsion side appears dull when compared with the shiny, nonemulsion side. The duplicating film has a direct positive emulsion; therefore if more film density is needed (darker film), the exposure time is shortened. Conversely if decreased film density is desired (lighter film), the exposure time is increased. This is the opposite of time requirements for exposing dental film to x-rays. The key to remembering this fact is to think the opposite of what would be done normally. Duplicating films do not have an orientation dot as standard intraoral films do, and so the films must be labeled "right" and "left." When an office receives a duplicate full series from another dental office and it is not labeled for right and left orientation, one should not assume that labial mounting has been used until confirmed by a clinical examination.

When duplication is being done in the darkroom, some white light may leak from the duplicator and may affect exposed film before it is placed in the

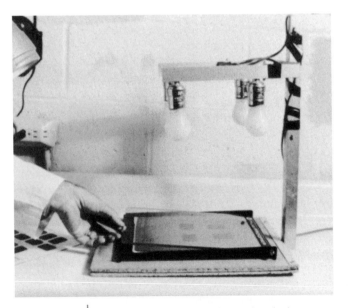

Figure 4-6. "Homemade" setup for radiographic duplication.

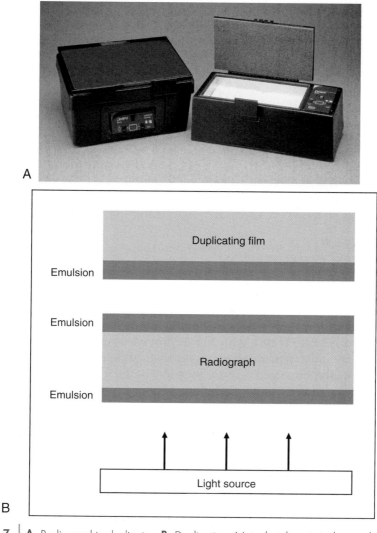

Figure 4-7. **A,** Radiographic duplicator. **B,** Duplication. Note that the originals are placed between the light source and the emulsion side of the duplicating film. *(Courtesy DENTSPLY Rinn, Elgin, IL.)*

solutions. Care should be taken when film processing and duplication are being done at the same time.

Procedure

Under safelight conditions the radiographs to be duplicated are placed in close contact with the emulsion side of the duplicating film positioned so that the light strikes the original or so that the raised part of the mounting dot faces the light source first. A photographic printing frame or any of the commercially available devices will hold the original radiograph against the duplicating film. The films are exposed to light for about 6 to 8 seconds. The intensity of the light may vary depending on which device is used; therefore trial exposures should be made to standardize time and light source distances. After the exposure is made, the duplicating film is processed in the same manner as radiographs, by using either manual or automatic technique (see Chapter 8). An original radiograph can be copied without limits. Close positive contact between the original radiograph and duplicating film is essential, or image definition will be compromised. The top of the printing frame should supply this contact. The original films should always be removed from their mounts to achieve tight contact and therefore good definition.

When a commercial duplicating device is used, the manufacturer's procedures should be followed, especially concerning the time of light exposure.

FILM-SCREEN COMBINATION

The imaging system used in extraoral radiography is a film-screen system. The film is used in combination with *intensifying screens*. Previously in dentistry some extraoral projections were taken with film alone in the so-called nonscreen technique. Today with the improved film quality and heightened concern for radiation safety, all extraoral films should be taken using intensifying screens. The film used is more sensitive to the light emitted by the intensifying screens than it is to radiation. However, the film used has to be sensitive to the type of light emitted by the particular screen (e.g., blue light or green light).

Extraoral film is available in 5 × 7 or 8 × 10 inch sizes, as well as the panoramic sizes, 5 × 12 and 6 × 12 inches (Figure 4-8).

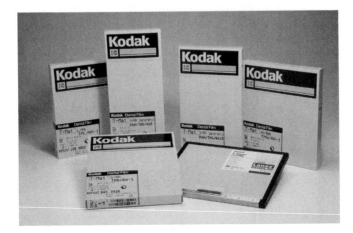

Figure 4-8. | Extraoral film. *(Courtesy Eastman Kodak Co., Rochester, NY.)*

Intensifying Screens

Metal and plastic cassettes used in extraoral and panoramic radiography contain intensifying screens (Figure 4-9). The rigid, nonflexible cassettes have the intensifying screens mounted on the inside of the front and back of the cassette, and the flexible screens are removable (Figure 4-10). As the name implies, these screens intensify or increase the radiation and thus decrease the exposure time needed. The screens are coated with a substance that has the property of *fluorescence*. Such a substance emits light when struck by x-radiation and is called a *phosphor*.

The intensifying screens produce light in the same pattern as the x-rays that have penetrated the object so that the film sandwiched inside the cassette between the intensifying screens is affected by both x-rays and light from the intensifying screen. However, a loss of image detail results from this intensification of the x-ray beam because the light produces a halo at the periphery of the field (Figure 4-11) that diffuses the borders of the image and thus decreases image sharpness.

Intensifying screens vary in their speed or exposure time requirements, just as does film. The speed of the screen depends on the type of phosphor and the size of the crystal: the larger the crystal, the faster the screen but the poorer the definition. Originally, the most common type of phosphor was *calcium tungstate*, which produces blue light. New phosphors, the *rare earth elements*, which produce green light, are now used in intensifying screens instead of calcium

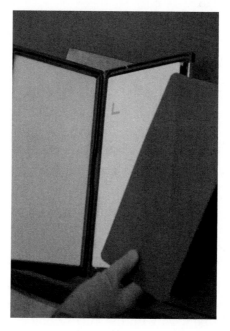

Figure 4-9. Cassette in open position showing front and back intensifying screens and piece of film.

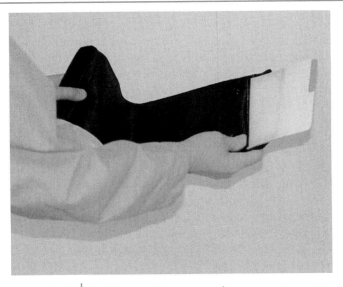

Figure 4-10. | Flexible intensifying screen of a panoramic cassette.

X-rays

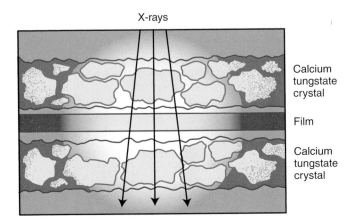

Calcium tungstate crystal

Film

Calcium tungstate crystal

Figure 4-11. | Effect of x-rays on intensifying screens. Note halo of light produced at the periphery that reduces radiographic definition.

tungstate. The rare earth elements are four times more efficient in converting x-ray energy into light than calcium tungstate crystals, and thus the screens are faster and require less exposure time. Rare earth screens must be used with a compatible film that is sensitive to the light in the green portion of the light spectrum. It is recommended that the rare earth screens with their corresponding film be used in preference to calcium tungstate screens. The appropriate film must be used with the intensifying screen.

Intensifying screens, even with the loss of definition, usually are used for extraoral work because the pathologic lesions, measurement points in

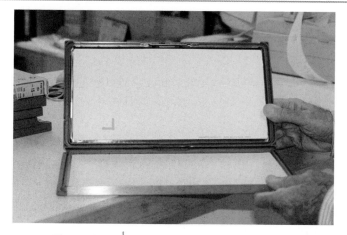

Figure 4-12. | Extraoral cassette left lead marker.

cephalometrics, or impactions being looked for are marked by gross changes of appearance. An extraoral projection using intensifying screens would not be the procedure of choice to look for recurrent decay or a thickened periodontal membrane, both of which require a high degree of definition.

When cassettes are loaded or unloaded in the darkroom, operators should take care not to scratch the intensifying screens with sharp objects such as film racks. If an intensifying screen is badly scratched and the phosphor removed, a dark streak will appear on the film taken with this screen. Damaged screens and cassettes should be discarded. Screens should be cleaned with a solution of soapy water. Maintenance and monitoring of screens are part of a quality-control program.

Because neither the film nor the intensifying screens have orientation dots, as the intraoral film does, metallic "R" and "L" markers are placed on the inside of the cassette (Figure 4-12).

SUGGESTED READINGS

American Academy of Oral and Maxillofacial Radiology: Recommendations for quality assurance in dental radiography, Oral Surg Oral Med Oral Pathol 55:421-426, 1983.

American Dental Association Council on Scientific Affairs: An update on radiographic practices: information and recommendations, J Am Dent Assoc 132:234-238, 2001.

Frommer HH, Jain RK: A comparative clinical study of group D and E dental film, Oral Surg Oral Med Oral Pathol 63:738-742, 1987.

Kantor ML, Reiskin AB, Lurie AG: A clinical comparison of X-ray films for detection of proximal surface caries, Erratum in: J Am Dent Assoc 112:310, 1986.

Ludlow JB, Platin E: Densitometric comparisons of Ultra-speed, Ekta Speed, and Ektaspeed Plus intraoral films for two processing conditions, Oral Surg Oral Med Oral Pathol Oral Radiol Endod 79:114-116, 1995.

New York City Health Code, Article 175, Feb 1998.

Platin E, Nesbit SP, Ludlow JB: The influence of storage conditions on film characteristics of Ektaspeed Plus and Ultra-speed films, J Am Dent Assoc 130:211-218, 1999.

Silha RE: Methods for reducing patient exposure combined with Kodak Ektaspeed dental x-ray film, Dent Radiogr Photogr 54:80-87, 1981.

Thunthy KH, Weinberg R: Sensitometric comparison of Kodak EKTASPEED Plus, Ektaspeed, and Ultra-speed dental films, Oral Surg Oral Med Oral Pathol Oral Radiol Endod 79:114-116, 1995.

White SC, Pharoah MJ: Oral radiology: principles and interpretation, ed 5, St Louis, Mosby, 2004.

CHAPTER 5

Biologic Effects of Radiation

EDUCATIONAL OBJECTIVES

1. Understand the biologic effects of ionizing radiation on human tissue.
2. Be able to relate these concepts to clinical dental radiology.

KEY TERMS

absorption
acute (short-term) effects
ALARA principle
attenuation
background radiation
cell recovery
chronic (long-term) effects

Compton effect
coulomb per kilogram
  (C/kg)
critical organ
direct effects
dose
dose equivalent

dose rate
dose-response curve
exposure
free radicals
genetic effects
gray (Gy)
indirect effects

interaction	radiation absorbed dose	somatic effects
ion	(rad)	threshold erythema dose
ionizing radiation	radiation caries	(TED)
latent period	risk estimate	tissue sensitivity
localized exposure	roentgen (R)	total body exposure
photoelectric effect	roentgen equivalent man	
progeny	(rem)	
quality factor	sievert (Sv)	

Much attention has been given, not only in scientific journals but also in the media, to the effects of *ionizing radiation*, both artificial and naturally occurring, on human beings and the environment. This continual concern about the biologic effects of ionizing radiation is not limited to the scientific community but is evident in the public sector and at all levels of government. On television patients view demonstrations against nuclear power plants and nuclear weapons. They read about radon gas in homes and hear discussions of arms treaties involving destruction of nuclear arsenals. Events such as the near-fatal nuclear accident at Three Mile Island, Pennsylvania, the catastrophe at Chernobyl in the former Soviet Union, and the more recent Japanese nuclear accident have heightened public awareness of the dangers of low-level radiation. The recent and ongoing concern with the high incidence of cancers in certain geographic areas, referred to as *clusters*, and revelations about human exposure to nuclear testing during World War II and the Cold War have kept radiation exposure in the headlines. To add to the mix is the fear of terrorism with its possible nuclear threat. A "dirty bomb" producing ionizing radiation is now considered a weapon of mass destruction (WMD). The uncertainty aroused by these events may lead some patients to refuse necessary diagnostic radiographic examinations or avoid dental visits completely. Health professionals must be informed about risks and benefits of dental radiation and the extent of its relationship to these events so that they may anticipate and allay unfounded fears.

Information about ionizing radiation that reaches the public from the media can be misleading and confusing. The latest data indicate that radiation from medicine and dentistry, including nuclear medicine, accounts for about 15% of the average annual dose equivalent to the U.S. population. This is the largest source of artificial radiation to which the population is exposed. At the same time, in learning about the risk of exposure, one should consider the diagnostic benefits and health-preserving or lifesaving consequences of radiation.

Patient reaction can vary from questioning the need for dental radiographs to outright refusal. The dental professional must face this patient reaction and, with the support of the dentist, be able to explain to the patient the biologic effects of dental x-ray exposure and the diagnostic benefits that are derived. Proper dentistry cannot and should not be done without adequate diagnostic radiographs. This is an accepted standard of care for dental practice. A patient may refuse to have radiographs, but the dentist also can and should refuse to treat that patient.

Ionizing radiation does produce biologic changes in living tissue, and patients should not be misled into believing that dental x-rays have no effect on human cells. The old reply to patient queries regarding radiation safety that "dental x-rays are safe because the dosage is so small it doesn't matter," no longer satisfies informed healthcare consumers.

The question is no longer whether dental x-rays pose a risk, but rather how much of a risk exists. In determining whether radiographs should be used, the dentist must weigh the potential harm of dental x-rays against the benefit that the diagnostic information will yield. In dental radiography performed under optimal conditions and when indicated, diagnostic benefits far outweigh potential risks.

The author's objective for the patient is to use the least possible amount of radiation to obtain the greatest diagnostic yield. For the dental professional and the dentist, the objective is to achieve occupational radiation exposure as close to zero as possible. To achieve these objectives, they must fully understand the subjects of radiation biology and protection. Explanations to patients then will be meaningful, and the dental professional will feel at ease working in an environment in which diagnostic radiation is used.

INTERACTION OF X-RAYS WITH MATTER

X-rays interact with all forms of matter. This *interaction* can result in *absorption* of energy and thus *attenuation* of the x-ray beam (a reduction in the intensity of the x-ray beam) and the production of secondary radiation. The x-ray energy absorbed by the tissue causes chemical changes that result in tissue damage. The two mechanisms for this change are ionization and free radical formation.

Primary radiation is radiation that emanates from the focal area that is the result of high-speed electrons hitting the target of the anode in the x-ray tube. Secondary radiation is the result of the interaction of primary radiation with any form of matter (see Figure 6-1).

When x-rays are absorbed by matter, positive and negative ions and secondary radiation are formed from previously neutral atoms. The amount and type of absorption that takes place depend on the energy of the x-ray beam (the wavelength) and the composition of the absorbing matter. The thicker the material that an x-ray beam must penetrate, the more x-rays will be absorbed. However, more than thickness determines x-ray absorption. The atomic configuration—the number of orbiting electrons and the numbers of protons and neutrons in the nucleus of the atom—also determine x-ray absorption. Heavy elements (those with greater mass) are better absorbers than lighter elements. The more electrons available in an absorbing material, the more x-ray photons are absorbed. Heavy metals with high atomic numbers (the atomic number indicates the number of protons in the nucleus of the atom), such as lead and gold, readily absorb x-ray photons.

An important detail is that when x-rays are absorbed by any material, that material does not become radioactive because x-rays have no effect on the nucleus of the absorbing atom, affecting only the atom's orbiting electrons. This means that the equipment or walls in a dental operatory do not become radioactive after continuous exposure to radiation. At the atomic level, four possibilities can occur when an x-ray photon interacts with tissue, and two of these will result in ionization, which is one of the basic mechanisms for the effect of radiation on tissue.

These possibilities are as follows:

1. *No interaction (pass through).* The x-ray photon can pass through the atom unchanged and leave the atom unchanged (Figure 5-1, *A*). This happens about 9% of the time in a bitewing examination.
2. *Thompson scatter (unmodified or coherent scatter).* In effect, the x-ray photon has its path altered by the atom. There is no change to the absorbing atom, but a photon of scattered radiation is produced (see Figure 5-1, *A*). This accounts for about 8% of the interactions that take place in dental radiography.
3. *Photoelectric effect.* The x-ray photon can collide with an orbiting electron, giving up all its energy to dislodge the electron from its orbit. The photo-electron that is produced has a negative charge, and the remaining atom has a positive charge. This, as mentioned, is ionization (Figure 5-1, *C*). This interaction takes place about 30% of the time with dental x-rays.
4. *Compton effect.* The x-ray photon can collide with a loosely bound electron in an outer shell of the atom and only give up part of its energy in ejecting the electron from its orbit. This results in a negatively charged, ejected Compton electron, a photon of scattered radiation, and a remaining atom that is now positively charged. This again is ionization (Figure 5-1, *B*). This interaction takes place about 62% of the time with dental x-rays.

In both the Compton and photoelectron interactions, the ejected high-speed electron interacts with other absorbing tissue and causes further ionization, excitation, or breaking of molecular bonds, all of which produce adverse tissue effects.

EFFECTS OF IONIZING RADIATION

Radiobiology is the study of the effects of ionizing radiation on biologic tissue. When a dental radiograph is taken, not all the x-rays reach the film, and some even penetrate beyond it. Some of the x-ray energy of the primary beam is absorbed by the skin, bones, teeth, and other body tissues that lie in its path. Tissues that do not lie in the path of the primary beam absorb the energy of the secondary radiation that comes from the patient as a result of the interaction of the primary beam. The differential absorption (density) of the x-ray photons by the hard tissues, teeth, and bones enables one to distinguish various structures on a diagnostic radiograph.

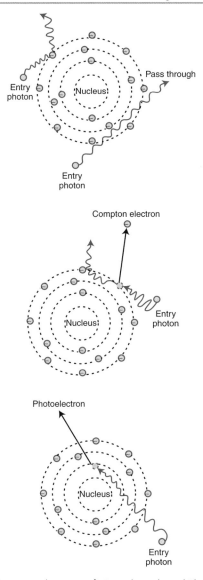

Figure 5-1. Interaction of x-rays with matter. **A,** Pass through and Thompson scatter. **B,** Compton effect. **C,** Photoelectric effect.

What then is the effect of this x-ray energy absorption on the various tissues, and how is it manifested? Human tissue is composed primarily of water (H$_2$O). X-ray photons separate the water into *ions* (HOH and an electron). These ions may recombine into water or go on to other reactions that result in free radical formation (OH, H, O). A *free radical* is an uncharged molecule with a single unpaired electron in its outer ring. These free radicals are very unstable and exist for only about 10^{-5} seconds before they stabilize themselves by (1) recombining to form a stable molecule that will not cause tissue damage or (2) combining with other free radicals, which causes changes or the production of a tissue toxin such as hydrogen peroxide.

Direct and Indirect Effects

Damage to biologic molecules by radiation can occur by either a *direct* or *indirect effect*, with indirect being by far the most prevalent mechanism. In the direct mechanism, the x-ray photons directly hit critical areas within the cell and cause damage to those particular cells (e.g., DNA). In the indirect mechanism, the free radicals that are formed as the result of the ionization of water go on to form toxins that injure or alter cells.

UNITS OF RADIATION MEASUREMENT

Before talking logically about the potential effects of dental radiation, there must be some means of measuring the radiation quantitatively. The settings on the control panel of the dental x-ray machine are not units of measure for the x-ray energy (ionizing radiation) produced. The kilovoltage and milliamperage are indications of the quality and quantity of the electric energy put into the x-ray machine, and the timer provides a reading of how long the ionizing radiation is produced. The half-value layer (HVL), although a characteristic of the x-ray beam, describes the penetration and quality of the beam, not its effect on tissue.

The units of measurement that commonly have been employed and are referred to as the conventional or traditional units are the *roentgen (R)*, the *radiation absorbed dose (rad)*, and the *roentgen equivalent man (rem)* (Table 5-1). To standardize units to the metric system, these conventional units have been replaced by those of the International System of Units (SI). In reality, however, the conventional units are still used widely both in presentations and the literature. The new units are the *coulomb per kilogram (C/kg)*, the *gray (Gy)*, and the *sievert (Sv)*. This text uses the conventional units, with the SI units in parentheses.

Table 5-1	Radiation Units			
Conventional Unit	**Definition**	**SI Unit**	**Definition**	**Conversion**
Roentgen (R)	1 ESU/cc^3 of air	Coulomb/kg	1 C/kg = 3876 R	
Rad	100 erg/g	Gray (Gy)	1 J/kg	1 Gy = 100 rad
Rem	rad × Q	Sievert (Sv)	Gy × Q	1 Sv = 100 rem

Exposure

The unit most commonly used to measure the amount of energy, or ionizing radiation, produced by the x-ray machine is the traditional unit called the *roentgen (R)*. The milliroentgen is $^1/_{1000}$ of a roentgen; because exposures in dental radiology are small, they are often expressed in milliroentgens, or mR (1000 mR = 1 R). The SI unit for exposure would be coulomb per kilogram (1 C/kg = 3.88×10^{-3} R) and is not often used.

The roentgen is a unit of measure of ionization in air. It is defined as the quantity of radiation that produces one electrostatic charge in 1 cm^3 of air. The roentgen is a measuring standard for radiation. Just as one must know what an inch is before comparing lengths, there must be a standard—the roentgen—to measure radiation exposure. Just as there are rulers and scales, there are ionization chambers calibrated in roentgens. An ionization chamber placed in front of a dental x-ray machine position-indicating device (PID) can indicate how many roentgens are produced per second (Figure 5-2). This is called the exposure rate or output of the machine. Because it is an expression of ionization in air, it is measured in roentgens per second. A well-calibrated dental x-ray machine will have an output in the range of 0.7 to 1 R/sec. If a patient had a radiograph taken with such a machine and the exposure time

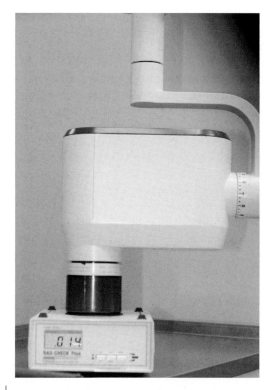

Figure 5-2. | Ionization chamber measuring the output of a dental x-ray machine.

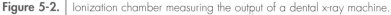

was 1 second, the facial exposure of the patient would be 0.7 R (0.7 R/sec × 1 = 0.7 R). This is a noninvasive method, as all measurements are made at the patient's skin.

Dose

The critical factor in discussing the effects of radiation is not the amount of radiation at a point in air, but rather the amount of energy absorbed by tissue at a specific point. To express the amount of energy absorbed by a tissue, the rad or gray is used. The rad is a unit of absorbed dose and is defined as 100 ergs of energy per gram of absorber (tissue). The millirad is $1/1000$ of a rad. The unit for the absorbed dose in SI units is the gray (1 rad = 0.01 Gy or 1 Gy = 100 rad). It is somewhat helpful in converting from the traditional system to the SI to just add the prefix "centi" to either the gray or sievert, and that will be equal to the traditional rad or rem (e.g., 1 rad = 1 centigray [1 cGy]).

Dose Equivalent

Different types of radiation on a rad-for-rad basis have different effects on living tissue. Neutrons, for example, have a greater effect on tissue than do x-rays or gamma radiation. A rad of x-radiation does not have the same effect on human tissue as a neutron rad. The term *dose equivalent* is meant to illustrate this difference; it is defined as the dose multiplied by the *quality factor, Q,* and is expressed in rem. The millirem is $1/1000$ of a rem. The unit for the dose equivalent in SI units is the sievert (1 rem = 0.01 Sv or 1 Sv = 100 rem). The quality factor by definition for x-radiation and gamma radiation is 1, so that the dose equivalent in rem (sieverts) is equal to the dose in rad (grays).

In terms of the effects of dental radiation, the rad (gray) and the rem (sievert) are identical, and the roentgen is approximately equal to both (roentgen = rad = rem).

BASIC CONCEPTS

Exposure and Dose

Although the terms are often interchanged, there is a very definite distinction between radiation exposure and dosage. *Exposure* is the amount of ionization in the air produced by x-rays or gamma radiation; it is the quantity of radiation in an area to which the patient is exposed. The radiation dose is the amount of energy absorbed per unit mass of tissue at a particular site. In dentistry, the patient is exposed to a certain amount of radiation, some of which is absorbed by tissue in different parts of the body; this is the *dose* to the area. Thus there is a skin dose, a thyroid dose, a gonadal dose, and so on. Exposure should be expressed in roentgens (C/kg), and dose should be expressed in rad (grays) or rem (sieverts).

Localized Radiation and Total Body Exposure

It is important to differentiate between localized radiation and total body radiation (Figure 5-3). When a dental radiograph is taken, the patient's face is exposed to an x-ray beam that is $2^3/4$ in in diameter (with circular collimation). This is a *localized exposure* and represents less than 1% of the total area of the body. A rad of radiation to the localized area means that each gram of body tissue in that area absorbs 1 rad. A rad of total body exposure means that each gram of tissue in the entire body absorbs 1 rad. In dentistry the x-ray machine delivers a localized exposure that results in a total body exposure much less than the facial exposure. In fact the *total body exposure* from a dental radiograph is approximately $1/10,000$ of the facial exposure.

When discussions of dental x-ray dosages appear in magazine articles or patients quote such articles, it is important to determine whether localized exposure or total body exposure is being discussed. For instance, what is the facial exposure of radiation to the patient from a full-mouth survey of radiographs? An average full-mouth survey at 70 kVp and 10 mA, using American

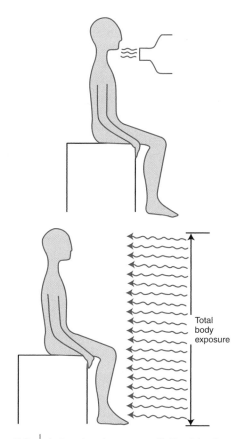

Figure 5-3. | **A,** Localized exposure. **B,** Total body exposure.

National Standards Institute (ANSI) group E film, produces a skin exposure to the patient's face of approximately 2 to 3 R (150 mR per film × 20 films). This is not the total body exposure but a localized exposure. If it were a total body dose, it would far exceed the patient's allowable maximum permissible yearly dose. The total body dose could be approximated by dividing the localized dose, 3 R, by 10,000. The most common misuse of such data occurs when people refer to the recommendation of the National Bureau of Standards that the total body dose for the general public for ionizing radiation should not exceed 500 mR in any 1 year. The misstatement is, "You are allowed 500 mR per year, and when your dentist x-rays your entire mouth, you are exposed to 3 R of radiation." The mistakes here are equating the total body dose to the localized dose and using a nonoccupational exposure for a patient exposure. The truer figure to compare the dental facial dose with the 500 mR standard would be 0.0003 R (0.3 mR).

Dose-Response Curve

The *dose-response curve* is an important concept because it illustrates the possible biologic responses to a harmful agent such as ionizing radiation. The responses can be linear or nonlinear, and they can be threshold or nonthreshold. In a linear dose-response relationship the response is directly proportional to the dose. In a nonlinear relationship the response is not proportional to the dose. Figure 5-4, *A*, is a threshold curve with both linear and nonlinear responses, indicating that below a certain level (the threshold) there is no response to the agent. Applying this concept to dental radiation would yield a level below which radiographs would be "perfectly safe" because there would be no biologic response below that level. This is not thought to be the case for ionizing radiation (Figure 5-4, *B*). This curve indicates that any dose of radiation, regardless of how small and whether the response is linear or nonlinear, will produce some degree of biologic response. Therefore dental x-rays do produce biologic changes in the tissues of patients who receive them, even though no signs or symptoms may be detected and no permanent damage is done to the tissue.

Most of the data that produce such a dose-response curve for humans come from studying the effects of large doses of radiation on such populations as atomic bomb survivors, patients with the dermatologic condition tinea capitis (ringworm of the scalp in patients treated with radiation), or the radium dial painters in New Jersey. In the low-dose range for humans, where dental x-rays fall, little has been documented. The line is therefore an extrapolation based on the limited human data and animal and cellular experiments. The prevailing consensus is that low-dose, ionizing radiation is a linear, nonthreshold relationship.

Somatic and Genetic Effects

All cells in the body, with the exception of the reproductive cells (sperm and ova), are included in the grouping of somatic tissue. Changes in these cells are

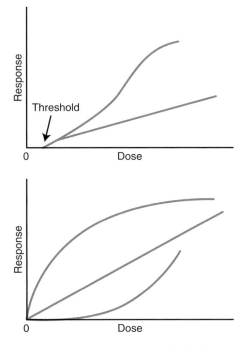

Figure 5-4. Linear and nonlinear dose-response curves. **A,** Threshold curve. **B,** Nonthreshold type. *(From National Council on Radiation Protection and Measurements: Ionizing radiation exposure of the population of the United States, Report No. 100, Washington, D.C. 1989.)*

not passed on to succeeding generations of the species. For example, a cancerous skin condition will not be passed on to an offspring. Somatic tissue can be affected by radiation, and some cells may die, be altered, or even recover, but none of these effects will be seen in the somatic tissue of the *progeny (offspring)*. This is known as the *somatic effect*.

Changes in genetic cells cannot be detected in the exposed patient but are passed on to succeeding generations. These are referred to as *genetic effects* or mutations. There are many agents other than ionizing radiation that have been found to be mutagenic, including a variety of chemicals, certain drugs, and even elevated body temperatures. *Background radiation* also accounts for a portion of naturally occurring mutations. Some of the mutations that have been manifested have been positive and have added to the so-called evolution of the species. A mutation may be recessive and carried in the progeny for many generations before becoming clinically evident.

With the increase in low-level, artificial radiation in recent years, concern focused originally on the possible genetic effects on succeeding generations. Recently the concern has turned to somatic tissue and cancer induction in the blood-forming organs in particular. Leukemia is now believed to be the major risk associated with chronic low-level radiation.

Acute and Chronic Effects

The *acute (short-term) effects* of radiation result from high doses of whole body radiation, usually more than 100 rad. The clinical effects of the exposure, which may vary from mild and transient illness to death, may occur minutes, hours, or weeks after the acute exposure. The median lethal whole body dose for humans is estimated to be 450 rad. Obviously, dentistry is not concerned with acute radiation doses.

Chronic (long-term) effects of radiation may be seen years after the original exposures. Acute and/or chronic exposures may produce cumulative effects on the somatic cells over the patient's lifetime, as well as genetic effects on future generations.

Latent Period and Cell Recovery

The *latent period* is the time that elapses between the exposure to ionizing radiation and the appearance of clinical symptoms. This time may vary from hours to years, depending on the magnitude of the exposure and the tissues involved. It is also difficult, if not impossible, to single out radiation as the cause of a specific pathologic change that takes years to develop. As noted, there is no specific long-term radiation disease, and the conditions associated with radiation (e.g., cancer) have multiple etiologic agents. Not all radiation-induced changes in tissue cells are permanent. Depending on the time interval, dose, and sensitivity of the affected cells to radiation, the cells' repair processes may be sufficient to effect *cell recovery* from the radiation.

Dose Rate

The *dose rate*, the rate at which exposure to ionizing radiation occurs and absorption takes place, is a critical factor in determining the effects. Because cells do recover from radiation, a specific dose produces less damage if it is fractionated over time. In dentistry the time interval between exposures, excluding retakes and working films is usually months or years, further minimizing the effects.

Long-Term Effects

The long-term effects of radiation manifest themselves years after the exposure. The latent period is very long. These delayed effects may be from an acute exposure or a series of low-level exposures. A low-level exposure is considered to be less than 5 rem (0.05 Sv).

Again, no specific disease is associated solely with the long-term effects of radiation. Cancer can be caused by radiation, but it is also caused by smoking, chronic irritation, and exposure to certain chemicals.

Because there is no specific radiation disease, the long-term effects of radiation express themselves in human populations as a statistical increase in the incidence of certain diseases. One can study the incidence of diseases in irradiated populations and compare it with that in nonirradiated groups. A study of atomic bomb survivors and the incidence of leukemias among them is a good example of this type of evaluation of long-term effects. Evaluating the long-term effects of dental x-rays, for which the dose is low, would require large populations over a long period because the latent period for radiation-induced cancer—even from large doses—ranges from years to decades.

Risk Estimates

There is no effective way of analyzing the cause of a radiation-induced cancer on a case-by-case basis, so dosages in irradiated populations are compared with the number of cancers in these populations. This number is then compared with that of nonirradiated populations, and the difference is expressed as the risk factor.

Risk factors are expressed as the number of cases or deaths from a specific disease per million persons. Estimates have been made of the number of cases of cancer for all body organs induced per 1 million dental examinations. For a full-mouth survey taken with round collimation, the estimate is 2.5 to 17 cases per million examinations. If rectangular collimation and E-speed film are used, the risk is reduced. With the F-speed film now being employed, this risk is further reduced.

These numbers may seem threatening, but they should be compared with risks that patients take in everyday life. Activities with a fatality risk of 1 in 1 million in everyday life include traveling 10 miles on a bicycle, 300 miles in an automobile, or 1000 miles on an airplane, or smoking 1.4 cigarettes per day. Obviously, people readily accept one-in-a-million risks in everyday living, even though in many cases there is no health benefit.

TISSUE SENSITIVITY

Tissue sensitivity is an important factor in determining the effects of ionizing radiation on the patient's tissue. Effective dose is a calculation that considers the difference in tissue sensitivity. It is the preferred method for comparing effective tissue sensitivity. The recent International Commission on Radiological Protection (ICRP) report is an example of use of this type of measurement. It is the basis for the American Dental Association (ADA) report that recommends the use of group F-speed film, digital sensors, rectangular collimation and the use of selection criteria in prescribing dental radiographs. Tissues vary widely in their sensitivity to ionizing radiation and thus the amount of radiation required to produce damage. The effect of radiation on certain tissues and organs has predictable disease manifestations, such as hematopoietic tissue giving rise to leukemia or exposure to the sun giving rise to skin cancer. The same dose of radiation has different degrees of effect on different types of cells in the same organism. Young, rapidly dividing, nondifferentiated cells,

Box 5-1   Effect of Radiation on Tissues and Organs

High sensitivity
- Lymphoid organs
- Bone marrow
- Testes
- Intestines
- Skin
- Cornea

Intermediate sensitivity
- Fine vasculature
- Growing cartilage
- Growing bone

Low sensitivity
- Salivary glands
- Lungs
- Kidneys
- Liver
- Optic lens
- Muscle cells
- Neurons

such as those found in the abdomens of pregnant dental patients, are more radiosensitive than older cells. In addition to the age of the cell and its rate of differentiation, tissues vary in their sensitivity to radiation. The grouping of tissues and organs in descending order of sensitivity to radiation is shown in Box 5-1.

Critical Organs

Certain organs and tissues have been designated as critical because they are exposed to more radiation than others when dental radiographs are taken. *Critical organs* and tissues, with their potential risks, are the skin, carcinoma; thyroid, carcinoma; eye lens, cataract; hematopoietic tissue, leukemia; and genetic tissue, congenital defects, or mutations.

Background Radiation

Background radiation is a form of ionizing radiation, both naturally occurring and artificial, present in the environment. Naturally occurring radiation always has been present on Earth, but the artificial component has been increasing as a result of nuclear accidents, fallout from nuclear testing, and radioactive wastes from industry. It would be helpful to know the level of background radiation and its sources so that dental radiation exposure can be put in its proper perspective. An estimate of the average personal exposure, weighted from different sources to approximate a "total body exposure," has been prepared and is shown in Table 5-2. This report shows an estimated average annual dose of 300 mrem (3 mSv) resulting from natural background sources. With the addition of the average contributions of medical and dental procedures, the total annual population exposure is about 360 mrem (3.6 mSv). This figure is increased at higher elevations, and the difference between these elevations and sea level is often used to make comparisons

Table 5-2	Annual Exposure of U.S. Population	
Source	**Dose (mrem)**	
Natural sources		
Radon	200	
Cosmic radiation	27	
Soil and building materials	28	
Internal radioactivity	39	
Occupational	0.9	
Nuclear fuel cycle	0.5	
Consumer products	9.0	
Miscellaneous	0.06	
Medical and dental	53.0	

for the dose from dental exposures. Of the total background exposure, 55% is from exposure to radon, and because not all geographic areas have large amounts of radon gases, background radiation is sometimes considered to be about 100 mrem per year.

These data are helpful in comparing dental exposure with background exposure. From the data and from known outputs of dental x-ray machines, it can be estimated that total body radiation from a four-film, bitewing examination using rectangular collimation and E-speed film is equivalent to about 12 hours of background radiation; this is the source of the often-quoted adage that "four bitewings is equal to 2 days in the sun." Using a round beam and D-speed film increases exposure to an equivalent of 82 hours of background radiation.

Patient Dosage

Ample evidence in the literature substantiates the adverse effects of radiation in high doses. The problem is that although no direct evidence exists of such effects from dental diagnostic doses, there is also no evidence for the absence of adverse effects. To treat a patient without current and diagnostic radiographs is a disservice to the patient and leaves the dentist unprotected against possible legal action for not adhering to the standard of care. Radiographs are an integral part of modern dental practice. The goal in dental radiography is to use the least amount of radiation to satisfy the patient's diagnostic needs; that is, minimize the exposure while maximizing the diagnostic yield. Efforts to minimize the amount of radiation must be guided by the *ALARA principle*, which means "as low as reasonably achievable." The radiation exposure to patients should be reduced as much as possible within the dental office without excessive cost or inconvenience to the patient.

How does one evaluate these effects of ionizing radiation and the weight of the dental component? There is no specific disease that can be attributed solely to the long-term effects of ionizing radiation. As mentioned, leukemia is not caused by x-ray exposure alone, but is probably the result of the interaction of several factors. Animal experimentation has been conducted, but direct extrapolation of the results to human populations is not always reliable. Data gained from acute exposures of humans, such as the victims of Hiroshima or industrial accidents, that are then extrapolated downward to low doses also have limitations. Furthermore the incidence of the diseases of concern is low; to relate an increased incidence to exposure to ionizing radiations, it is necessary to study large populations.

Dental professionals and dentists, because of their involvement with low-level ionizing radiation, should be aware of the consequences of chronic exposure for their patients. In this manner they are better equipped to make the essential risk-benefit decision before making x-ray exposures.

The following examples of specific tissue effects from dental x-ray exposure and the critical levels for these tissues support the conclusion that the benefits derived from dental x-ray exposure, when used judiciously under proper conditions, far outweigh any possible risk.

Skin

Erythema (reddening of the skin) is the usual effect of radiation and is not a major risk in dental radiography. Its importance lies in the fact that the skin dose is the most commonly reported value for dental x-ray examinations. The skin dose has limitations in that (1) skin is easily penetrated and does not reflect a dose to deeper tissues, (2) the skin dose varies greatly with the kVp used, and (3) the skin is less sensitive than many other tissues exposed during dental radiography. The *threshold erythema dose* (TED), the amount of radiation needed to produce an erythema or reddening of the most sensitive individual, is 250 R (250 cSv) in a 14-day period. A full-mouth x-ray series using 70 kVp, D-speed film, and round collimation produces a skin dose of 840 mrem (8.4 mSv). With E-speed film the dose would be approximately one half of that. Using ANSI group E film, more than 60 full surveys in a 14-day period would be necessary to produce an erythema in the most sensitive patient. These values would be further reduced with the use of F-speed film. Clinically this is an absurd possibility, and it is not surprising that no cases of erythema have been reported as a result of exposure to dental radiographs. Risk for the earliest type of skin cancer is not evident below dose levels of 25,000 mrem (250 mSv). However, skin erythema may be seen on patients who have undergone radiation therapy for head and neck cancer. These patients receive total doses in the range of 6000 rad in a 6-week period.

Eyes

Exposure of the lens of the eye to ionizing radiation in high doses can induce cataract formation. The required dose to produce this change has been reported to be in the range of 200,000 to 500,000 mrem (2000 to 5000 mSv), whereas the mean corneal surface dose for a full-mouth series is about 60 mrem (0.6 mSv). The lens of the eye is exposed to radiation during intraoral radiography, but the risk of cataract formation is extremely low.

Thyroid

The thyroid gland, which is particularly radiosensitive, may lie in the beam of primary radiation in some dental views. Malignant changes have been reported in the thyroid glands in a group of patients who received x-ray therapy for tinea capitis (ringworm of the scalp). The dose to the thyroid in these patients was estimated to be 6 rad. Presently the thyroid exposure for a full-mouth series is about 94 mR (0.94 mSv). This exposure is approximately one sixth of the thyroid exposure from a radiographic examination of the cervical spine. The dose to this radiosensitive tissue should be kept to an absolute minimum, especially in children. This can be accomplished, as shall be seen in the next chapter, by the use of a thyroid collar and the paralleling technique.

Bone Marrow

It is now thought that the greatest somatic hazard to patients from dental x-rays is leukemia induction. The red bone marrow is one of the blood-forming organs of the body. The significant hematopoietic bone marrow exposed to dental x-rays is located in the mandible, the calvarium of the skull, and the cervical spine. The calvarium and cervical spine are exposed to primary radiation in extraoral and panoramic radiography. The bone marrow of the mandible and maxilla is the major dental concern and, when exposed to radiation in a full-mouth survey, still represents only 5% of the total body bone marrow.

White and Rose published a report that will help the dental professional and dentist discuss the risk of leukemia with patients. They compared the higher background radiation in Denver, Colorado, caused by high elevation and thus increased cosmic ray exposure with bone marrow exposure from dental examinations. The report states:

> If a person in an average location in the United States were to receive a full-mouth intraoral periapical and panoramic examination every 4 months for the rest of his life, he would incur only the same risk, in terms of bone marrow exposure, as a person living in Denver who was not exposed to dental radiography.

The leukemia risk, then, is very low but still exists. However, with judicious use of radiation and proper technique, the diagnostic benefit derived outweighs the slight risk.

Numerous demonstrations have produced no changes in the complete blood count (CBC) after dental x-ray examination. This finding refutes an outdated report, still often cited in the lay press, that claimed significant blood changes after dental x-rays.

Gonads

The reproductive cells (sperm and ova) are very radiosensitive. Sterilization from an acute exposure from the dental x-ray beam is an impossibility; 400 R is needed in the male and 625 R in the female to cause sterility. The dose to the gonads from dental radiographic procedures is in the form of secondary radiation. For a full-mouth series without the use of a lead apron, the gonadal dose is 0.5 mrem (0.005 mSv). With the use of a lead apron, this dose can be reduced by about 95%. The gonadal exposure for a full-mouth series with a lead apron is about one-seventh the average daily gonadal exposure of the U.S. population from background radiation. This background dose, of course, nearly doubles at higher elevations, such as Denver.

Pregnancy

As mentioned, the nondifferentiated rapidly dividing fetal cells are extremely radiosensitive; therefore there is a concern about pregnant patients. A panel of dental radiologists in the early 1980s considered the appropriateness of dental radiography for pregnant patients. They concluded that the guidelines for taking radiographs (discussed in Chapter 6) need not be altered for the pregnant patient. They pointed out that the concept of avoiding radiography during pregnancy generally applies to procedures in which the fetus or embryo would be in or near the primary x-ray beam. In dentistry the primary beam is limited to the head and neck region, and the only radiation the fetus would be exposed to would be secondary radiation. Uterine doses for a full-mouth series without use of a lead apron have been shown to be less than 1 mrem. As shown, the uterine dose from naturally occurring background during the 9 months of pregnancy can be expected to be about 225 mrem (2.25 mSv) based on the background dose of 300 mrem (3 mSv) per year. So with the uterine dose being a fraction of background and no reported birth abnormalities linked to background elevations, there seems to be no scientific reason to preclude any indicated dental x-ray examination during pregnancy. Radiographs in some cases may have to be deferred during pregnancy for purely psychological reasons or ill-founded recommendations of physicians. If this is the case, then no dental treatment should be rendered that would violate the standard of care, as stated previously.

Recently a study was published that indicated a possible link between dental x-rays taken of women during their pregnancy and low birth weight deliveries. This raises the possibility that x-ray exposure of the thyroid area could be linked to low birth weight. The dental profession through its many organizations was quick to point out that the use of a thyroid collar on any patient is routine procedure and restates its position that only radiographs that are essential to proper treatment should be taken for pregnant patients, and that patients should be encouraged to return for complete treatment after they deliver. Again, it is a risk-benefit concept because the overall health of the patient and the fetus can severely be affected by dental disease.

As shown in Chapter 7, no occupational hazard for the pregnant dental professional exists. When appropriate precautionary procedures are followed, the occupational dose is zero.

Radiation Caries

One of the accepted modalities for treatment of head and neck cancer is radiation. The high doses of radiation used (6000 rad) affect not only the malignant cells, but also the soft tissue of the oral cavity, the mandible and maxilla, and the salivary glands, if they are in the field of radiation. The saliva production of the irradiated salivary glands is diminished and is more viscous; thus it loses its lubricative function, leading to xerostomia (dry mouth). The altered quality and quantity of saliva make the patient more susceptible to a rampant type of *radiation caries* that is characterized by its circumferential pattern as it affects all surfaces of the teeth at the cervical area. A well-taken health history and therapeutic measures such as fluoride treatments, artificial saliva, and frequent recall visits are all part of an accepted means to cope with this condition.

Another sequela that dentists must contend with is osteoradionecrosis. It is not the dental exposure that is the major cause of this infectious condition, but the lowered resistance of the irradiated tissue. One should understand that it is not the small dental dose of radiation that causes dental caries and osteoradionecrosis of bone, because the actual dental exposure is a minor etiologic factor.

SUGGESTED READINGS

Budowsky J, et al: Lack of effect of exposure to radiation during intraoral roentgenographic examination as evidenced by post examination blood studies, J Am Dent Assoc 55:199, 1957.

Gibbs SJ: Radiation dose to sensitive organs from intraoral dental radiography, Dentomax Radiol 17:15-23, 1987.

Hujoel PP, et al: Antepartum dental radiography and infant low birth weight, JAMA 291 (16):1987-1993, 2004.

National Academy of Sciences, National Research Council: The effects on population of exposure to low levels of ionizing radiation (Beir V), Washington, D.C., National Academy Press, 1990.

National Council on Radiation Protection and Measurements: NCRP Report No. 145, Radiation in dentistry, 2004.

Nolan WE: Radiation hazards to the patient from oral roentgenography, J Am Dent Assoc 47:681, 1953.

U.S. Department of Health and Human Services, Public Health Service FDA: The selection of patients for dental radiographic examinations, HHS/PHS/FDA, 88-827310-21, 1987.

White SC: 1992 assessment of radiation risk from dental radiography, Dentomax Radiol 21:118-126, 1992.

White SC, Pharoah MJ: Oral radiology: principles and interpretation, ed 5, St Louis, Mosby, 2004.

Patient Protection

EDUCATIONAL OBJECTIVES

1. Understand and be able to practice dental radiography in a safe, efficient manner so that the patient receives the smallest possible dose of radiation as the maximum diagnostic information is acquired.

KEY TERMS

administrative
   radiographs
exposure technique
exposure time
film-holding device
film viewing
filtration

lead apron
operator concern
patient concern
primary radiation
radiation history
rectangular collimation
retake

secondary radiation
selection criteria
thyroid collar
timer
tube head drift
tube head leakage

Now that the mechanism of ionizing radiation and its effects on human tissue have been discussed, these principles can be applied to the clinical dental environment. The issue of radiation exposure and protection can be discussed from the perspectives of the two major concerns: *patient concern* and *operator concern*. Of the two, concern for radiation exposure of the operator is the easier to deal with because the radiation can be quantified and measured and the recommended exposure can be easily employed.

PATIENT PROTECTION

In patient protection the objective is to use the least amount of radiation to achieve the maximum diagnostic results. The patient must be protected from excessive or unnecessary primary radiation and the resulting secondary radiation. This goal can be met by adhering to the ALARA principle, "as low as reasonably achievable," through the use of safe, well-calibrated x-ray machines, rectangular collimation, film-holding devices, D-, E-, or F-speed film or digital imaging, lead aprons, rare earth intensifying screens and thyroid collars, proper shielding, good chairside and darkroom techniques, and sound professional judgment in selection criteria.

Primary radiation is the x-rays that come directly from the target of the x-ray tube. The primary radiation is collimated by the lead diaphragm, and its softer, less penetrating wavelengths are removed by aluminum filters; it then can be referred to as the *useful beam*. All other radiation can be considered secondary radiation. *Secondary radiation* is defined as radiation that comes from any matter struck by primary radiation. The scattered radiation that results from the interaction of the useful beam and the patient's face is a form of secondary radiation (Figure 6-1). Secondary radiation, besides being harmful to

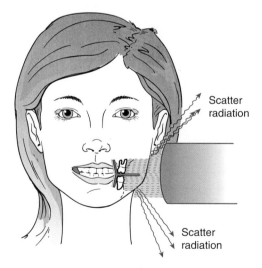

Scatter radiation

Scatter radiation

Figure 6-1. Production of scatter radiation of primary beam by interaction with a patient's face.

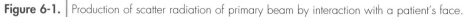

both patient and operator, degrades the diagnostic image of the film because the scattered rays produce film fog on the radiograph.

EQUIPMENT

All dental x-ray machines manufactured after 1974 must meet federal diagnostic equipment performance standards. No federal standards existed for x-ray machines before that year, yet there are many x-ray machines still in use that were manufactured or installed before 1974, although the number of these continues to decrease. It is important to remember that the federal standards do not regulate diagnostic equipment users, such as dentists, dental hygienists, and dental assistants, but only the equipment itself. However, most state or local governments also regulate equipment and have radiation health codes that pertain to the use of radiation. The federal government regulates the manufacture and installation of x-ray machines, whereas state and local governments may regulate the equipment and how the x-ray units are used. Depending on the local radiation code, dental offices, clinics, and dental schools may be inspected every 1 to 3 to 5 years to monitor equipment performance, processing, and the barriers and procedures used when radiographs are taken. Usually a fee is charged for this inspection, and many jurisdictions also require a fee for licensure to use x-ray machines.

Tube Head and Arm

Head Leakage
The term *tube head leakage* refers to radiation that escapes through the protective shielding of the x-ray tube head. The only radiation that should leave the tube head is the primary beam. Radiation leakage exposes the patient unnecessarily and should not occur in a properly functioning x-ray unit. Leakage is a violation of the federal performance standards and local radiation codes. It is not a common problem because x-ray units are well built, and if the unit is not abused in use or moving, head leakage is unlikely to occur.

Drift
Tube head drift (Figure 6-2) is a common problem that is easily corrected. The tube head of the dental x-ray machine should not move, or drift, in any direction after positioning for an exposure (see Figure 1-3). The movement can cause a blurred image or position the central ray off the film, resulting in a collimator cutoff ("cone cut"). If the tube head drifts, the arm should be repaired immediately. This usually entails just tightening the bolts that attach the tube-head to the yolk. The patient or the dental professional should never hold the tube head in place during an exposure to correct for tube head drift.

Checking for tube head drift in all directions is an important step in an office quality assurance program.

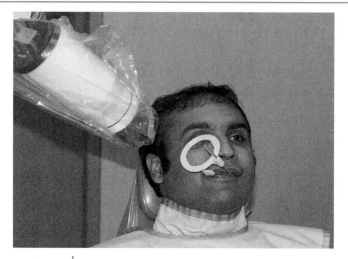

Figure 6-2. | Tubehead drift places the x-ray beam far from the film.

Kilovoltage and Milliampere Seconds

The equipment-related factors of kVp and mAs control proper penetration and film density and contrast. As explained in Chapter 3, film speed and focal-film distance (FFD) determine the contribution of mAs to the patient's radiation exposure. However, the choice of kVp affects the contrast of the film and radiation dose. The patient's skin exposure decreases as the kVp increases, but the dose to deeper tissues and the amount of scatter radiation increase. At present some debate focuses on the best kVp within the 65 to 90 range that should be used in dentistry. A kilovoltage that is best suited to the diagnostic requirements should be chosen. There is no question that kVp below 65 should not be used; although it is possible to produce a diagnostic image, the exposure to the patient per film is nearly doubled when a kVp below the acceptable range is used (Figure 6-3).

Filtration

Because of the enactment of federal performance standards and the enforcement of local health codes, filtration is no longer a major concern in patient protection; compliance is almost 100%. The purpose of *filtration* is to remove the long (soft), nonpenetrating x-ray photons from the x-ray beam (see Chapter 2). These photons either would be absorbed by the overlying tissues or give rise to secondary radiation to the patient and degrade the diagnostic image.

Collimation

The collimation of the x-ray beam limits the size of the area exposed by the primary beam and the amount of scatter produced. The beam size is discussed in Chapter 2, and at present a $2^3/_4$-in (7-cm) circular beam measured at the skin is required. If the size and shape of the x-ray beam were changed to a

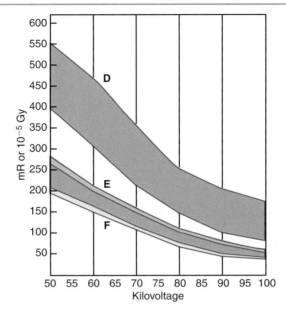

Figure 6-3. Acceptable x-ray exposure ranges for group D, E, and F films. Note the increased exposure in the low-kVp range and that the exposure with group E is about half that of group D. *(Courtesy Department of Health and Human Services. Modified by S. White.)*

rectangle that is slightly larger than the film, the volume of tissue exposed could be reduced by more than half. The American Dental Association (ADA) and the American Academy of Oral and Maxillofacial Radiology strongly recommend the use of *rectangular collimation* (Figure 6-4). Rectangular collimation is the single most effective factor in reducing radiation to the patient.

Timing Device

The use of more sensitive x-ray film with extremely short exposure times makes the use of electronic *timers* imperative (see Figure 2-5). All new x-ray machines come equipped with these devices.

The mechanical timers existing on older machines are inaccurate at short exposures. These timers are usually calibrated down to $1/4$ second and can have a $1/4$-second margin of error. It is impossible to use a mechanical timer with group D, E, and F films and make accurate exposures. Unfortunately those still using mechanical timers often compensate for the unavoidable overexposure by underdeveloping and in this way produce a diagnostic radiograph at the expense of patient exposure. Only an electronic-type timer should be used as the standard of care.

Position-Indicating Devices

Open-ended, lead-lined (shielded) rectangles (Figure 6-5, *A*) or cylinders (Figure 6-5, *B*) are the only types of position-indicating devices (PIDs) that should be used. The use of closed-end, pointed cones is contraindicated

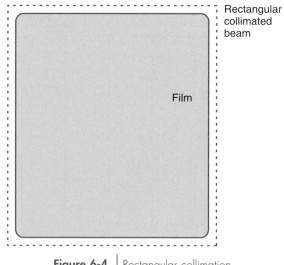

Rectangular
collimated
beam

Film

Figure 6-4. | Rectangular collimation.

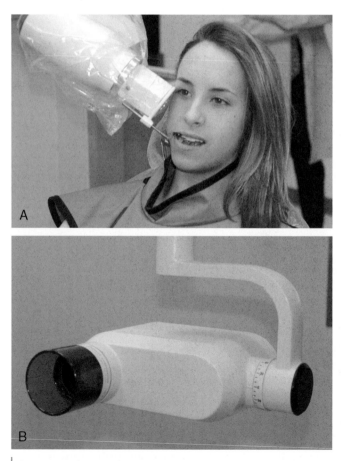

Figure 6-5. | **A,** Open-ended metal rectangular collimator. **B,** Open-ended lead-lined cylinder.

(see Chapter 2). These cones increase scatter radiation to the patient because of the interaction of the primary beam with the closed end of the cone (see Figure 2-10). It is somewhat disconcerting to note that in an era of concern for radiation, radiation surveys of practicing dentists have reported use of the pointed cone. Many state or local health codes prohibit the use of closed-end, pointed PIDs. Any existing closed-end, pointed cones should be replaced by the recommended PIDs.

Receptor (Film) Holders

Film holders that align the x-ray beam with the film in the patient's mouth should be used. These *film-holding devices* reduce the possibility of "cone cutting." Some of these devices also produce rectangular collimation (Figure 6-6). A film holder should never be held in place for the patient by the operator. Some of the more commonly used film-holding devices are shown in Figure 10-12.

Film, Intensifying Screens, and Digital Sensors

Decreasing the *exposure time* by the use of a more sensitive receptor (film, film-screen combinations, digital detectors) is one of the most effective factors in reducing radiation exposure to the patient. As discussed in Chapter 4, film slower than group D should never be used. Group E film, when compared with group D film, reduces the radiation exposure by 50% (see Figure 6-3). At present the American Dental Association recommends the use of E-speed or faster film. The E film and new F film are major advances in patient

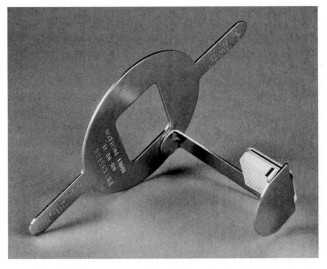

Figure 6-6. | Precision device used for rectangular collimation. *(Courtesy Masel Enterprises, Bristol, PA.)*

protection. Their use requires an electronic timer and strict adherence to time-temperature processing because there is very little leeway for error. The new film has not been accepted universally by practitioners because of claims of lost diagnostic ability. Many recent reports of clinical tests of D versus E film show that no significant clinical difference between the films exists. The Eastman Kodak Company changed the shape of the silver halide grains of their E-speed film to increase the sharpness and give higher-contrast images with less dependence on processing conditions. This improvement was designed to overcome the profession's reluctance to universally accept the use of E-speed film. In response to the market, Kodak has discontinued the manufacture of its E-speed film but continues to market D-speed (Ultra speed) as well as its new F-speed (Concise) film. Clinical trials of the new F-speed film have found that its contrast and resolution are equal to that of D-speed film.

As discussed in Chapter 15, the use of digital imaging can reduce the patient's radiation exposure by up to 90%. Extraoral projections (e.g., pantomograms, lateral skull projections) should always be done using the fastest intensifying screen available.

Lead Aprons and Thyroid Collars

All patients should be draped with a *lead apron* and wear a *thyroid collar* for every intraoral exposure (Figure 6-7). This rule holds regardless of the patient's age or the number of films exposed. The use of lead aprons and thyroid collars can reduce radiation to the thyroid and gonads by up to 94%. The apron should cover the patient from the thyroid to the gonadal area. Lead aprons with attached cervical (thyroid) shields are available. Separate thyroid collars can be purchased to use with existing lead aprons. The aprons

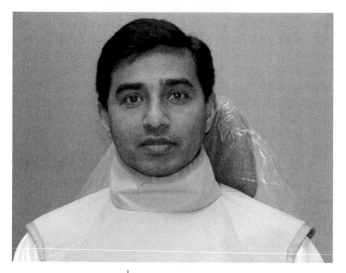

Figure 6-7. | Lead apron with thyroid collar.

available are usually the equivalent of 0.25-mm lead, relatively light and flexible, and not uncomfortable for the patient. The dose to the gonads is very small during dental exposures but can be reduced even further with the lead apron. The thyroid gland, except with rectangular collimation and more specifically the bisecting-angle technique, may lie in the path of the primary beam. The dose may be small but can be decreased significantly with the use of the thyroid collar. There is no valid reason not to use the lead apron and collar for every intraoral exposure. Many states have enacted legislation that makes this procedure mandatory. Patients react favorably to the apron as they feel protected and are reassured that the dental office is up-to-date and concerned about radiation safety.

Lead aprons should not be folded but rather hung up or draped over a rounded surface when not in use. Folding eventually cracks the lead and allows leakage. For taking panoramic films, the positioning of the front and back lead aprons must be modified, as discussed in Chapter 12.

TECHNIQUE

Retakes

As discussed in Chapter 16, one of the major sources of unnecessary exposure to radiation in the dental office is retaking films as a result of poor technique in either taking or processing films. Every *retake* represents an unnecessary doubling of radiation exposure to the patient for that film. Both the dental professional and the dentist are obligated to perfect their intraoral technique so that retakes are unnecessary. This professional improvement can be accomplished by taking continuing education courses or intraoffice training. Every error should be analyzed regarding its cause and rate of occurrence and what must be done to correct the error. Colleagues should critique each other's work and help to correct errors of technique.

Exposure

Films should be exposed properly. A technique that employs overexposure with underdevelopment subjects the patient to unnecessary radiation. If exposed films come out too dark with time-temperature processing, the exposure time or the kVp, not the developing time, should be reduced. An overexposure and a shortened processing time used to expedite patient treatment are unconscionable in relation to good patient radiation hygiene. Figure 6-8 shows an acceptable range of x-ray exposure. The exposures are expressed in milliroentgens and not impulses or seconds. If one knows the output of the dental x-ray machine (mR/s), then the exposure can be expressed as milliroentgens instead of impulses to see whether the exposure falls within the acceptable range. Film packets or boxes also come with recommended exposure times, so there is no excuse for overexposure.

D-Speed Film ★			E-Speed Film ★ ★		
kVp	Lower Limit	Upper Limit	kVp	Lower Limit	Upper Limit
50	425	575	50	220	320
55	350	500	55	190	270
60	310	440	60	165	230
65	270	400	65	140	200
70	240	350	70	120	170
75	170	260	75	100	140
80	150	230	80	90	120
85	130	200	85	80	105
90	120	180	90	70	90
95	110	160	95	60	80
100	100	140	100	50	70

*Exposure Conditions

10 mA
  8" S.S.D.
50−70 kVp − 1.5 mm A1
71−100 kVp − 2.5 mm A1

**Exposure Conditions

10 mA, 12" S.S.D.
50−70 kVp − 1.5 mm A1
71−100 kVp − 2.5 mm A1

Figure 6-8. Acceptable range of x-ray exposure. *(From Department of Health and Human Services:* Dental exposure normalization technique [DENT] instruction manual.*)*

Paralleling Technique

In addition to a more accurate diagnostic image, the paralleling technique results in lower dose levels to the thyroid gland and the lens of the eye (Figure 6-9). In the paralleling method the x-ray beam for all projections is very close to being parallel to the floor, whereas the bisecting method results

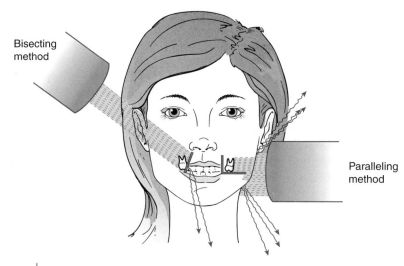

Figure 6-9. X-ray beam in the paralleling and bisecting methods and scatter radiation to the thyroid gland.

in an x-ray beam that has steep vertical angulations that may put the thyroid gland and lens of the eye in the path of the primary x-ray beam as well as the secondary radiation.

Focal-Film Distance

Increased focal-film distances (FFDs), up to 16 in, are recommended with the paralleling technique to compensate for the magnification of the image caused by the increased object-film distance (see Chapter 3). Another important advantage of an increased FFD is that less total tissue volume is in the path of the primary beam at 16 in than at 8 in. As the distance increases from 8 in to 16 in (Figure 6-10), the x-ray beam becomes less divergent and less total body area is irradiated by the primary beam after it penetrates the skin. The shorter FFD, with a more divergent beam, irradiates a far greater volume of tissue. The diameter of the primary beam is still 2³/₄ in at the skin in both cases. The difference is in the beam divergence after the skin entry and film exposure.

Darkroom

Every effort should be made to establish darkroom procedures that produce films with the maximum diagnostic yield. As mentioned, underdevelopment should not compensate for overexposure. There is no excuse for darkroom errors that cause film retakes. This subject is discussed thoroughly in Chapter 8.

Viewing Finished Radiographs

To obtain maximum diagnostic yield for the radiation expended, the manner of *film viewing* for interpretation is extremely important. The only proper way to view a radiograph is in front of an illuminator (viewbox), preferably with a variable light source (see Figure 3-14). Using sunlight in front of a window or

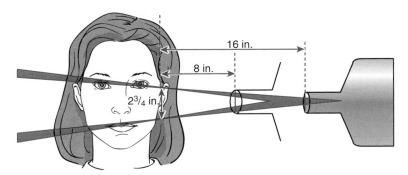

Figure 6-10. Focal-film distance (FFD) and tissue volume exposed. Shaded areas represent tissue exposed at 8-inch FFD but not in the beam at 16-inch FFD because of the more parallel and less divergent x-rays.

the lamp on the dental unit is unsatisfactory. The film mount used for the full-mouth survey should cover the entire illuminator, and empty windows in the mount should be covered with an opaque material. This prevents light that escapes around the periphery or through the mount from distracting the viewer. Ideally, radiographs should be viewed in a darkened room to avoid excessive reflection, but this is not practical in the average dental facility.

CLINICAL JUDGMENT

Radiation History

Specific questions regarding the patient's previous radiation exposures should be part of every history. This *radiation history* should include medical, dental diagnostic, and therapeutic radiation. Patients may not voluntarily divulge such information because they may not realize its importance. Questions of this type may help determine whether dental radiographs have been taken recently that might be available and still diagnostically valid. Such radiographs also provide historical data, show previous dental disease, and indicate the result of treatment. Such historical data will influence the selection criteria evaluation, in which certain positive historical findings will indicate a need for radiographs. A history of radiation therapy is important not so much because of risk of the added dental dose but because of interest in the areas irradiated. As mentioned in Chapter 5, radiation to the head and neck region may leave the patient susceptible to xerostomia, radiation caries, and osteoradionecrosis, and a postradiation preventive protocol should be instituted. The radiation history contains valuable and pertinent information in treatment planning.

Selection Criteria

Selection criteria are descriptions of clinical conditions (signs and symptoms) and historical data that identify patients who are most likely to benefit from a particular radiographic examination. The selection criteria aid the dentist, as this is the dentist's decision, to select which patients need radiographs and determine which radiographs are needed. The final decision rests with the individual dentist and is determined by professional judgment.

An expert panel of dentists sponsored by the Public Health Service had developed guidelines for the prescription of dental radiographs. The guidelines have been revised recently by another select panel of the ADA and Food and Drug Administration (FDA) (Figure 6-11). Using these guidelines, the dentist can decide when, what type, and how many radiographs should be taken. The practice of taking dental radiographs based on a time interval rather than on patient needs, as determined by clinical examination and dental history, is not considered an appropriate way to practice dental radiography. The dentist should decide whether to take radiographs after examining the patient. There are no routine dental radiographs. Radiographic needs are not determined by the calendar but rather by evaluating the overall health needs of a patient after a clinical examination and history. Positive findings in these categories would change the radiation needs of a patient and reclassify the patient from the asymptomatic to the symptomatic category, for which radiographs would be indicated and the guidelines would not be operative. This is true for new patients, emergencies, and recall visits.

These guidelines for patients who are asymptomatic are shown in chart form in Figure 6-11 and are from a report that covers three general categories of patients: patients with positive historical findings, those who are symptomatic, and those who are asymptomatic. Asymptomatic patients are divided into three main categories: (1) children with primary or transitional dentition, (2) adolescents with permanent dentition, and (3) adults, including dentulous and edentulous patients. Each patient category is further divided into new patient and recall patient categories. In addition, the recall patient category is subdivided into clinical caries or high-risk factors for caries, no clinical caries or high-risk factors, periodontal disease, growth and development assessment, and patients with other circumstances.

Using these guidelines, it is clear that all new patients should have a recent full-mouth survey of some type on file before treatment is instituted. The radiographs may be taken by the current dentist or may be duplicates of those taken by a previous dentist. The full-mouth survey is essential for case planning, baseline data for future reference, and medicolegal reasons.

Recall radiographs should not be taken for all patients as a matter of routine. As seen in Figure 6-11, very few patients need radiographs at 6-month intervals. Caries susceptibility, for example, is a major factor in determining the time frame for recall radiographs. The diagnostic radiographic needs of a decay-prone teenager are quite different from those of a middle-aged periodontal recall patient whose last filling was placed 20 years earlier. Using the Guideline Chart, apply it to some clinical examples.

Patient #1: A 59-year-old edentulous patient presents to a dental office seeking new dentures. The patient's dentures were made in that office 5 years ago after radiographs revealed the necessity of multiple extractions. Following the extractions the tissue healed uneventfully, and the dentures were fabricated. At the present time the clinical examination yields negative results and the patient's only concern is the lack of retention of the dentures. What would be the radiographic prescription for this patient?

The correct answer would be **no radiographs necessary**. According to the chart, an asymptomatic edentulous patient does not need recall radiographs. If there were signs, symptoms, or a positive history, then radiographs would be indicated.

Patient #2: A 14-year-old patient presents for a 6-month recall examination. At the last visit, three teeth needed restorations. What would be the radiographic prescription?

The correct answer would be **take posterior bitewings**. The chart indicates that this patient should have bitewing radiographs every 6 to 12 months until he is caries-free.

The recommendations in this chart are subject to clinical judgment and may not apply to every patient. They are to be used by dentists only after reviewing the patient's health history and completing a clinical examination. Because every precaution should be taken to minimize radiation exposure, protective thyroid collars and aprons should be used whenever possible. This practice is strongly recommended for children, women of childbearing age, and pregnant women.

TYPE OF ENCOUNTER	PATIENT AGE AND DENTAL DEVELOPMENTAL STAGE				
	Child with Primary Dentition (prior to eruption of first permanent tooth)	Child with Transitional Dentition (after eruption of first permanent tooth)	Adolescent with Permanent Dentition (prior to eruption of third molars)	Adult, Dentate or Partially Edentulous	Adult, Edentulous
New patient* being evaluated for dental diseases and dental development	Individualized radiographic exam consisting of selected periapical/occlusal views and/or posterior bitewings if proximal surfaces cannot be visualized or probed. Patients without evidence of disease and with open proximal contacts may not require a radiographic exam at this time.	Individualized radiographic exam consisting of posterior bitewings with panoramic exam or posterior bitewings and selected periapical images	Individualized radiographic exam consisting of posterior bitewings with panoramic exam or posterior bitewings and selected periapical images. A full-mouth intraoral radiographic exam is preferred when the patient has clinical evidence of generalized dental disease or a history of extensive dental treatment.		Individualized radiographic exam, based on clinical signs and symptoms.
Recall patient* with clinical caries or at increased risk for caries†	Posterior bitewing exam at 6- to 12-month intervals if proximal surfaces cannot be examined visually or with a probe		Posterior bitewing exam at 6- to 12-month intervals if proximal surfaces cannot be examined visually or with a probe	Posterior bitewing exam at 6- to 18-month intervals	Not applicable
Recall patient* with no clinical caries and not at increased risk for caries†	Posterior bitewing exam at 12- to 24-month intervals if proximal surfaces cannot be examined visually or with a probe		Posterior bitewing exam at 18- to 36-month intervlas	Posterior bitewing exam at 24- to 36-month intervals	Not applicable

Figure 6-11. Guidelines for prescribing dental radiographs. *(From American Dental Association, U.S. Food & Drug Administration: The Selection of Patients for Dental Radiograph Examinations, November 2004. Available at www.ada.org.)*

TYPE OF ENCOUNTER	PATIENT AGE AND DENTAL DEVELOPMENTAL STAGE				
	Child with Primary Dentition (prior to eruption of first permanent tooth)	Child with Transitional Dentition (after eruption of first permanent tooth)	Adolescent with Permanent Dentition (prior to eruption of third molars)	Adult, Dentate or Partially Edentulous	Adult, Edentulous
Recall patient* with periodontal disease	Clinical judgment as to the need for and type of radiographic images for the evaluation of periodontal disease. Imaging may consist of, but is not limited to, selected bitewing and/or periapical images of areas where periodontal disease (other than nonspecific gingivitis) can be identified clinically.				Not applicable
Patient for monitoring of growth and development	Clinical judgment as to the need for and type of radiographic images for evaluation and/or monitoring of dentofacial growth and development		Clinical judgment as to the need for and type of radiographic images for evaluation and/or monitoring of dentofacial growth and development. Panoramic or periapical exam to assess developing third molars	Usually not indicated	
Patient with other circumstances including, but not limited to, proposed or existing implants, pathologic conditions, restorative/endodontic needs, treated periodontal disease, and caries remineralization	Clinical judgment as to the need for and type of radiographic images for evaluation and/or monitoring in these circumstances				

*Clinical situations for which radiographs may be indicated include but are not limited to the following:

A. Positive Historical Findings
1. Previous periodontal or endodontic treatment
2. History of pain or trauma
3. Familial history of dental anomalies
4. Postoperative evaluation of healing
5. Remineralization monitoring
6. Presence of implants or evaluation for implant placement

Figure 6-11—cont'd

B. Positive Clinical Signs/Symptoms
1. Clinical evidence of periodontal disease
2. Large or deep restorations
3. Deep carious lesions
4. Malposed or clinically impacted teeth
5. Swelling
6. Evidence of dental/facial trauma
7. Mobility of teeth
8. Sinus tract ("fistula")
9. Clinically suspected sinus pathologic condition
10. Growth abnormalities
11. Oral involvement in known or suspected systemic disease
12. Positive neurologic findings in the head and neck
13. Evidence of foreign objects
14. Pain and/or dysfunction of the temporomandibular joint
15. Facial asymmetry
16. Abutment teeth for fixed or removable partial prosthesis
17. Unexplained bleeding
18. Unexplained sensitivity of teeth
19. Unusual eruption, spacing, or migration of teeth
20. Unusual tooth morphology, calcification, or color
21. Unexplained absence of teeth
22. Clinical erosion

†**Factors increasing risk for caries may include but are not limited to:**
1. High level of caries experience or demineralization
2. History of recurrent caries
3. High titers of cariogenic bacteria
4. Existing restoration(s) of poor quality
5. Poor oral hygiene
6. Inadequate fluoride exposure
7. Prolonged nursing (bottle or breast)
8. Frequent high sucrose content in diet
9. Poor family dental health
10. Developmental or acquired enamel defects
11. Developmental or acquired disability
12. Xerostomia
13. Genetic abnormality of teeth
14. Many multisurface restorations
15. Chemo/radiation therapy
16. Eating disorders
17. Drug/alcohol abuse
18. Irregular dental care

Figure 6-11—cont'd

Patient #3: A new edentulous patient presents seeking new dentures and dental care. Intraoral examination suggests the presence of retained root tips. What would be the radiographic prescription?

The correct answer would be a **full-mouth intraoral series** or a **panoramic examination**. All new patients should have a radiographic examination.

Administrative Radiographs

Administrative radiographs are those required for reasons not related to the patient's immediate health needs. Included in this category are teaching films, those required by state examination and licensing authorities, and radiographs taken to verify treatment for compensation by insurance companies or other third-party carriers. Radiographs should never be taken for administrative reasons. If it produces no diagnostic benefit to the patient, the radiograph should not be taken. This is not to say that radiographs should not be submitted to insurance carriers; films taken for diagnostic purposes, or their duplicates, can be submitted because no unnecessary radiation is used. Many states have laws that prohibit the use of administrative radiographs, and the FDA recommends that insurance carriers and others refrain from requiring administrative radiographs.

Postoperative radiographs are indicated only when they have diagnostic value, such as for confirming the retrieval of a root tip in surgery or the placement of filling materials in endodontic procedures. The use of radiographs to check the fit, contact, contour, and seating of restorations or seating of implant fixtures is strongly discouraged. These checks are best done with mirror, explorer, and floss, thus saving the patient the radiation exposure.

Working films in endodontics, surgical implant placement, and restorative post and pin preparations may be necessary for proper treatment, but every effort should be made to keep the number of exposures to a minimum.

SUGGESTED READINGS

American Dental Association Council on Scientific Affairs: An update on radiographic practices: information and recommendations, J Am Dent Assoc 132:234-238, 2001.

Code of Federal Regulations, 21 subchapter J Radiol Health part 1000, Washington, D.C., Office of the Federal Register, General Services Administration, 1994.

National Council on Radiation Protection and Measurements: NCRP Report No. 145, Radiation in dentistry, 2004.

Recommendations on administratively required dental examination, Fed Reg 45:40976-40979, 1980.

U.S. Department of Health and Human Services, Public Health Service FDA: The selection of patients for dental radiographic examinations, HHS/PHS/FDA, 88-827310-21, 1987.

White SC, Pharoah MJ: Oral radiology: principles and interpretation, ed 5, St Louis, Mosby, 2004.

Operator Protection

Operator Dosage and Protection
   Maximum Permissible Dose
   Exposure Technique
   Radiation Monitoring

Protective Barriers
Pregnancy
Patient Concerns and Education

1. Understand and feel comfortable working with ionizing radiation.
2. Perform all necessary precautions to obtain a maximum permissible dose of zero.

barrier
exposure technique
film badge

maximum permissible
   dose
monitoring devices
pocket dosimeters

pregnancy
   primary radiation
secondary radiation

OPERATOR DOSAGE AND PROTECTION

As was noted earlier about the concerns of protecting the operator and patient from radiation, it is much easier to deal with the protection of the radiographer. The sources of potential exposure to the dental professional are the primary beam, head leakage from the tube, and secondary radiation originating from the patient, x-ray machine, or objects in the operatory. Through the use of careful technique in a well-designed, well-equipped, and well-monitored office, the occupational exposure of dental professionals and dentists to ionizing radiation can be kept to a minimum; in effect, the occupational dose should be zero.

Maximum Permissible Dose

At present the *maximum permissible* dose (MPD) of whole body radiation for persons occupationally concerned with ionizing radiation, such as dental professionals and dentists, is 5000 mrem (50 mSv) per year, or 100 mrem/week. This is in contrast to the recommended MPD of 500 mrem (5 mSv) for the general public. In addition, the operator should not receive more than 3000 mrem (30 mSv) in any 13-week period. Dental personnel also should not exceed a maximum accumulated lifetime dose of $(N - 18) \times 5000$ mrem. In this formula, N is the operator's age.

The current stated MPD for the operator is 5000 mrem/year, but historically the MPD has been higher, and this figure may be revised downward. The International Commission on Radiation Protection (ICRP) has recommended that the yearly MPD be reduced to 2000 mrem (20 mSv). This recommendation is based on new information that has been released concerning the amount of x-radiation in the atomic bombs at the end of World War II and their effects on the Hiroshima and Nagasaki populations. However, the National Council on Radiation Protection and Measurements (NCRP) in its most recent report has chosen to maintain the present MPD. Dental professionals and dentists should strive for an occupational dose of zero. If one's occupational dose is zero, any downward change in the MPD would produce no cause for concern because zero is zero. Zero exposure is not difficult to achieve in an office whose members have an awareness of radiation hygiene. A dental professional should not fear working with x-rays, but he or she should be knowledgeable regarding their use and abuse.

Exposure Technique

The dental professional or dentist should never be in the path of the primary beam. Film packets should never be held in the patient's mouth, nor should a drifting tube head be held by the person making the exposure. There are *no exceptions* to this rule. The operator should not make the mistake of saying, "I'll just hold the film for the patient this one time." Ideally for proper *exposure technique*, the operator should be a minimum of 6 ft away from the tube head and behind a suitable barrier (i.e., a wall) when the exposure is made. At 6 ft the minimum occupational exposure does not exceed the MPD, but at 6 ft and behind the barrier the occupational exposure is zero.

Federal and state regulations require that every x-ray machine be equipped with either a 6-ft retractable exposure cord or a remote switch that permits such operator positioning. The remote switch is preferable because it prevents lapses in operator technique. Though not as crucial as distance and shielding, knowing the areas of minimum scatter is important to the operator. These areas are at right angles to the x-ray beam and toward the back of the patient (Figure 7-1). The areas of highest scatter are in back of the tube head and behind the patient. Correct positioning of the operator still necessitates the minimum 6-ft distance and adequate barrier protection (Figures 7-2 and 7-3).

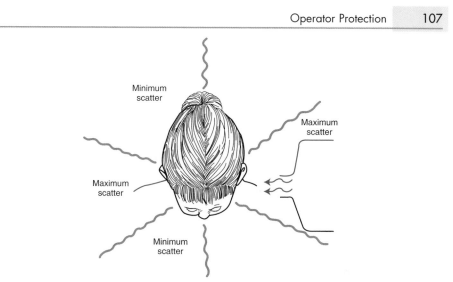

Figure 7-1. Areas of minimum and maximum scatter during dental x-ray exposure.

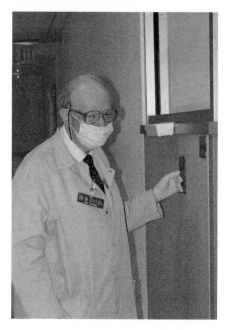

Figure 7-2. Operator standing outside operatory and viewing patient through protective window.

Radiation Monitoring

How can dental professionals and dentists know the amount of occupational exposure of radiation they receive? Concerned personnel can use two methods to measure the levels of radiation and potential exposure. First, a CRESO

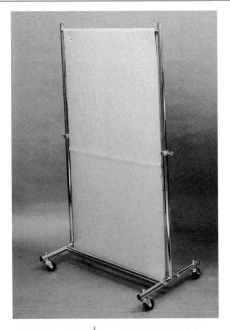

Figure 7-3. | Portable x-ray shield.

(Certified Radiation Equipment Safety Officer) can perform a radiation survey using ionization chambers to determine radiation levels during exposures at all locations in the office. This type of survey, which is very much like a survey done by local or state agencies, checks the reliability of the x-ray machine and protective barriers. It does not monitor the day-to-day activity of the concerned personnel.

The second method is to have personnel wear *monitoring devices*, such as *pocket dosimeters* or *film badges*. Of the two methods, film badges are less expensive and more widely used. Film badge service is readily available from many radiation survey companies at a nominal monthly cost. The badge (Figure 7-4) is usually worn for a 3- or 4-month period and contains a sensor that is embossed with the wearer's name and identification number. At the end of the prescribed reporting period, the film packet is returned to the survey company, where it is processed; the density on the film is compared with standards and the exposure is determined. The report returned to the dental office contains not only the exposure for the reporting period, but also the accumulated quarterly, yearly, and lifetime exposure of the individual (Figure 7-5). Using the 100-mrem weekly MPD limit, the dental professional's radiation exposure can be evaluated easily. The film badge should be worn in the office at all times to provide an accurate reading of occupational exposure. If clipped to a pocket, it should not be covered with a pen or piece of jewelry that might shield the film. Dental professionals should not wear the badge outside the office, especially in sunlight, and they should remove it if they are having medical or dental x-rays exposed because it is intended to measure only occupational exposure.

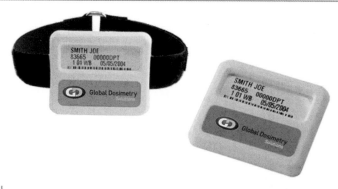

Figure 7-4. A film badge can be attached to a belt or uniform. *(Courtesy Global Dosimetry Solutions, Irvine, CA.)*

Protective Barriers

The walls, floor, and ceiling of the x-ray operatory must be of such construction that the surrounding areas are shielded from both *primary* and *secondary radiation*. This does not mean that they must be lead-lined. Many materials used in construction today in the proper thickness provide protective shielding. Because of the relatively low workload and the low x-ray energies used (65 to 90 kVp), dental offices with concrete or cinder block walls have enough inherent shielding in wall construction materials. Drywall construction, if of proper thickness, is also sufficient for dental shielding.

The shielding or *barrier* requirements are based on such factors as workload, use and occupancy factors, maximum kilovoltage, and distance from the tube head. The formula $W \times U \times T$ is used to calculate the guide number. In this formula, W is the workload (in milliampere minutes per week) and U is the use factor. The walls in dental radiography have a higher use factor (1/4) than the floors or ceiling (1/16) because the central ray is never directed straight up or down. T is the occupancy factor, which accounts for whether a person is behind the barrier all the time, as one seated at a desk ($T = 1$); sometimes, as in a waiting room ($T = 1/4$); or occasionally, as in a passageway ($T = 1/8$). The guide number is correlated with the proper kVp and distance in reference tables found in Report 35 by the NCRP. These tables give the specifications of materials necessary for adequate shielding for the given conditions.

Pregnancy

The pregnant dental professional, in relation to occupational exposure, should not be compared with the pregnant patient, discussed in Chapter 5. In a well-designed and well-monitored dental office, the occupational exposure is zero. If a pregnant dental professional or dentist follows proper procedure in such an office, there is no risk to the fetus. A pregnant worker who is apprehensive should wear a film badge to document occupational exposure and allay any fears. The courts have held that there is no reason to change chairside or other

Occupational Radiation Exposure Report

Accredited by the "National Institute of Standards and Technology through NVLAP for the specific scope of accreditation under lab code 100555-0"

REPORT NO: **01224** ACCOUNT NO: **30426S** LOCATION: **30426DPT**

DATE BADGES RECEIVED:	01/17/2001
DATE BADGES REPORTED:	JAN 19, 2001
PAGE: 1 OF: 1	Copy 1 of 2
LICENSE NO:	
PURCHASE ORDER NO:	

NOTIFICATION LEVELS		
DEEP	SHALLOW	EXTREMITY
400	*600*	*600*

S/I: 1

REPORT TO:
ABC Corporation
LOUIS

3300 Hyland Avenue
RSO
COSTA MESA, CA 92626

SHIP TO:
ABC Corporation
LOUIS

3300 Hyland Avenue
RSO
COSTA MESA, CA 92626

WEARER NUMBER	SLOT NUMBER	PROCESS CONTROL NUMBER	NAME (LAST) OR OTHER DESIGNATION	F I	M I	ID TYPE	SSN / ID	BIRTH DATE	SEX	BADGE TYPE	BODY REGION	BODY PART	SERVICE	MONITORING PERIOD FIRST DAY	MONITORING PERIOD LAST DAY	DOSE EQUIVALENT IN MILLIREMS FOR PERIODS INDICATED BELOW: CURRENT DEEP	CURRENT EYE	CURRENT SHALL.	CURRENT NEUT.	CURRENT PROC. NOTES	QUARTER TO DATE DEEP	QUARTER TO DATE EYE	QUARTER TO DATE SHALL.	YEAR TO DATE DEEP	YEAR TO DATE EYE	YEAR TO DATE SHALL.	YEAR TO DATE NO. RPTS	LIFETIME TO DATE DEEP	LIFETIME TO DATE DOSE HISTORY ADJUSTMENTS	LIFETIME TO DATE INCEPTION DATE LIFETIME TOTAL
		0055631	CONTROL-DAILY							01			M	01/01/2001	01/31/2001															
		0026349	CONTROL-DAILY							03			M	01/01/2001	01/31/2001															
		0026349	CONTROL-DAILY							18			M	01/01/2001	01/31/2001															
		0026349	CONTROL-DAILY							19			M	01/01/2001	01/31/2001															
70004		0055631	JONES	C		1	124567890	19900701	M	01	EW		M	01/01/2001	01/31/2001	10	10	10			10	10	10	10	10	10	1	888		09/01/1998
70004		0055631	JONES	C		1	124567890	19900701	M	01	WB	CL	M	01/01/2001	01/31/2001	200	200	200			200	200	200	200	200	200	1	1474		11/01/1998
			EDE Calculation													23					23			23			1	23		
70004		0026349	JONES	C		1	124567890	19900701	M	18	NSE	FN	M	01/01/2001	01/31/2001			1752					1752			1752	1			09/01/1998
70005		0055631	SMITH	T		1	135678901	19881212	M	01	EW		M	01/01/2001	01/31/2001	20	20	20			20	20	20	20	20	20	1	869		10/01/1998
70005		0055631	SMITH	T		1	135678901	19881212	M	01	WB	CL	M	01/01/2001	01/31/2001	300	300	300			300	300	300	300	300	300	1	1573		11/01/1998
			EDE Calculation													42					42			42			1	42		
70005		0026349	SMITH	T		1	135678901	19881212	M	18	NSE	FN	M	01/01/2001	01/31/2001			15250					15250			15250	1			10/01/1998
70006		0055631	SMITH	J		1	145673215	19800901	M	01	EW		M	01/01/2001	01/31/2001	30	30	30			30	30	30	30	30	30	1	890		10/01/1998
70006		0055631	SMITH	J		1	145673215	19800901	M	01	WB	CL	M	01/01/2001	01/31/2001	400	400	400			400	400	400	400	400	400	1	1659		11/01/1998
			EDE Calculation													61					61			61			1	61		
70007		0026349	JAMES	S	J	1		19800101	F	03	WB		M	01/01/2001	01/31/2001	1257	1350	1475			1257	1350	1475	1257	1350	1475	1	1257		02/01/1999
70007		0026349	JAMES	S	J	1		19800101	F	19	NSE	FN	M	01/01/2001	01/31/2001			21					21			21	1			02/01/1999
1	2	3	4	5	6	7	8	9	10	11	12	13	14	15	16	17	18	19	20	21	22	23	24	25	26	27	28	29	30	31

SEE REVERSE SIDE FOR COMPLETE REPORT DETAILS BY COLUMN NUMBER

IT IS RECOMMENDED THAT YOU KEEP THIS REPORT FOR YOUR RECORDS

Global Dosimetry Solutions

2652 McGaw Avenue, Irvine, CA 92614
U.S./Canada: (800) 251-3331
http://www.dosimetry.com e-mail: info@dosimetry.com

REPORTS APPROVED FPM/TPM FRM4047 09/22/04

Figure 7-5. Film badge report. This monthly report gives current and cumulative exposure for the listed personnel. *(Courtesy Global Dosimetry Solutions, Irvine, CA.)*

duties during *pregnancy* because of concern about radiation exposure. However, there are specially designed lead aprons available for pregnant operator usage if they are deemed necessary.

PATIENT CONCERNS AND EDUCATION

Dental professionals and dentists should understand and be sensitive to patients' concerns about and possible fear of dental radiographs. Recent years have been marked by a rise in consumerism and an increasing mistrust of healthcare providers. The media have been replete with stories warning of the danger of medical and dental radiographs.

Dental professionals, through knowledge and understanding, must be able to allay fears and explain the necessity of radiographs for proper dental treatment. A patient is likely to question the dental professional rather than the dentist about the danger of radiography. It may be helpful to explain to the patient how essential radiographs are in the detection and management of diseases and treatment planning. Patients also can be informed of federal and local laws enacted for their protection. Patient educational material, such as the American Dental Association's pamphlets *Dental X-ray Examinations, Your Dentist's Advice,* and *The Benefits of X-Rays,* or the Food and Drug Administration's *X-rays: Get the Picture on Protection,* can be placed in the waiting room or given to interested patients.

Comparisons of common sources of radiation to dental dosage can also be helpful. The patient can be reminded that the dose from four bitewing films can be as little as 0.038 mSv (3.8 mrad), which is the equivalent of about $1\frac{1}{2}$ days of background radiation, and a full-mouth series of 0.150 mSv (15 mrad) is about equal to 7 days of background radiation exposure. Comparisons can be made between a lower gastrointestinal series dose of 4.06 mSv (406 mrad) and yearly background radiation of 3.6 mSv (360 mrad).

SUGGESTED READINGS

American Academy of Dental Radiology, Quality Assurance Committee: Recommendations for quality assurance in dental radiography, Oral Surg 55:421-426, 1983.

American Dental Association: The benefits of x-rays, Chicago, 1993, The Association.

Goren AD, Lundeen RC, et al: Updated quality assurance self assessment exercise in intraoral and panoramic radiology, American Academy of Oral and Maxillofacial Radiology, Radiology Practice Committee, Oral Surg Oral Med Oral Pathol Oral Radiol Endod 89:369-374, 2000.

Macdonald JCF, Reid JA, Berthory D: Dry wall construction as a dental radiation barrier, Oral Surg 55:319-326, 1983.

National Council on Radiation Protection and Measurements: NCRP Report No. 145, Radiation protection in dentistry, 2004.

National Council on Radiation Protection and Measurements: NCRP Report No. 116, Limits of exposure to ionizing radiation, 1993.

Plunket L: When an employee becomes pregnant, N Y State Dent J 62:9-11, 1996.

CHAPTER 8

Film Processing: The Darkroom

EDUCATIONAL OBJECTIVES

1. Understand the theory of film processing and how to operate and maintain a darkroom.
2. Be able to process radiographs and identify and correct errors made in the darkroom.

KEY TERMS

automatic processing	film roller	stop bath
clear film	fixer	thermometer
coin test	latent image	thermostatic valve
dark image	light leak	thin image
darkroom	light-tight	time-temperature
daylight loader	manual processing	development
dense image	overdeveloped	torn emulsion
developer	rapid processing	underdeveloped
developer cutoff	replenisher	water bath
drying	reticulation	wet reading
electrostatic artifact	safelight	
film hanger	sight development	

The processing of exposed x-ray film either manually or automatically is an important but often neglected and abused step in the radiographic chain of events. It is at this point that a visible image is produced, from which a diagnosis can be made. The x-rays that have penetrated the hard and soft tissue in the patient's mouth have created a latent image on the exposed x-ray film. The processing of this film converts the latent image to a visible diagnostic image. It should be noted that with increased use of digital radiography, the need for a *darkroom* has become less necessary (as discussed in Chapter 15). However, the knowledge of manual and automatic film processing continues to be included in dental radiology education.

The darkroom is one of the areas in a dental office for which the dental professional has complete responsibility. In addition to processing film, the dental professional must keep the darkroom clean, change solutions regularly, keep accurate records of processed radiographs, and maintain a quality-assurance program. Only through meticulous attention to detail can proper darkroom technique be maintained. It is important to realize that the processing of films is vital in the production of the diagnostic radiograph. Errors in the darkroom can easily ruin what would otherwise have been diagnostic radiographs, making it necessary to retake the films with the resultant loss of time and increased radiation exposure to the patient. It is important to remember that every film that requires retaking doubles the patient's radiation exposure for that film. Good chairside radiographic technique must be coupled with good darkroom technique.

The lack of attention to detail and concern for film processing in many dental offices has been reported in the literature. A study of radiographs submitted to an insurance company for reimbursement reported that a majority of the radiographs were substandard. Of these substandard radiographs, 20% were judged unsatisfactory because of poor density or improper processing. More than 20 years ago, another study done in Nashville, Tennessee, reported equally disturbing findings. About 15% of the facilities changed their processing solutions less frequently than recommended, and severe light leaks in the darkroom were found in 10% of the facilities. More than 40% of the darkrooms did not have a thermometer, and more than 20% did not have a timer. The most alarming finding was that offices using *sight development* techniques showed a much higher milliroentgen exposure per film than offices using the time-temperature technique. Unfortunately, more recent studies have shown that this lack of attention and priority to processing continues. It is much easier to prevent darkroom errors than chairside errors, yet many dental patients receive excessive radiation because of poor processing technique. It is important for the dental professional to have a working knowledge of the chemical reactions taking place in film processing. This understanding helps prevent and correct errors. To process films without understanding is a "cookbook" technique that leads to errors and a lack of appreciation for the importance of the processing task. The importance of eliminating darkroom errors, with the consequence of increased radiation dose to the patient if there is a need to retake films, should be uppermost in the minds of dentists and dental professionals.

DESIGN AND REQUIREMENTS OF THE DARKROOM

The *darkroom* is a room in the dental office set aside for radiographic processing. It should be designed and used only for that purpose, and it should not be combined with a dental laboratory, used as a lounge or a place to hang clothing, or used as a place where the coffee pot is kept. The essential requirements and components of a darkroom are that it should be light-tight and have safelight and white light illumination, processing tanks, a thermostatically controlled supply of water, thermometer, timer, film hangers, *drying* racks, and storage space.

Location and Size

A properly planned and located darkroom is an important but often overlooked feature in a dental office. Darkrooms are placed in unused spaces, closets, and laboratories without proper concern for the function or importance of the procedures to be conducted there.

Dental professionals should have some knowledge of planning, although in most instances they work in previously established facilities. However, office renovation or relocation of a practice occurs often, and the knowledgeable dental professional can have valuable input in the planning and design of a new office.

The darkroom should be a space unto itself, located near the rooms in which the x-ray units are placed. This eliminates the necessity of personnel walking the length of the office with wet readings, thereby saving time, eliminating dripping of processing solutions, and reducing office traffic.

The location of a darkroom should not be determined by the existing plumbing; rather, the darkroom should determine the location of the plumbing.

The darkroom should be a minimum of 16 square ft (4 × 4), allowing enough room for one person to work comfortably. The factors that should be considered in determining the space needed are (1) the volume of radiographs to be processed; (2) the number of dental professionals handling the processing; (3) the type of processing to be done (manual, automatic, or both); and (4) the space required for duplicating, drying, and storage.

The walls of the darkroom should be a light color that reflects the safelighting; darkroom walls do not have to be black. The surfaces of the walls and floor should be of materials that are resistant to staining and can be cleaned of the processing solutions that inevitably spill or splash onto them.

The darkroom must be completely *light-tight* so that when the safelight is on, it is the only illumination in the darkroom. Because x-ray film is sensitive to white light, any light leaks fog the film. A fogged film is less diagnostic and in some cases may be useless. The easiest way to check for *light leaks* is to stand in the darkroom in complete darkness; any leaks around the door or in other areas will be apparent and can be corrected with either black masking tape or weather stripping. The darkroom door should have an inside lock so that the door cannot be opened from the outside while films are being processed.

The darkroom should be well ventilated to exhaust the moisture from the drying films or the heat, if a dryer is used, and maintain comfortable working conditions. Keeping the darkroom at a reasonable temperature makes it easier to maintain desired processing solution temperatures. Another consideration is film quality; if unexposed film is stored in the darkroom cabinets, high temperatures (greater than 90° F) will cause film fog.

Lighting

A well-designed darkroom has five different light sources: (1) an illuminating safelight, (2) an overhead white light, (3) a viewing safelight, (4) an x-ray viewbox, and (5) an outside warning light.

Illuminating Safelight
When film packets are opened, film is attached to hangers, or film is being processed, safelight conditions must be maintained. As mentioned, white light fogs x-ray film. *Safelight* is any illumination that does not affect the x-ray film (Figure 8-1). It is a low-intensity light composed of long wavelengths from the orange/red range of the spectrum. As shown in Chapter 4 in the discussion of intensifying screens, x-ray films are more sensitive to the blue/green region of the light spectrum, where the wavelengths are relatively short. Red lighting was used previously as safelighting, but it has been replaced by yellow because one can see better with yellow lighting. Not all yellow and red lights are safe. The determining factors are the sensitivity of the x-ray film to the type of light used and the position and intensity of the light source. Usually a 7½- to 10-W bulb with a yellow filter (e.g., Kodak yellow Morlite M-2) placed 3 to 4 ft from

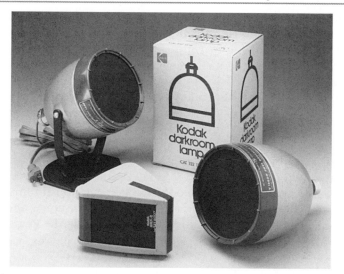

Figure 8-1. A variety of safelights are available for use in the darkroom. *(Courtesy Eastman Kodak Co., Rochester, NY.)*

the work surface is used for working with intraoral film. If extraoral screen film is used, a Kodak GBX-2 Safelight Filter with a 15-W bulb is needed because of the film's increased sensitivity to light. This filter also can be used for intraoral film.

A simple and reliable way to check a safelight is by the *coin test,* in which a coin is placed on an unwrapped, unexposed piece of dental film on the bench top under safelight conditions. After 3 minutes of exposure to the safelight, the film is developed. If the film shows an outline of the coin, the light is not safe; the uncovered part of the film should have been as unaffected as the part covered by the coin (Figure 8-2).

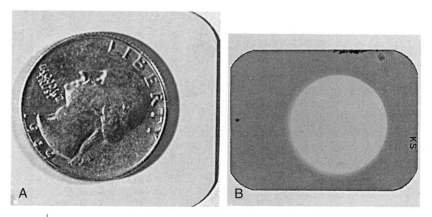

Figure 8-2. Coin test for safelighting. **A,** Coin placed on unexposed film. **B,** Processed radiograph showing an outline of the coin, indicating that safelight intensity is too great and not safe.

Cell Phones

The recent increase in the use of cell phones has produced another possible source of light that could fog or completely expose and ruin the film. When the cell phone is opened, the instrument produces light that affects the film. This is more likely to happen with extraoral and panoramic film, as they are more sensitive to light and have a larger film surface area. The more people who are using their cell phones in the darkroom, the more likely is the possibility of affecting the film; therefore cell phones should not be used in the darkroom.

Panoramic and other extraoral films used with intensifying screens are more sensitive to light than periapical films. As mentioned, screen film must be used with a different filter (e.g., Kodak GBX-2). Periapical films can be processed with the GBX filter or in offices in which both screen and nonscreen (periapical) films are used, and the darkroom can have two safelights, each of a different intensity.

Overhead White Light

The only requirement for overhead white light is that it must provide adequate illumination for the size of the room. The switch for this light should be placed outside the darkroom or in a position inside the darkroom where it cannot be bumped accidentally and turned on, exposing films to white light.

Viewing Safelight

Most dental offices use wet readings for emergencies and working films. In these cases it is convenient to have a viewing safelight mounted on the wall behind the processing tanks. Then films can be removed from the *fixer* after 3 minutes and checked by safelight to see if they have cleared enough for washing and reading. If a viewing safelight is not located behind the processing tanks, the operator would have to hold the wet film up to the overhead safelight with the obvious problem of the dripping and staining of the fixer solution. Dental professionals should never check for clearance or the lack of murkiness on fixed film by holding it to the overhead white light or viewbox; in the uncleared state, the film still can be affected by the white light.

X-Ray Viewbox

The ability to read wet films in the darkroom is a great convenience. A proper diagnosis can be made only by having an adequate viewing mechanism. The darkroom should have a viewbox to suit these needs. A diagnosis should not be made by holding a wet radiograph up to the overhead light.

Outside Warning Light

This light should be wired so that when the safelight is on in the darkroom, the warning light is on outside the darkroom. This is a double check on the inside lock on the door and helps to prevent entry into the darkroom when safelight precautions are in effect.

Plumbing

The darkroom should have intake lines of hot and cold water with an adequate drainage line. There should be a *thermostatic valve* controlling intake to maintain constant temperatures of the solutions. The disposal line should be made of materials that resist the action of the processing chemicals. If automatic processors are used, the flow rate of the incoming water should be considered in planning darkroom plumbing. Automatic processors have individual requirements for flow rates of water, and this should be a factor in darkroom planning and choosing an automatic processor.

A sink with a gooseneck faucet is extremely convenient for tank cleaning and solution changing. This is often overlooked in darkroom planning, and dental personnel will realize that oversight the first time they carry processing tanks to the nearest sink for cleaning and replenishing. The gooseneck faucet is essential because a normal-size faucet neck does not allow enough room to place the tanks under the faucet for cleaning.

Contents

Processing Tanks

Most dental offices have processing units that contain either 1- or 2-gal developer and fixer insert tanks suspended in a tank of running water (Figure 8-3). The unit should be made of stainless steel, and the *water bath* should have a thermostatically controlled flow valve to keep the solutions at the desired temperature. Each tank is equipped with a lid that should be kept on at all times. The cover protects developing films from accidental exposure to white light and prevents oxidation and evaporation of the processing solutions.

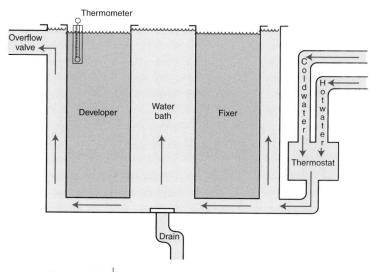

Figure 8-3. | Typical processing tanks in a dental office.

Solutions

Table 8-1 lists the main ingredients of developer and fixer and their functions. The developer and fixer solutions are usually supplied as liquid concentrate that must be diluted. Some commercial services deliver prepared solutions in 1-gal containers. Extra amounts of prepared solutions should be stored in either dark bottles or opaque plastic containers away from heat and light sources.

Under normal working conditions, developer and fixing solutions should be changed at a minimum of every 2 to 3 weeks. A normal workload is considered to be 30 intraoral films per day. If many panoramic films are processed, solutions should be changed more often because more chemical is needed per film area. The chemical solutions lose strength when exposed to air and should be replaced even if normal workload maximums have not been met. This means that the times that an office is closed for vacation still are counted in determining time to change solution. Remember that film development is a chemical reaction: every time the developer and fixer solutions affect a film emulsion, the solutions become weakened. In a busy office, solutions may have to be changed more frequently than every 2 weeks. Weak developer and fixing solutions do not bring out the optimum image on the film and thus do not provide the maximum diagnostic information for the radiation exposure.

Replenishing

Developer and fixer solutions should be replenished daily. Commercially prepared replenishment solutions are available, but it is usually easier to

Table 8-1   Chemicals for Development Process

Ingredient	Function
Developer	
Elon or Metol and hydroquinone (developing agent)	Reduces the energized silver bromide crystals to silver
Sodium sulfite (preservative)	Prevents oxidation of developer
Sodium carbonate (activator)	Provides alkaline medium and softens gelatin to allow developing agents to reach silver bromide crystals
Potassium bromide (restrainer)	Controls activity of developing agents and prevents chemical fog
Fixer	
Sodium thiosulfate (clearing solution)	Removes undeveloped or unexposed silver bromide crystals from the emulsion
Sodium sulfite (preservative)	Prevents the decomposition of the thiosulfate clearing agent
Potassium aluminum sulfate (hardener)	Shrinks and hardens gelatin
Acetic acid (acidifier)	Maintains acid medium

use the standard developer and fixer solutions to fill the tanks. Approximately 8 oz of replenishment are required each day for the developer and fixer solutions. Commercial replenishers include manufacturer's instructions. The *replenisher* is added directly to the existing solutions in their respective tanks to bring them to the proper fluid levels. The levels of solutions always should be kept at the top of the tank to ensure that the immersed films are covered with solution. Water should never be added to the solutions to bring them to tank-top level; this dilutes the strength of the chemicals.

Timer and Thermometer

No darkroom is complete without a timing device and a thermometer (Figure 8-4). The most modern radiographic equipment cannot produce optimum results without time and temperature control in the darkroom. There is no other correct way to process films. The timer is used to determine the length of time the films stay in the developer solution. This depends on the temperature of the developer, not the temperature of the water in the surrounding tanks or that of the water entering through the flow valve. To determine the temperature of the developer, a *thermometer* must be suspended in the developer tank. Early in the day, developer solutions may be cold or hot, depending on the overnight office temperature. It may take some time for equalization of temperatures between the water tank and the developer tank. For this reason, the temperature of the developer bath is read, not the temperature of the water entering the surrounding water tank. It is ironic that some dental offices have thousands of dollars invested in radiographic equipment but are missing a timer and a thermometer, which together cost

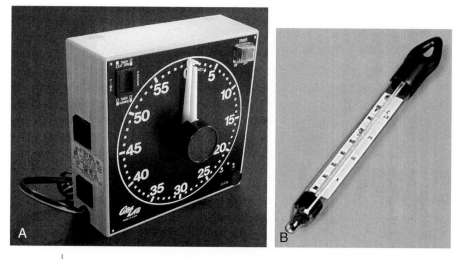

Figure 8-4. Darkroom timer **(A)** and thermometer **(B).** (Both are essential parts of time-temperature technique.) *(A, Courtesy Dimco-Gray Co., Centerville, OH. B, Courtesy DENTSPLY Rinn, Elgin, IL.)*

approximately $40. A time-temperature chart, similar to the following, appears on every package of developer-fixer solution. These charts may vary slightly from manufacturer to manufacturer. A chart like the following should be posted in every darkroom.

Time and Temperature Chart
80° F   2½ minutes in the developer
75° F   3 minutes in the developer
70° F   4 minutes in the developer (optimum)
68° F   4½ minutes in the developer
60° F   6 minutes in the developer

Film Hangers
Intraoral *film hangers* come in various sizes and contain clips for 2 to 20 films (Figure 8-5). In all cases the films should be unwrapped and attached to the clips by using the techniques described in Chapter 9 (Figure 8-6). It is important that the film not be touched with contaminated gloves. This can be accomplished easily by using the wrapping paper in the film packet. The working surface on which the hanger is loaded should be clean and dry to prevent film staining. Film hangers should be numbered or have the patient's name written on them to avoid mix-ups. The implications of a film series with the wrong patient's name are obvious. Hangers with defective clips should be discarded because a defective clip can scratch films on adjacent hangers in the

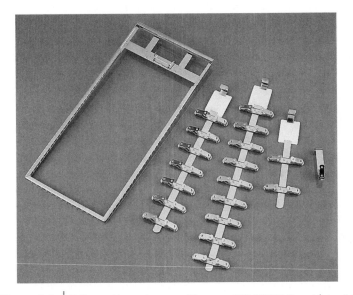

Figure 8-5. Different film rack sizes. *(Courtesy DENTSPLY Rinn, Elgin, IL.)*

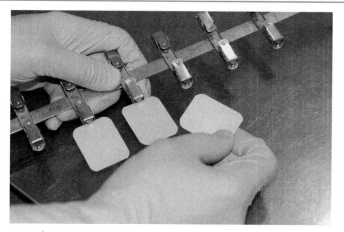

Figure 8-6. Placing film in hangers in the darkroom under safelight conditions.

solution. Defective clips also lead to lost film in the solutions. The idea that one would remember which clip is defective and avoid using it is not realistic. A film hanger that is defective in any way should be discarded.

Dryer
After films have been washed for 20 to 30 minutes, they are ready for drying. This can be accomplished with the use of an x-ray dryer or simply by hanging them on towel racks in the darkroom and letting the films air dry. In either method the films should not touch one another or they will stick together; separating them will rip the emulsion. Drying racks should be out of the way in a clean room. One of the major objections to laboratory-darkroom combinations is that the dust and dirt of the grinding and polishing done in the laboratory contaminate the dental films.

THE DEVELOPMENT PROCESS

Explanation and Discussion

Latent Image
Radiographs after having been exposed are said to contain a *latent image.* The silver halide on the radiographic emulsion is energized by the x-ray beam. The pattern of this energizing of the silver halide depends on the densities of the objects being radiographed. For instance, the silver halide crystals on the film that lie behind a metallic restoration receive almost no radiation because the density of the metal absorbs all the x-ray energy. Silver halide crystals on the film that correspond to an area such as the pulp of the tooth or a cavity receive more radiation energy because these areas are less dense and absorb little x-ray energy (Figure 8-8).

PROCEDURE 8-1

MANUAL PROCESSING

1. Lock the darkroom door from the inside, and record on the film hanger the names of the patients whose films are to be processed.
2. Stir the solutions to equalize the temperature and the chemical distribution of the processing solutions. Use a different stirring paddle for each solution to prevent cross-contamination. Check the levels of solutions and replenish if necessary.
3. Check the temperature and set the timer. The temperature of the developer solution should be checked with an accurate thermometer. Refer to the time-temperature chart, which should be posted in the darkroom, and set the time for the desired interval.
4. Turn off the white light and turn on the safelight.
5. Put on gloves and open the film packets, dropping the films onto the working surface. Discard contaminated film packets and/or barrier wraps, remove gloves, and load the film hangers. Work carefully, avoiding finger marks or film scratches. Be sure the film is securely fastened to film hanger clips.
6. Immerse the film hanger in developer and activate the timer. After immersing the film, immediately raise and lower the hanger a few times so that the film surfaces are covered totally by solution.
7. Remove the film rack from the developer when the timer sounds (under safelight conditions).
8. Rinse thoroughly for 20 seconds in the water bath (under safelight conditions).
9. Place the film rack in the fixer solution. Agitate the rack up and down immediately after the initial placement. Films should remain in the fixer for a minimum of 10 minutes (approximately twice the developer time) for permanent fixation but may be removed after 3 or 4 minutes for use as a wet reading. After fixing, with the tank lids firmly in place, normal lighting can be resumed in the darkroom. Safelighting is not needed after the timer signals that fixation is complete and films are moved from the fixer to the water bath.
10. Place the films in the running water bath for 20 minutes.
11. Dry the films. Remove the films from the water bath and suspend them from rack holders to dry.

Helpful Hint: While the film is in the developer it is preferable for you to remain in the darkroom. If necessary, you can leave the darkroom, but be sure to check that the tank lids are securely in place before you leave.

AUTOMATIC PROCESSING (Figure 8-7)

1. If there is no daylight loader, lock the darkroom from inside and record the name of the patient whose films are to be processed.
2. Turn on the processor or switch from the standby to the ready mode.
3. Turn off the white light and turn on the safelight.
4. Put on gloves and open the film packets, dropping the films onto the working surface of the automatic processor. Discard contaminated film and/or barrier wraps, remove gloves, and load the film into the processor. Be sure that the films are aligned with the film tracks and that they are not put in so quickly as to produce overlapping.
5. Retrieve the dried films and place them in a mount.

> **Helpful Hint:** When loading film into the automatic processor, it is a good idea to alternate tracks to avoid errors.

PROCEDURE 8-2

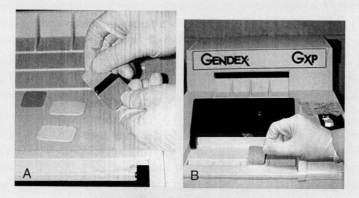

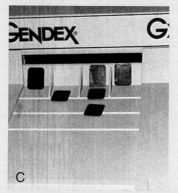

Figure 8-7. | Steps in automatic processing. **A,** Remove film from packets. **B,** Feed film into tracks. **C,** Finished films leaving processor.

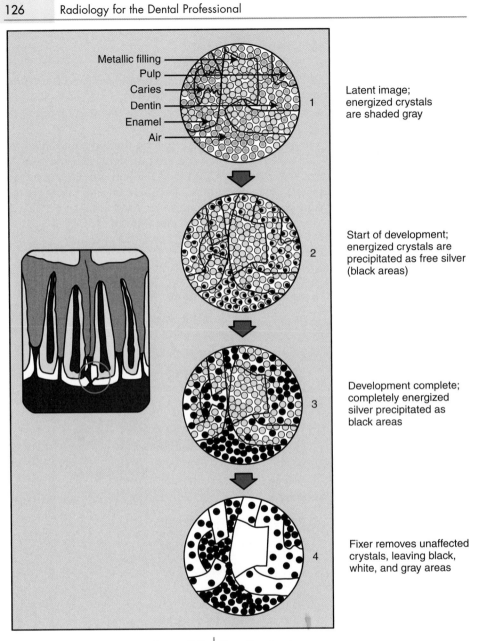

Figure 8-8. | X-ray film development.

Developing

Exposed dental film packets should be processed as soon as possible. In the darkroom under safelight conditions, the x-ray films are removed from the packets and placed on film racks. The developer is the first solution into which these film racks are placed. The *developer* has a pH above 7 and thus is basic compared with the acidic fixing solution. The developer softens the gelatin and allows the solution to chemically reduce the energized silver halide crystals by precipitating silver on the film base. This precipitation corresponds to the black (radiolucent) areas on the radiograph. An area of less density, such as the pulp, allows greater penetration of x-rays; therefore more x-rays reach that part of the film. The silver halide crystals are more greatly energized, and more silver precipitates to give a black, or radiolucent, outline to the pulp chamber.

This is a chemical reaction. The optimum precipitation of silver for the amount of x-ray energy delivered to the object takes place in a specified amount of time with the developing solution at a certain temperature. This is the basis and importance of the time-temperature technique.

If films are left in the developing solution too long, more silver precipitates than was intended, and dense and less dense structures lose their distinctions. A completely *overdeveloped* film results when all the silver is precipitated by the developer and the film is totally black.

Crystals of silver halide that have received small amounts of radiation have correspondingly less silver precipitated and appear gray. The silver halide that was unenergized by radiation, such as the area on the film behind a gold crown, precipitates no silver and appears white, or radiopaque, on the x-ray film.

Washing (Stop Bath)

The main purpose of washing is to remove the developer from the film so that the development process stops. In photographic developing, a chemical *"stop bath"* is used to stop the developing and also remove the basic developer so that it does not contaminate the acidic fixer.

In dental radiography, this is usually accomplished by agitating the film hanger in a water bath for about 20 seconds. Safelight conditions must be maintained when the films are transferred from the developer to the wash tank and then to the fixing solution.

Fixing

The acidic fixing solution (fixer) removes the unexposed and undeveloped silver halide crystals from the film emulsion and rehardens the emulsion, which has softened during the development process. For permanent fixation the film is kept in the fixing solution for a minimum of 10 minutes. However, films may be removed from the fixing solution after 3 minutes for viewing. This procedure is known as the *wet reading* and is useful when films are needed immediately. For example, a wet reading of a film would be used to check that all of the root tip has been removed in an extraction before dismissing the patient. As previously mentioned, a film is ready for a wet reading if it has cleared enough for washing and reading. Operators should always check for clearance or the lack of murkiness under safelight conditions.

Because all films should be made part of the patient's permanent record (archival), they should be returned to the fixing solution to complete the required 10 minutes. Films not fixed properly fade and turn brown in a short time. Excessive fixing (i.e., 2 to 3 days) can completely remove the image from the film.

Washing and Drying

The film is washed for about 20 minutes in the water tank to remove the fixing solution from the emulsion. The film is then dried in a clean, dust-free area. Excessive washing will remove the image from the film.

TIME-TEMPERATURE VERSUS SIGHT DEVELOPMENT

The only correct way to process dental x-ray films is by *time-temperature development*, as described in this chapter. This scientific method produces optimum information on the film. Even so, many dental offices develop x-ray films by sight. The usual technique is to immerse the film hanger in the developer, removing it at frequent intervals to hold it up to the safelight, until fillings or root shapes are visible. At that point the films are washed and placed in the fixer. This is obviously an inexact, unacceptable technique. The usual reason given for the use of the sight development method is, "We have always done it this way, and it works well." This continual acceptance of lower standards for the quality of radiographs leads dentists and dental professionals to believe that this is the way the radiograph should appear. Sight development is unfair to the patient because it does not provide the maximum diagnostic information for the radiation exposure. The time-temperature method, performed either manually or by automatic processors, is the only acceptable way to process dental radiographs.

Rapid Processing

Rapid processing of dental radiographs is done with the use of higher solution temperatures, concentrated solutions, agitation of the film, or a combination of these. It is sometimes called "hot processing," a term that refers to the temperature of the solutions. Rapid processing does not require an increase in radiation to the patient, but the images produced by this technique are not comparable in density and definition to films processed by standard methods. The use of *rapid processing* is clinically indicated when time is more important than exacting detail of the image. For example, it may be used when a patient has just had an extraction and a radiograph is taken to make sure no debris is left in the socket before suturing. The degree of definition needed to visualize anything in the socket is not great, and it is desirable to begin suturing as soon as possible.

The use of regular-strength developing solutions at 92° F with agitation of the film can produce acceptable diagnostic images in less than 1 minute (20 seconds developing, 3 seconds washing, and 30 seconds fixing). Concentrated processing solutions are also available that can be used at room temperature. The increased chemical activity of these solutions makes the rapid processing possible. Some of these solutions use a two-bath technique, developer and fixer; others use a single-bath technique, or monobath, that contains the developer and the fixer (Figure 8-9).

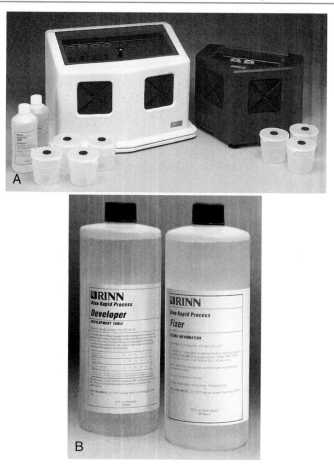

Figure 8-9. A rapid processing system includes **A,** a chairside darkroom (available in regular and compact sizes) and **B,** rapid processing chemicals. *(Courtesy DENTSPLY Rinn, Elgin, IL.)*

Rapid processing can be helpful with endodontic working films and postoperative films in oral surgery when a high degree of definition is not essential. It should not be used for routine processing of films.

EXTRAORAL AND PANORAMIC FILMS

Extraoral and panoramic films are processed in the same manner as intraoral films, using the time-temperature technique with the same solutions. As mentioned, the only precaution that must be taken is to check safelight intensity. Those extraoral films that are used in combination with intensifying screens (screen films) are more sensitive to light than nonscreen films. Darkroom illumination that may be safe for intraoral films may adversely affect screen films. The safety of the light can be checked by using the coin test discussed earlier.

CARE AND MAINTENANCE OF THE DARKROOM

Although darkroom maintenance may seem like a housekeeping chore, it is really a means of ensuring quality control. Maintenance should be likened to our regard for sterility to avoid contamination and subsequent infection. Contaminants in the darkroom or other errors resulting from sloppy techniques may ruin diagnostic radiographs and require retaking of films, which leads to an unnecessary increase in the patient's radiation burden.

Cleanliness

The working surface, where films are stripped and placed on hangers, always should be clean and dry. Developer, fixer, and water produce the most common stains. Drying films should not be placed above the working surface without catch pans. If the working surface is made of Formica, it can be cleaned easily with a mild detergent. Film hangers should be clear and dry when films are loaded. Hangers used for wet readings are the most likely ones to be insufficiently washed and contain residual fixer that can stain the next film. Hangers should be washed after each use, and clean, dry hangers should always be used.

Processing tanks should be cleaned thoroughly when solutions are changed. This includes not only the insert tanks that hold the developer and fixer, but also the water reservoir. The water tank accumulates sludge and algae, especially under the metallic lip and in the overflow tube. Operators can use a bland detergent or preferably one of the tank cleaners made specifically for this purpose. It is in this routine tank cleaning that one appreciates the sink and gooseneck faucet in the darkroom.

Solutions

Solutions should be brought to the optimal temperature at the beginning of the working day and kept at that temperature by the thermostatic control on the mixing valve.

Tanks should be kept full by the use of replenishers rather than by the addition of water because water dilutes the concentration and weakens the solutions. If the tanks are not kept full, the films or portions of the films on the top clips of the film rack may not be immersed fully in solution and will not be developed (Figure 8-10).

As mentioned, both the developer and fixer solutions should be changed at least every 2 to 3 weeks regardless of use. In some practices with heavy film volume, it may be necessary to change solutions as often as once a week. The practice of not changing solutions until the radiographs are too thin (light) to read is incorrect. Processed films should always be compared with a reference film (Figure 8-11) of desired density and contrast that is kept posted on the darkroom viewbox. When the processed films start to show a *thin image*, the solutions should be changed even if it is before the scheduled change date.

The lids of the processing tanks always should be closed when the tanks are not in use to prevent oxidation and weakening of the solutions.

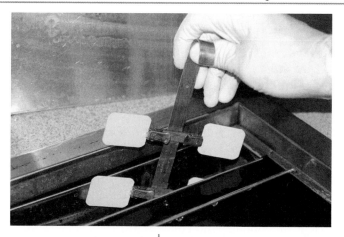

Figure 8-10. | Low solution levels.

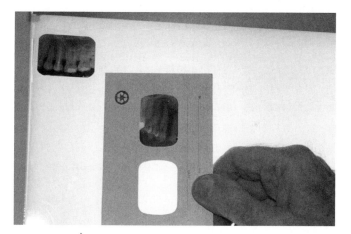

Figure 8-11. | Processed film being compared with a reference film.

Record Keeping

Two types of records are important in the darkroom. The first is the supply inventory, including the date of the next scheduled solution change. It is helpful to post the date of the next scheduled solution change in a prominent place.

Film identifications are the second important type of records in the darkroom; accurate records are essential to processing radiographs. The patient's name, chart number (if applicable), the number of films, the number or letter of the hanger on which the films were placed, and the date should be recorded. This eliminates the likelihood of lost films or mixed radiographs.

ENVIRONMENTAL CONCERNS

Dental professionals must be aware of and comply with a growing number of environmental laws that regulate the management of waste materials. It is our professional responsibility to be aware of these federal and local regulations as they apply to our office and to comply.

Dental radiology generates the following three types of waste: (1) waste solid, (2) x-ray processing solution effluent, and (3) medical waste. Waste solid is the x-ray film packaging, including the lead foil but not the outside packet wrapping. The effluent is the liquid waste coming from the x-ray processing chemicals. The medical waste consists of the intraoral dental packets that have been contaminated by blood or blood components and saliva.

The federal statute that regulates discarded material is the Resource Recovery Act of 1976. Professionals who create hazardous wastes are referred to in this statute as *generators*. Most dental offices in the United States would be classified as "conditionally exempt small-quantity generators" because the small amount of hazardous waste they generate is exempt from federal regulations. State and local laws vary, and exemption from federal regulation does not mean automatic exemption from local laws. Under most local laws the hazardous waste must be removed by a certified carrier (in red bags) in the same way that used gauze pads or cotton rolls are removed. Large dental clinics and dental schools, because of their volume, may be classified as "small-quantity generators" and may be subject to federal regulation.

Silver

There are two sources of silver retrieval in the dental office. In the category of waste solid are the old, no longer needed, or unusable processed radiographs. The second source is the exhausted fixer solution, which falls under the effluent category.

Silver can be recovered from the processed radiographs by ashing the film above the melting point of silver. The economic benefit of this endeavor is limited, but it is an environmentally sound practice and is preferred to ordinary disposal. A pound of radiographs is worth less than $25. In a litigious society, dental offices may be better off saving old radiographs, even beyond the statute of limitations, than using the ashing process. Discarded film is generally not a regulated waste. The discharge of fixer processing solution effluent into a sewer system or a septic tank is not recommended and in many localities is prohibited by law, depending on the concentration of silver in the effluent. The concentration depends on the volume of films processed. Chemical precipitation or electrolysis can retrieve residual silver from the fixer and the wash water. There is no residual silver in developer solution, and hence it can be discharged into the sewage system. Electrolysis units that can be inserted into dental processing tanks or connected to automatic processors cost about $100 (Figure 8-12). Exhausted silver solutions can be removed by a certified carrier.

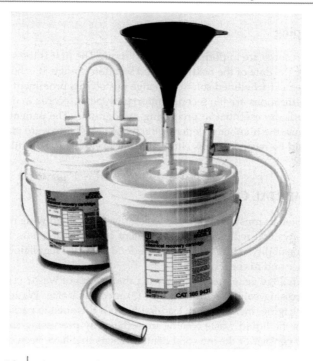

Figure 8-12. | Silver retrieval unit. *(Courtesy Eastman Kodak Co., Rochester, NY.)*

Throwing the lead foil inserts of film packets in regular trash is not environmentally sound; although there is very little lead in each packet, the total amount of lead entering the environment because of the discarding is significant. Eastman Kodak offers to their film users, for the cost of the pre-paid shipping label, cardboard holding boxes for collecting and shipping the foil to qualified disposal facilities (Figure 8-13).

Medical waste must be removed by a certified carrier in the same manner as for disposal of used gauze pads, cotton rolls, and so on.

AUTOMATIC PROCESSING

In recent years, automatic dental x-ray film processing units have become more popular. They are not an essential component of a darkroom but a sub-stitute for manual time-temperature processing. The major advantage of *automatic processing* is the maintenance of standardized procedure; these units provide solutions of proper strength, correct temperature, and regulated pro-cessing time. In short, they provide automated time-temperature processing. Other advantages of the units are the time saved and the increased volume of films that can be processed when compared with the manual method. However, these units are costly, and they still require maintenance and a

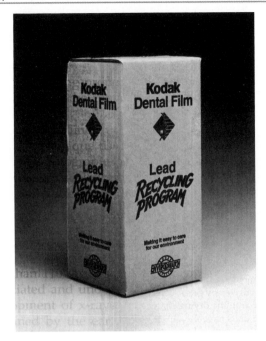

Figure 8-13. | Mailing package for lead foil disposal. *(Courtesy Eastman Kodak Co., Rochester, NY.)*

quality-control program. Some offices that use automatic processing still maintain a backup system of *manual processing* tanks.

The typical automatic processor has three solutions—developer, fixer, and wash—and a drying chamber (Figure 8-14). The wash between developer and fixer solution is eliminated in most automatic processors. A transport system of either rollers or tracks driven by gears, belts, or chains moves the film

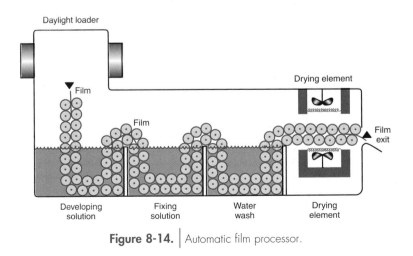

Figure 8-14. | Automatic film processor.

from solution to solution and then into the drying chamber. Finished film is produced in 4 to 7 minutes, and some units have the capacity to process even faster by elevating the temperature of the solutions.

Automatic processors vary in the size of film they can accept, their safelight and plumbing requirements, and the option of automatic replenishment. Free-standing units are not connected to water and waste lines and may be kept in the operatory, as films are fed into the unit through a *daylight loader*.

Size of Film

Some units accept only periapical and bitewing size film (#0, #1, #2, #3) (Figure 8-15), whereas others can accommodate all sizes, including 8 × 10-, 5 × 12-, or 6 × 12-inch panoramic film (see Figure 8-15).

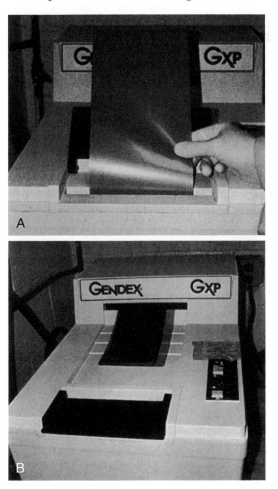

Figure 8-15. | **A,** Panoramic film being inserted into processor. **B,** Finished panoramic film leaving the processor.

Safelight

Some processors must be located in the darkroom because safelight procedures are required for stripping and inserting the film (Figure 8-16). Units with daylight loaders do not have to be in the darkroom because they have light-tight baffles into which the hands are placed during stripping and inserting of the film into the rollers (Figure 8-17). The problems of infection control with daylight loaders are discussed in Chapter 9.

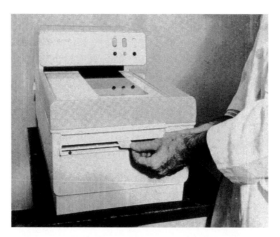

Figure 8-16. | Film being inserted into an automatic processor in the darkroom under safelight conditions. Note that gloves have been removed after film was taken from packet.

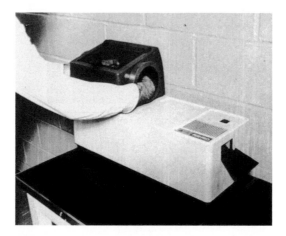

Figure 8-17. | Automatic processor with a daylight loader being used in the operatory. Gloves have been removed inside the daylight loader.

Plumbing

If there is a constant flow of water in the wash chamber, plumbing is required to bring in the water and a waste line for recapturing the fixer to remove the silver. This arrangement is more desirable than a freestanding chamber, in which the water level may drop and constant change is necessary.

Automatic Replenishment

More sophisticated processors maintain solution concentration and levels by automatic replenishment. Each time a piece of film is fed into the unit, a few drops of fixer and developer are added automatically to the baths to maintain solution strength.

Care and Maintenance

Automatic processors require daily or weekly cleaning, depending on the volume of films processed. The *film rollers* should be cleaned at the beginning of the day by running an extraoral size film or clean-up film that is designed to clean through the rollers. This removes any residual debris or dirt from the rollers. The rollers should be removed weekly from the processor and soaked in a water bath for about 20 minutes.

Solution levels should be checked at the beginning of every day and replenished when necessary. Quality-assurance checks are also necessary. The processors are only as good as the care their operators give them.

Technique remains important and cannot be neglected just because the machine runs automatically. Films should not be fed into the rollers too quickly. Operators should maintain at least a 10-second interval between films on the same track. This prevents overlapping of films in processing and failure of chemicals to reach overlapped portions of the film. Carelessness in feeding the films too quickly may lead to the films overlapping in the automatic processor.

Quality assurance for the darkroom is discussed in Chapter 17.

DUPLICATE RADIOGRAPHS

After the exposure to light in the duplicating device, duplicate radiographs (see Chapter 4) are processed in the same manner, either manually or automatically, as other films are processed.

THE DARKROOM (see also the Appendix)

Fogged film (Figure 8-18). Fogged film has an overall gray appearance because of diminished contrast. This can be caused by light leaks in the darkroom, improper safelighting, or improper film storage, as well as exposure to secondary radiation.

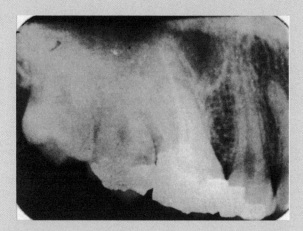

Figure 8-18. | Maxillary molar radiograph that has been fogged. Note lack of definition and contrast.

Remedy. Safelight conditions can be tested with a coin (see p. 117). All doors should be checked for possible leaks, and old film should be used first.

Underdeveloped film: thin image (Figure 8-19). Underdeveloped film is light (thin) in appearance and does not contain all possible diagnostic information. This results when the optimum amount of silver has not been precipitated because of weak or cold developing solutions or insufficient developing time. This type of film is identical to the thin image produced by such chairside technique errors as incorrect mA or increased focal film distance. If all films taken with different machines are light, then the error probably was in the processing. If, however, an occasional film is light, the error probably was at the chair.

Remedy. The developer and fixing solutions should be changed every 2 to 3 weeks, and the time-temperature method should be used. That is, the temperature of the developer should be checked before films are immersed in the solution, and the timer should be set for the appropriate time as given in the manufacturer's specifications, with the operator referring to the density comparison standard mounted on the view box. Daily quality-assurance checks should be performed to determine solution strength.

Overdeveloped film: *dense image* (Figure 8-20). Overdeveloped film may vary from dark to totally black, depending on the degree of overdevelopment. This type of film is of no diagnostic value. A dense image, or *dark image*, results when too

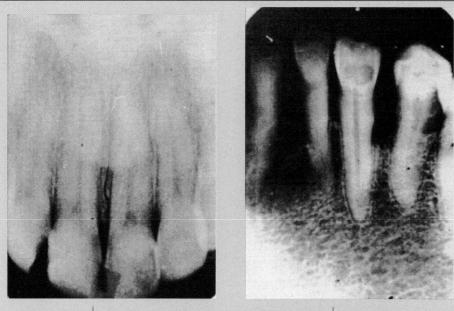

Figure 8-19. | Underdeveloped film.   **Figure 8-20.** | Overdeveloped film.

much silver has been precipitated on the film base; in the case of the totally black film, all the silver from the silver bromide has been precipitated. This error can be caused by hot developing solutions or prolonged developing time. As mentioned with light films, chairside errors also can produce this error.

   Remedy. The time-temperature method of processing always should be used. The timer should have a bell or buzzer that rings when the developing time has elapsed. This enables the dental professional to leave the darkroom while the films are being processed. Without the bell the dental professional may be distracted by other duties and forget to remove the films from the developer at the proper time. Operators should perform daily quality-assurance checks on solution strength.

   Developer cutoff (Figure 8-21). Cutoff film shows a straight radiopaque border on what was the upper edge of the top film on the processing hanger. This is an undeveloped area of the film. When the solutions are allowed to deplete in the processing tanks, the films on the top positions on the racks may not be covered by solution when the racks are placed in the tanks. This error should be differentiated from "circular collimation" (collimator cutoff), which may give a curved radiopaque border. In collimator cutoff the film portion is unexposed; in *developer cutoff* the film portion is undeveloped.

   Remedy. One should always make sure that processing tanks are full. If the levels of solutions have dropped, water should not be added; this will only dilute

COMMON ERROR 8-1

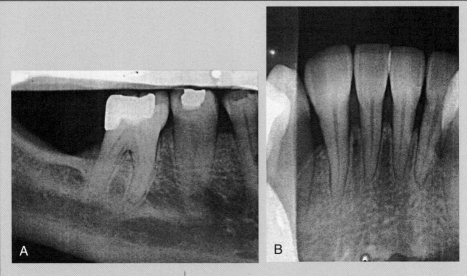

A   B

Figure 8-21. | Radiographs with developer cutoff.

the solution and result in *underdeveloped* films. Proper replenisher solutions should be added to maintain the desired level.

Clear films (Figure 8-22). Films are clear because the entire emulsion has been washed off. This occurs when films are overfixed or left in running water baths for 24 to 48 hours. *Clear film* is identical to an unexposed film that is developed and processed. With unexposed film the fixer removes all the unaffected silver bromide crystals. Clear films can also result if a film is placed in the fixer solution before the developing solution.

Figure 8-22. | Clear film can result from excessive washing or fixing or an unexposed film.

COMMON ERROR 8-1

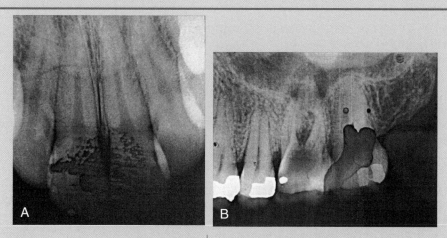

Figure 8-23. | Stained radiographs.

Remedy. Films should never be left in water baths overnight. Processing should be complete before one leaves the office. Films should not be left in the fixer overnight or for prolonged periods beyond the recommended 10 minutes; the fixer will lighten and ultimately remove the image. A common misconception is that films cannot be overfixed. Do not place exposed films in the fixer before the developer.

Stained films (Figure 8-23). If the working surface in the darkroom is wet and dirty, films can be stained either before or after processing. There is no excuse for this error.

Remedy. Darkroom work surfaces must be kept clean and dry.

Discolored films (Figure 8-24). Films that have not had adequate fixation (approximately twice the developing time) turn brown after a period and are

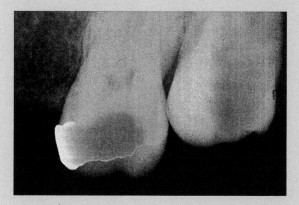

Figure 8-24. | Insufficient fixing results in a partially discolored film.

useless as part of the patient's permanent record. A radiograph should have an archival life of at least 7 years.

Remedy. All films must have adequate fixation time (10 minutes). All wet readings should be returned to the fixation tank after the patient has been treated.

Torn emulsion (Figure 8-25). If films that are drying are allowed to touch and overlap, they stick together, leading to *torn emulsion.* When one separates the films, the emulsions are usually torn off the film base in the overlapped area, rendering the film useless for diagnosis.

Remedy. Film racks should be checked to ensure that drying films from different racks are not touching.

Scratched films (Figure 8-26). A radiopaque line on a film is usually an artifact caused by scratching the emulsion on the film base in film processing. Most often it is the result of putting a second film rack into a tank that already contains a film rack. It also can be caused by fingernails scratching the film while it is being unpacked and placed on a rack.

Remedy. When film racks are put into the processing solution, care should be taken to avoid touching those already immersed. Any film racks should be discarded if they have sharp edges or broken clips that could scratch other films.

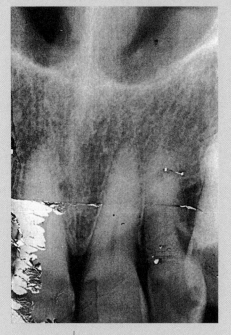

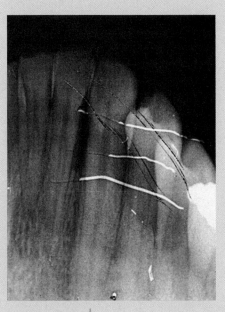

Figure 8-25. | Radiograph with torn emulsion.   **Figure 8-26.** | Scratched radiograph.

Lost film in tanks. If films are not firmly clipped onto the hangers, they may fall off in any of the three processing baths. A lost film necessitates a retake or results in a "wet elbow" in an attempt to retrieve it from the processing solution.

Remedy. All films should be checked to see that they are clipped securely to the hangers before processing.

Fluoride artifacts (Figure 8-27). Some fluorides, especially stannous fluoride, produce black marks on radiographs.

Remedy. After working with fluoride, the dental professional should wash hands thoroughly with soap and a weak acid, such as vinegar or lemon juice, or change gloves before handling films in the darkroom.

Reticulation (Figure 8-28). If film is developed at an elevated temperature and then placed in a cold water bath, the sudden change in temperature causes the swollen emulsion to shrink rapidly and give the image a wrinkled appearance called *reticulation*.

Remedy. Sharp contrasts in temperatures between processing and the water bath should be avoided.

Air bubbles (Figure 8-29). If air bubbles are trapped on the film as it is placed in the processing solutions, the chemicals cannot affect the emulsion in that area.

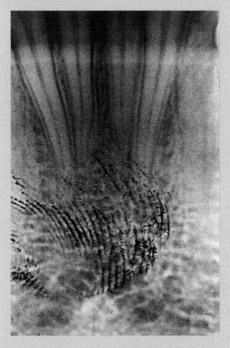

Figure 8-27. Fluoride artifact. Operator's fingertip, contaminated by fluoride, touched film during stripping and placing of film on hanger.

COMMON ERROR 8-1

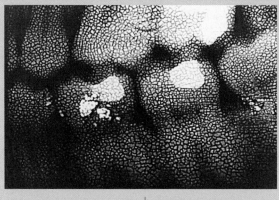

Figure 8-28. Reticulation.

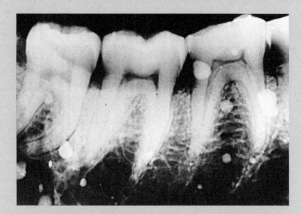

Figure 8-29. Artifact caused by air bubbles trapped on the film, preventing processing solution from touching film in the area.

Remedy. The film hangers always should be agitated when they are placed in the processing solutions to dislodge any trapped air bubbles.

Static marks (Figure 8-30). Static electricity can be produced when intraoral film packets are opened forcefully in the darkroom. This is not common for intraoral film in today's film packets. The static electricity produces multiple black linear streaks (*electrostatic artifacts*) on the radiograph. The same effect occurs much more often on extraoral films. With these films, static electricity may result when the piece of film is removed from a full box; the sliding of the film out of the tightly packed box may produce static electricity. Static electricity also may be produced during loading and unloading of flexible cassettes in panoramic machines as the film is slid in or out between the intensifying screens. In addition, walking

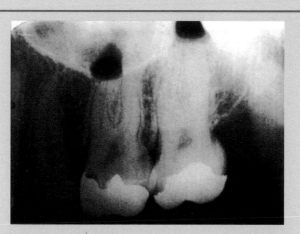

Figure 8-30. | Periapical radiograph with static marks.

around a carpeted office may produce static electricity. If the dental professional does not touch a conductive object before unwrapping the film, charge marks may result. Static electricity occurs most often on cold, dry days.

Remedy. Operators should ground themselves by touching any conductive object in the darkroom before handling film and should avoid friction of any kind against the film that will produce static electricity.

Automatic & Processing

Daylight loaders: light leaks (Figure 8-31). Film fog, a ruined film, or unusual artifacts can be caused by removing one's hands from the baffle (see Figure 8-17) before the film has entered the processor.

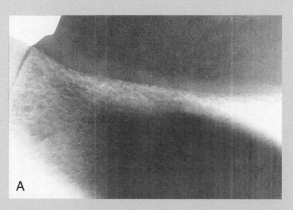

A

Figure 8-31. | **A,** Artifact caused by a light leak in the daylight loader, resembling a large pathologic area in bone.

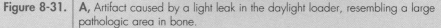

Continued

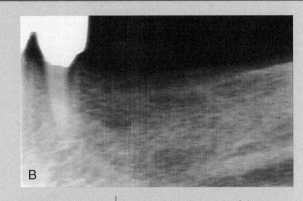

Figure 8-31—cont'd. | **B,** Normal radiograph of the same area.

Remedy. The operator's hands must be kept on the film until it has been completely taken up by the rollers. The material that makes up the baffle should fit tightly around the hands. Rips and tears should be repaired immediately and stretched elastic replaced. It is a good idea to remove wristwatches and bracelets because they tend to tear the baffle material.

Dirty rollers (Figure 8-32). If the rollers are not cleaned periodically, radiolucent bands or other forms of debris will appear on the finished film.

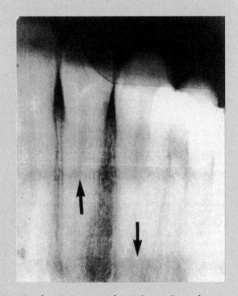

Figure 8-32. | Bands of stain (*arrows*) from dirty rollers of an automatic processor.

COMMON ERROR 8-1

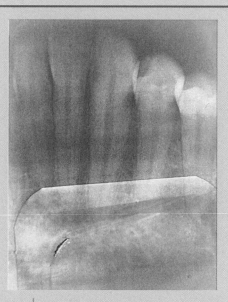

Figure 8-33. | Overlapped films during automatic processing.

Remedy. Rollers should be cleaned periodically by removing and soaking them in accordance with the manufacturer's recommendations. A piece of extraoral film should be run through at the beginning of every work day to clean the rollers.

Overlapped films (Figure 8-33). If the films are fed into the processor too quickly, they overlap and the processing solutions cannot reach the emulsion.

Remedy. The operator should wait 10 seconds before putting a following film into each processing track.

SUGGESTED READINGS

Alcox RW, Jameson WR: Rapid dental x-ray film processor for selected procedures, J Am Dent Assoc 8:517-519, 1969.

Beideman RL, et al: A study to develop a rating system and evaluate dental radiographs submitted to a third party carrier, J Am Dent Assoc 93:1010-1013, 1976.

Eastman Kodak Co.: Quality assurance in dental radiography, Rochester, NY, 1989, Health Science Division.

Eastman Kodak Co.: Waste management guidelines, Rochester, NY, 1994, Health Science Division.

National Council on Radiation Protection and Measurements: NCRP Report No. 145, Radiation in dentistry, 2004.

Suleiman OH, et al: Radiographic trends of dental offices and dental schools, J Am Dent Assoc 130:1104-1110, 1999.

Swanson RL, et al: Reuse of lead from dental X-rays, N Y State Dent J 65:34-36, 1999.

Infection Control in Dental Practice

EDUCATIONAL OBJECTIVES

1. Take and process all radiographs, adhering to and understanding the accepted infection control policy.
2. Prepare and break down a dental operatory after completing patient radiographs.
3. Feel comfortable and assured in treating a patient with an infectious disease by following infection control protocol.

KEY TERMS

acquired
   immunodeficiency
   syndrome (AIDS)
antibiotic prophylaxis
antiseptic
autoclaving
barrier
Centers for Disease
   Control and
   Prevention (CDC)

cross-contamination
disinfection
hepatitis
human immunodeficiency
   virus (HIV)
immunization
infection
microorganism

Occupational Safety and
   Health Administration
   (OSHA)
pathogen
sterilization
universal precautions
vaccination

Infection control has become a major concern of patients, regulatory agencies, and healthcare workers in the practice of dentistry. The dental profession has been or should have been practicing infection control at all times because dental personnel have always been at risk from pathogens. A pathogen is a microorganism capable of causing disease. Pathogens can be transmitted by infection from cuts, breaks in the skin, and contact with body secretions and inhalants. The emergence and identification of *acquired immunodeficiency syndrome (AIDS)* in 1981, the highly infectious hepatitis B and C viruses (HBV and HCV), and the resurgence of tuberculosis have brought the issue to the forefront. Diseases such as tuberculosis, *hepatitis*, and herpes always have been a risk for dental professionals, but it took the fatal consequences of AIDS to heighten the interest and awareness of the public, the government, and the profession to the importance of infection control in the dental office. Dentistry came into the spotlight of public and media attention with the report of an incident in Florida of possible *human immunodeficiency virus (HIV)* infection during an invasive dental procedure. A female patient, whose lifestyle may or may not have put her in a high-risk category, was reported to be infected with a strain of HIV closely related to that of her HIV-infected dentist. The resulting inquiry by state and local health officials, including congressional testimony, revealed that seven other patients in the practice were HIV-positive, and five of them carried a strain similar to that of the infected dentist. The exact nature of the transmission, if it occurred at all, is still unknown and debatable to this day; however, the public has become alarmed, and federal and state agencies at all levels are imposing requirements for office procedures and required courses in infection control.

INFECTION CONTROL IN DENTAL PRACTICE

Any comprehensive infection control policy in dentistry must include protocols for radiology, including both chairside technique and darkroom procedures. Radiology is not exempt from infection control, even though radiographic procedures do not involve the aerosol spray produced by the dental handpiece, needles, or the cutting of tissue and splatter of blood. Infectious disease can be transmitted by the *cross-contamination* of equipment, supplies, and film packets and cassettes used to take or process radiographs. In addition, dental radiographic procedures are in almost all cases performed in the same dental chairs and units that are used for more invasive procedures, with the potential for cross-contamination. Also, lead aprons and thyroid collars should be disinfected after each use to avoid contamination from one patient to the next. The American Dental Association, the Centers for Disease Control and Prevention (CDC), and the Occupational Safety and Health Administration (OSHA) all state that gloves must be worn when contact with blood, saliva, or other potentially infectious material, items, or surfaces is anticipated. Masks, eyewear, and protective clothing are required only when splatter is anticipated, and their use should be left to the judgment of the dentist. We believe that masks, eyewear, and gowns should also be used at all times because these precautions fall under the rule of ALARA (as low as reasonably achievable). The use of gowns, masks, and gloves is easily achievable. (It is better to be safe than sorry.)

If infection control is understood and practiced, then patients, fellow workers, and dental workers themselves can be protected from harm. The objective is to be educated so that work can be conducted in a concerned manner as opposed to a fear-induced, hysterical manner. As educated professionals, dental workers should act in a manner befitting the profession.

The following is a list of terms and definitions that are used in this discussion of infection control in the dental setting:

antiseptic: a substance that inhibits the growth of bacteria

autoclaving: the process of sterilization using steam

barrier: a substance used to protect the patient or worker from infective or contaminated substances

blood-borne pathogen: a pathogen present in blood that can cause infection in humans

critical instrument: an instrument used to penetrate soft tissue or bone

disinfection: the process of destroying disease-causing microorganisms by physical or chemical means, e.g., hand washing

noncritical instrument: an instrument that does not come in contact with mucous membranes, e.g., position-indicating device, exposure button, control panel

occupational exposure: contact of the skin or mucous membranes by blood or other infectious material that results from performing dental procedures

parental exposure: exposure to blood or other infectious material that results in skin puncture

semicritical instrument: an instrument that comes in contact with the mucous membrane but does not penetrate, e.g., x-ray film-holding device

sterilization: the process used to destroy all pathogens, including highly resistant bacteria and spores

universal precautions: an infection control protocol that is followed for all patients regardless of their history and clinical condition

Patient History

Every patient should have his or her current medical history documented. The dentist or the dental professional should obtain this history at the initial or recall visit, using a questionnaire and/or direct questioning of the patient. Information gained by the history will alert the dental team to the presence or history of infectious disease or to potentially high-risk situations. Unfortunately, many potentially infectious patients cannot be identified by history or examination. Thus a rational infection control policy should not distinguish between patients who are known to be infected and those who are not. Every patient should be treated in the same manner, with universal precautions procedures carried out at all times. There are no exceptions and therefore no surprises.

SOURCES OF INFECTION

Through contact with saliva, blood, and nasal and respiratory secretions, many instruments and pieces of equipment can become the means of pathogen transmission. A *pathogen* is a *microorganism* that can cause disease. After the dental professional's gloves are contaminated by oral cavity fluids during radiographic procedures, everything that person touches is a possible transmitter of pathogens. Our concern then is with film-holding devices, instruments, film, x-ray machine, position-indicating device (PID), tube head, control panel and exposure switch, clothing, countertops, dental chair, lead apron, light handle, walls, doorknobs, processors, and patient records. In short, any object that the operator touches after placing the packet in the patient's mouth can be considered contaminated and a source of transmission to the operator or other patients. On the other hand, any object the operator touches before working in the mouth is a potential source of transmission to the patient. Thus barriers to the transmission of infective microorganisms must be used. Barriers include gloves, masks, protective eyewear, gowns, and surface coverings. If contamination does occur, as it does in the dental office, steps must be taken to remove or destroy the pathogen and the contaminated item to prevent further transmission.

PERSONNEL

Dental personnel always should wear gloves, masks, and protective eyewear and clothing when working on patients (Figure 9-1). Just as there is no excuse for not standing 6 ft away from the x-ray machine, there is no excuse for not protecting oneself from infection. Blood is the most common and easily recognized transmission route of HIV and of HBV and HCV. Although HIV has been isolated in the saliva of some patients, saliva alone is not considered to be a risk for HIV transmission, but because saliva is often contaminated with blood, there is a potential for transmission. It is true that no cases of HIV transmission have been documented via the salivary route by casual contact, but this should not serve as an excuse for not wearing gloves, masks, and eyewear. Saliva can be contaminated by blood and therefore poses the potential for transmission.

Gowns

Any dental professional involved in direct patient care should wear a clean, long-sleeved, three-quarter length uniform, jacket, or gown with a closed collar. Gowns should not be worn outside of the office and should ideally be laundered immediately after professional use.

Masks/Eye Protection

Face masks and protective eyewear with solid side shields should be worn by dental professionals whenever they perform any intraoral radiographic

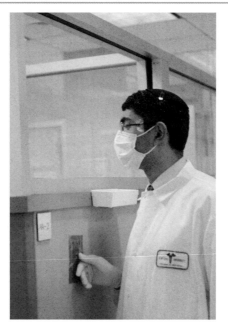

Figure 9-1. | Operator making exposure while wearing gloves, eyeglasses, mask, and protective clothing.

procedure. Masks and eyewear should be in place before a practitioner washes hands and dons gloves, and should not be removed until the unit is cleaned after the completion of patient care.

Gloves/Hand Washing

Dental professionals must wear gloves when they perform intraoral procedures, and there is no exception to this rule. Before putting on gloves, one should wash their hands with an antimicrobial soap or instant hand sanitizer (Figure 9-2), and this process should be repeated after gloves are removed at the completion of the patient's treatment. Hand jewelry and watches should be removed before hand washing, and fingernails should be clean and filed short and smooth. While gloved, one should not touch items such as pens, pencils, x-ray mounts, charts, or telephones. Paper towels may be used as barriers between these items and the gloved hands.

BARRIERS

Any object that the operator touches after placing the film in the patient's mouth must be covered with a removable barrier or disinfected after the patient leaves. A good maxim to remember is, "The less you touch, the less you have to worry about." There is now a complete line of dental wrap with

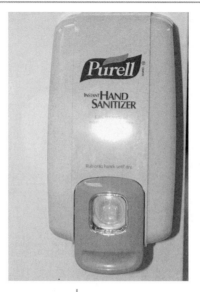

Figure 9-2. | Instant hand sanitizer

adhesive backing made specifically for barriers. The material should be placed over the chair headrest, the countertop, the arm and PID ("cone") of the x-ray machine, control panel, and exposure button before the patient is seated (Figures 9-3 to 9-6). The barriers are easily removed after the radiographic procedure is completed. If barriers are not used, these objects must be disinfected after the radiographic procedure is completed. Disinfecting solutions such as iodophor or any other Environmental Protection Agency–registered chemical germicide have the drawback that they may not reach irregular

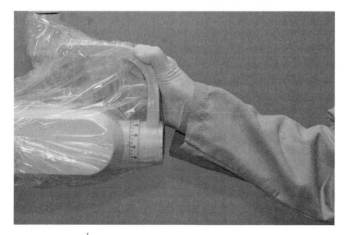

Figure 9-3. | Plastic wrap covering yoke of the x-ray machine.

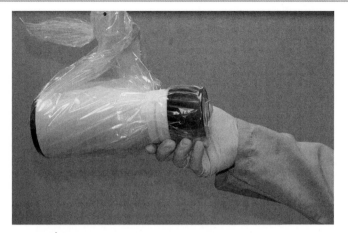

Figure 9-4. | Plastic wrap covering the position-indicating device (cylinder).

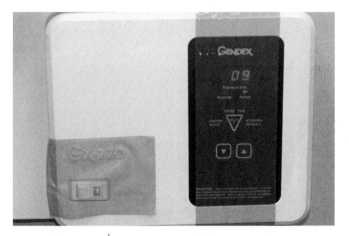

Figure 9-5. | Plastic wrap covering the control panel.

surfaces of the dental x-ray machine and have the potential to affect electrical connections in the head of the machine (Figure 9-7).

Sterilization and Disinfection

Sterilization produces the absence of all microorganisms, including spores. The most common methods of sterilization used in the dental office are steam autoclaving and the use of the dry-heat oven. The radiographic instruments are sterilized in bags in the same manner as other dental instruments.

Disinfection is the process that results in the absence of pathogenic organisms but not spores. Disinfecting agents are usually employed on surfaces

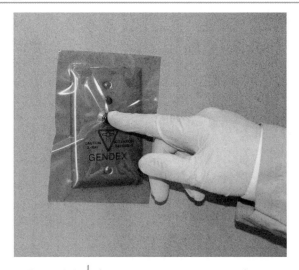

Figure 9-6. | Plastic wrap covering exposure button.

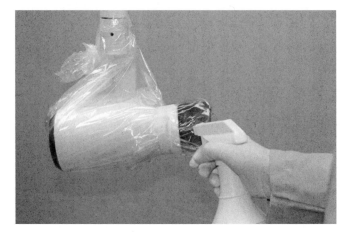

Figure 9-7. | Disinfecting the x-ray machine.

but not on human tissue. Iodophors, chlorines, and synthetic phenolics are examples of disinfectants commonly used in the dental office.

"Cold sterilization" of instruments with quaternary ammonium compounds or glutaraldehyde is still used in the dental office but requires up to 6 hours of immersion to achieve sterilization. This method does not seem practical in a busy office and might lead to shortcutting time requirements. Some instruments, such as plastic film holders, bite blocks, or localizing rings, may be damaged if not handled correctly during heat sterilization. Dental professionals either should stop using these instruments or should place them in protective plastic wrap covers. However, the majority of radiographic devices manufactured today are autoclavable and are clearly marked as such.

Antiseptics are agents used on human tissue that are either bacteriostatic or bacteriocidal. In dentistry they are used mainly for hand washing. In dental radiography, the use of sterilization, disinfection, and antiseptic agents results in a rational, workable infection control policy.

Film Packets

Other than the operator's hands, the film packet is the main vector of cross-contamination. The packet remains in the patient's mouth, and when removed it is coated with saliva or possibly with blood. The film packet is handled in the operatory and then transported to the darkroom. The following three methods can theoretically prevent transmission of microorganisms by the film packet to other parts of the operatory or the darkroom: (1) sterilization or disinfection of the exposed packet, (2) use of barrier protection for the packet, and (3) proper handling technique.

1. Sterilization and disinfection of the film packet are impractical and time-consuming and may degrade or ruin the radiographic image; therefore these methods are not recommended. Autoclaving or sterilizing by dry heat destroys the image. Immersing the packet in a disinfecting solution for the required time results in penetration of the solution to the film emulsion. Thus neither sterilization nor disinfection is recommended.

2. Barrier envelope for film packets are now available in the dental marker. D-, E- and F-speed films (sizes #0, #1, and #2) may be purchased with the film packet already inserted into barrier envelopes, or the barrier envelopes may be purchased separately and individual film packets (sizes #0 through #2) may be inserted in them before exposure (Figure 9-8).

   The film packet is placed and sealed in the barrier envelope before the radiographic procedure is begun. All film packets to be used are prepared in this manner. The film packet is exposed in the barrier envelope, dried of saliva, and then brought to the darkroom in some type of a receptacle

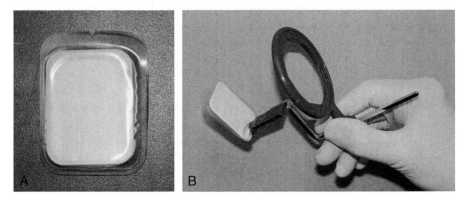

Figure 9-8. │ Barrier envelope. **A,** With film packet. **B,** In film holder.

without the barrier envelope. The operator wears gloves to open the barrier envelope, taking care not to touch the film packet, and the packet is allowed to drop onto a clean surface. The gloves and the barrier envelope are then discarded, and the operator opens the film packet and processes the film.

3. If the barrier film packet technique is not used, after the exposure is made, the film packet that is contaminated by saliva or blood should be wiped dry and placed in a receptacle that is outside the operatory or in a lead receptacle in the operatory and carried to the darkroom when all the exposures have been made. Operators should always remember that the gloves they wear are contaminated, so they should not touch anything on the way to the darkroom. They can change gloves after the exposures have been made if touching surfaces and objects such as a doorknob is unavoidable. Once operators are in the darkroom under safelight conditions, they can open film packets, taking care not to touch the films as they are allowed to drop onto a clean surface (Figure 9-9). The contaminated gloves are then discarded, and the films are processed either manually or automatically. If there are two people in the darkroom (admittedly, this is not common in most offices), one gloved person can open the contaminated packet and the other can remove the film from within the packet without touching the outside (Figure 9-10). This process will also prevent contamination of the film.

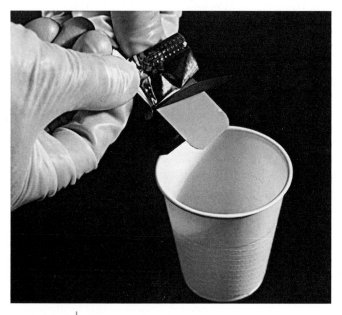

Figure 9-9. | Opening contaminated film packet in the darkroom.

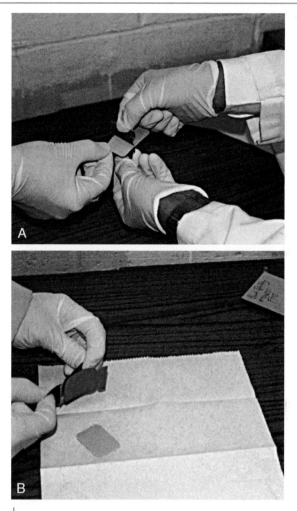

Figure 9-10. Two-operator technique for removing film from a contaminated packet.

Processing Solutions

The developing and fixing solutions used in the darkroom have not been shown to act as sterilizing agents. It is a common misconception that they do. Any contaminated film that is processed emerges from the processing still contaminated. It has been shown that microorganisms can remain viable on radiographic equipment for at least 48 hours. In automatic processors the rollers and tracks can be contaminated by the film, as can the film hangers in manual processing.

CHAIRSIDE EXPOSURE PROCEDURES

1. Cover all appropriate surfaces with plastic wrap. This should include but not be limited to the PID and arm of the x-ray machine, the control panel, the exposure button, and the working surfaces where unexposed films are placed (Figure 9-11). Plan in advance, setting out all anticipated supplies (film, film holders, cotton rolls, etc.).
2. Seat the patient and drape with the lead apron and thyroid collar in the appropriate manner.
3. Wash hands with antiseptic soap and put on gloves.
4. Make the required exposures, taking care to touch only the covered surfaces. If the procedure is interrupted and you have to leave the room and touch anything (e.g., the telephone), remove the gloves, dispose of them, and put on a new pair before resuming work. Each exposed film packet should be wiped dry of saliva and put in a disposable cup outside the operatory.
5. If no other dental procedures are to be done, dismiss the patient. Dispose of all contaminated barriers and supplies in the operatory and then disinfect the lead apron and other appropriate surfaces.
6. Remove contaminated gloves and carry the film container to the darkroom.

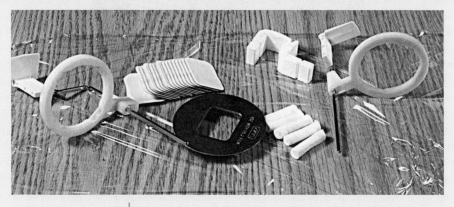

Figure 9-11. | Plastic wrap covering necessary items on work surface.

PROCESSING PROCEDURES

1. Put on new gloves.
2. Under safelight conditions with gloved hands, remove the films from the film packet or the film packets from the barrier envelopes by allowing them to drop onto a clean surface. Do not touch the film with gloved hands. The gloves are considered to be contaminated because they touched the film packet.
3. Dispose of the film packet wrappers and carrying cup and remove and dispose of the gloves.
4. Process the uncontaminated film on the clean surface either manually or automatically.
5. The film is not contaminated, so gloves are not needed for processing or mounting.

PROCEDURE 9-2

Automatic Processing

Operators should load film into an automatic processor with the same concern and method for avoiding cross-contamination as with manual processing film hangers. The problem is with the automatic processors used with daylight loaders. Use of daylight loaders should be discouraged because it is very difficult to avoid contamination as a result of the tight-fitting hand baffles, which serve as a source of cross-contamination (Figure 9-12). This is not the case if one is using the barrier packs. It is also very difficult to remove the film from the film packet

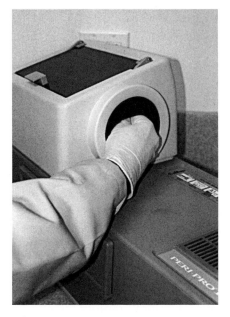

Figure 9-12. The sleeves of an automatic processor have been contaminated by the operator's contaminated gloves.

PROCEDURE FOR DAYLIGHT LOADERS

1. Prepare the interior of the daylight loader by placing a barrier on the bottom surface. Place the cup with the exposed film packets, a pair of gloves, and a second cup on that surface, and then close the top of the daylight loader.
2. Place clean hands through the sleeve baffle and put on the gloves.
3. Open packets, allowing the films to drop into the second cup.
4. Remove gloves and place the uncontaminated films in the processing slots, and then remove ungloved hands through the sleeves.
5. Open top of loader and wrap all trash in the barrier and remove.
6. Wash hands.

and to put on one's gloves within the confined space of the daylight loader and then take off the contaminated gloves and feed the film into the uptake slots. An operator who must use a daylight loader when the barrier packets are not available should follow the protocol found in Procedure Box 9-3.

Panoramic X-ray Units

Because panoramic radiography is an extraoral procedure, fewer areas are contaminated by the patient's saliva. The patient bite block should be covered by a plastic barrier cover or autoclaved if possible. Plastic barrier wrap should be used on the chin rest, ear rods, and patient handgrips. Processing presents no problems because the cassette does not contact the patient; thus the procedure for preventing film contamination is not necessary. The only possible contaminant in the darkroom would be the operator's gloves. These gloves should be removed before the cassette is taken from the panoramic unit.

ANTIBIOTIC PROPHYLAXIS

It is an accepted and required procedure to provide prophylaxis for certain patients with antibiotics before invasive dental procedures. Patients with positive medical histories of prosthetic cardiac valves, previous infective endocarditis, specific cases associated with congenital heart disease (CHD), cardiac transplantation recipients who develop cardiac valvulopathy, artificial joint replacement (within the first 2 years after replacement), and immunocompromised patients (i.e., those with HIV, uncontrolled diabetes, autoimmune disease, etc.) fall into this category. Any procedure, including probing, that might produce bleeding should be considered invasive. The question then arises regarding whether intraoral radiography is an invasive procedure because in rare instances it may produce bleeding. A recent survey shows no consensus on this subject, although the American Medical Association suggests that no prophylaxis is necessary before taking radiographs. Because of the immense risk to the patient, it is prudent to provide prophylaxis if any bleeding is expected. Patients with advanced periodontal disease with positive medical histories are a good example of this type of need. In clinical practice, however, most patients needing *antibiotic prophylaxis* will have been provided with prophylaxis because it is rare that the only procedure done at a specific appointment is the taking of radiographs.

Immunization

All dental personnel should have the appropriate *immunizations* (e.g., tetanus, influenza, varicella), including that for the Hepatitis B virus. OSHA's standard covering blood-borne pathogens requires healthcare employers to offer a three-injection HBV *vaccination* series free to all employees exposed to blood or other potentially infectious fluids or materials. The OSHA standard also states that if routine booster doses of the hepatitis vaccine are recommended at some future date, then the employer also should make these boosters available to employees at no cost.

SUGGESTED READINGS

American Academy of Oral and Maxillofacial Radiology infection control guidelines for dental radiographic procedures, Oral Surg Oral Med Oral Pathol 73:248-249, 1992.

ADA Council on Scentific Affairs and ADA Council on Dental Practice: Infection control recommendations for the dental office and the dental laboratory, J Am Dent, Assoc 127:672-680, 1996.

Bartoloni JA, Chariton DG, Flint DJ: Infection control practices in dental radiology, Gen Dent 51:264-271, 2003.

Eastman Kodak Co.: Infection in modern practice, Rochester, NY, 1999, Health Science Division.

Glass BJ: Infection control in dental radiology. Current and future, N Y State Dent J 60:42-45, 1994.

Jones GA, et al: Radiographic protocol for patients needing antibiotic prophylaxis: dental schools report no consensus, J Am Dent Assoc 125:602-604, 606, 1994.

Kohn WG, et al: Guidelines for infection control in dental health care settings—2003, J Am Dent Assoc 135:33-47, 2004.

Kohn WG, et al: Guidelines for infection control in dental health-care settings—2003, MMWR Recomm Rep, Dec 19; 52(RR-17):1-61, 2003.

Hastreiter RJ, Jiang P: Do regular dental visits affect the oral health care provided to people with HIV, J Am Dent Assoc 133:1343-1350, 2002.

CHAPTER 10

Intraoral Technique: The Paralleling Method

EDUCATIONAL OBJECTIVES

1. Understand the geometry of the x-ray beam direction and film placement.
2. Be able to apply these principles to take a full-mouth survey of radiographs for dentulous or edentulous adult or pediatric patients.
3. Recognize unacceptable radiographs and their causes and know how to correct the errors.

KEY TERMS

bite block
bitewing
chair position
cone cutting (collimator
    cutoff)
dimensional accuracy
dimensional distortion

double exposure
elongation
exposure routine
extension paralleling
    technique
film position
film reversal

foreshortening
full-mouth survey
hemostat
horizontal angulation
localizing ring
long axis
occlusal plane

overexposure	point of entry	vertical angulation
overlapping	right-angle technique	vertical bitewings
patient movement	sagittal plane	
periapical film	underexposure	

THE FULL-MOUTH SURVEY

The full-mouth intraoral radiographic survey is one of the cornerstones of a complete oral diagnosis. No dental examination or treatment plan can be considered complete without current or valid radiographs, and in some cases the *full-mouth survey* is the radiographic procedure of choice. The full-mouth survey is a difficult procedure to do correctly and requires time and meticulous attention to detail. It bears with it the responsibility of exposing the patient to the least amount of ionizing radiation to obtain the maximum diagnostic yield. Unnecessary radiographs or those of poor quality that have no diagnostic value do not serve the patient's needs and only add to the patient's radiation burden. Whether the dentist, or dental professional takes the radiographs is not important, as long as the same quality standards are maintained.

The full-mouth radiographic survey is usually composed of 14 or more periapical films and, where possible, four posterior bitewing films (Figure 10-1, *A* and *B*). The bitewing films can be held vertically or horizontally. This text discusses a 14-periapical and a four-horizontal bitewing film technique. Some series of more than 14 periapical films include distal maxillary molar projections, vertical bitewings, anterior bitewings, and individual radiographs using #1 size film of the six maxillary and four mandibular anterior teeth.

The number of radiographs in a full-mouth survey can be modified to include extra or fewer projections, depending on the size of the patient's mouth or tooth position. In all cases the minimum number of films that satisfies the diagnostic requirements of a full-mouth survey should be used. Film mounts are available in various combinations of numbers and sizes of films. The radiographic survey should not be determined by the film mount available, but by the diagnostic needs of the patient. The recommended film projections are listed in Box 10-1.

A periapical film shows the entire tooth from occlusal surface or incisal edge to the apex and 2 to 3 mm of periapical bone. This film is necessary to diagnose normal or pathologic conditions of tooth crowns and root, bone, and tooth formation and eruption (Figure 10-2).

The bitewing film can be taken only if there are opposing teeth to hold the film in position with their occluding surfaces. This film projection shows the upper and lower teeth in occlusion. Only the crowns of the teeth are seen. It is used for detecting interproximal decay, periodontal bone loss, recurrent decay under restorations, and faulty restorations (Figure 10-3). Bitewing films can be taken of the anterior teeth, but are usually unnecessary if the

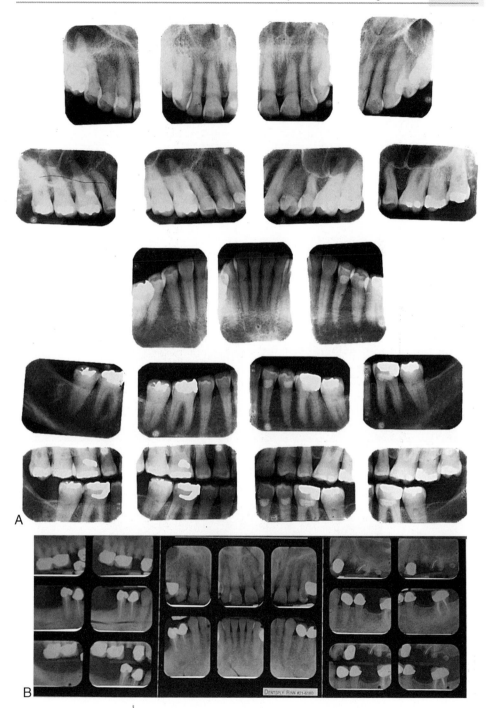

Figure 10-1. | **A,** A 19-film full-mouth survey. **B,** An 18-film full-mouth survey.

Maxillary	Mandibular
Central and lateral incisors	Central and lateral incisors
Right and left canines	Right and left canines
Right and left premolars	Right and left premolars
Right and left molars	Right and left molars
Bitewing	
Right and left premolars	
Right and left molars	

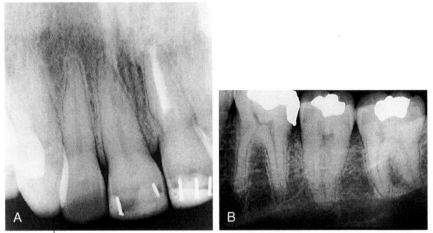

Figure 10-2. Anterior **(A)** and posterior **(B)** periapical radiographs. Note that the entire tooth and surrounding periapical bone are shown.

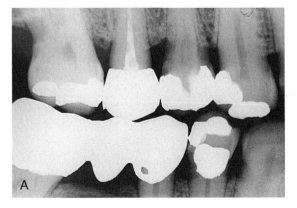

Figure 10-3. **A,** Bitewing radiograph. Note that only the crowns, alveolar ridge, and a small part of the roots of opposing teeth are seen.

Continued

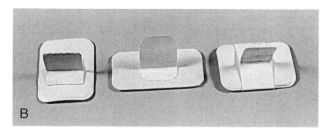

Figure 10-3—cont'd. **B,** Types of bitewing films: *left,* vertical; *middle,* long posterior; and *right,* standard.

paralleling method is used. Proponents of the use of vertical bitewings point out that in this film position, more root is seen and thus can be more diagnostic for root caries and alveolar bone levels.

The full-mouth survey shows all of the teeth in the mandible and maxilla, as well as the surrounding bone. Each tooth is shown at least twice in the survey; that is, the maxillary second premolar can be seen on the premolar periapical film and on the premolar bitewing film. Some teeth may be seen in three or four views. This gives the diagnostician an opportunity to view the tooth from different radiographic angles and eliminates the possibility that an artifact could be mistaken for caries or other pathologic conditions.

All the teeth-bearing areas of the jaws are covered in a full-mouth survey. However, the survey includes more than teeth. A clinically edentulous area may have residual root tips, unerupted teeth, impacted teeth, foreign bodies, or other pathologic conditions in the bone. One should not assume that because no teeth are present, everything is all right. The full complement of periapical films should be taken for all patients where indicated.

Pediatric Full-Mouth Series

Depending on the child's age and the size of the child's mouth, the composition of the full-mouth series may vary. A report of the Selection Criteria Panel recommends that for the asymptomatic clinically negative pediatric patient with closed posterior contacts, only two bitewing films be taken. For asymptomatic and clinically negative pediatric patients with open posterior contacts, no radiographs are necessary.

For patients up to age 5 who need a full-mouth series, the operator should use the pediatric-size film #0 for anterior, posterior, and bitewing projections (Figure 10-4). The full-mouth series at this age entails 12 films: three maxillary anterior films, three mandibular anterior films, four mandibular and maxillary molar projections, and two bitewing projections. Only one molar bitewing film is taken on each side.

In the 6- to 9-year-old group, the pediatric film or narrow adult film size #1 can be used for anterior projections because the child's arch shape at this age can still be very narrow. For posterior projections, adult size #2, narrow adult,

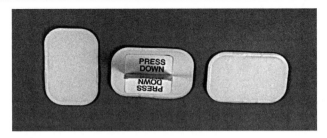

Figure 10-4. Size #0 pediatric film for anterior, posterior, and bitewing projections.

or pediatric film is used, depending on the size of the arch. At this age, two posterior periapical films in each quadrant are taken because the 6-year molars have erupted and the dental arch has lengthened. One bitewing film on each side also is used.

After age 9 the full adult series is taken, with the narrow adult film being used where necessary. These age guidelines are flexible and depend on the growth and development of the child. As a rule, it is best to use the largest film size that the patient can accommodate comfortably (Figure 10-5).

In the pediatric series, the chair position, film placement, point of entry, and vertical and horizontal angulations follow the same rules as in the adult series.

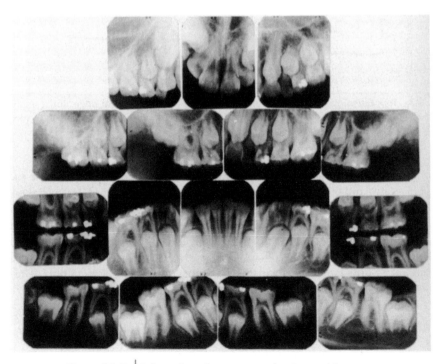

Figure 10-5. Full-mouth pediatric survey of a 9-year-old patient.

Edentulous Series

A radiographic examination must be performed even though the patient may be wholly or partially edentulous. The absence of teeth in an area of clinical examination does not preclude the possibility of retained roots, impacted teeth, cysts, or other occult pathologic conditions that may be present in the bone. The edentulous examination may use periapical projections, occlusal projections, or a panoramic radiograph. The intraoral edentulous series is usually composed of 13 periapical films. The bitewing films are not taken because there are no opposing teeth to support the film tabs, and only one film is used in the maxillary central, lateral, and canine areas (Figure 10-6). In small edentulous mouths, an 11-film survey may suffice by use of only one mandibular periapical film and extension of the premolar projection anteriorly to include the canine area.

The films are positioned in the same way as in a regular dentulous series but with certain modifications. The crest of the edentulous ridge replaces the occlusal plane of the teeth as the plane of orientation. The film is positioned either 1/8 in above or 1/8 in below the ridge. Because there are no teeth and there may be a great deal of ridge resorption, it may be difficult to parallel the *long axis* of the film with the long axis of the edentulous ridge, and so the film will lie flatter against the palate or in the floor of the mouth. In these cases it may be possible to support the film with cotton rolls to achieve parallelism or, if necessary, to increase the vertical angulation. The best guideline in the edentulous series is to adjust the vertical angulation so that the central ray is almost perpendicular to the film. Any slight foreshortening that may result will not affect the diagnosis of any intrabony conditions.

The exposure times should be reduced by a factor of one fourth for the edentulous series. There are two possible alternatives for the edentulous periapical survey. The first is a panoramic survey (Figure 10-7). The second is the use of topographic occlusal projections (Figure 10-8, *A* and *B*), the technique of which is discussed in the next chapter. The entire maxillary and mandibular

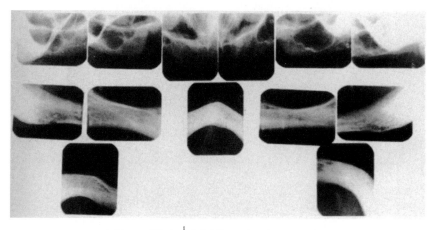

Figure 10-6. | A 13-film edentulous survey.

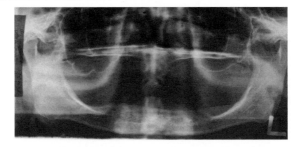

Figure 10-7. │ Edentulous panoramic survey.

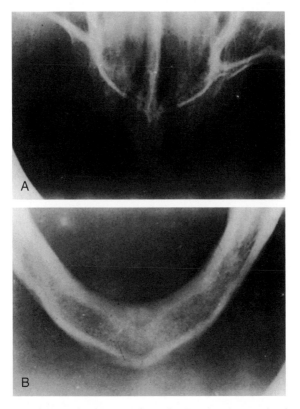

Figure 10-8. │ **A,** Edentulous occlusal survey of maxilla. **B,** Edentulous occlusal survey of mandible.

ridges usually can be seen on their respective occlusal projections. Both the panoramic and the occlusal are survey films, and if any suspicious areas are seen, a periapical projection of the area can be done to obtain better definition for making a definitive diagnosis.

The criteria for judging whether a single radiograph or a full-mouth survey is diagnostically acceptable are listed in Box 10-2.

| Box 10-2 | Criteria for Intraoral Radiographs |

1. The radiograph should show proper definition and detail and a degree of density and contrast so that all structures can be delineated easily.
2. The structures should not be distorted either by elongation or by foreshortening.
3. The radiograph should show the teeth from the occlusal or incisal edges to 2 to 3 mm beyond their apices.
4. In a full-mouth survey, the entire alveolar processes of the mandible and maxilla must be seen, as far distal as the tuberosity in the maxilla and the beginning of the ascending ramus in the mandible.
5. All interproximal surfaces of the teeth should be seen without overlapping, providing the teeth are not overlapped in the mouth.
6. The x-ray beam should be centered on the film so that there are no unexposed parts of the film ("cone cuts" or "collimator cutoff").
7. The radiograph should not be cracked or bent or have any other artifacts.
8. The radiograph should be processed properly (see Chapter 8).

If a single radiograph does not meet these criteria and provide diagnostic value, it must be retaken. In a full-mouth survey, those areas and structures that do not appear on the primary film may be seen on adjacent films in the series. Although a technically perfect full-mouth survey is ideal, retakes should not be done unless they are necessary for proper diagnosis.

Quality Assurance

These criteria should be used to evaluate radiographs taken by dentists and dental professionals as part of a quality assurance program. This can be accomplished either by self-analysis and criticism of one's work or by peer review. In this manner, technical errors can be corrected and high-quality diagnostic radiographs produced. Quality assurance is discussed further in Chapter 17.

PARALLELING TECHNIQUE

The basic principle of the paralleling technique for intraoral periapical films is that the film packet and the long axis of the tooth being radiographed must be parallel to each other, and the central ray of the x-ray beam must be directed perpendicular to both (see Figure 3-15). To accomplish this parallelism, the object-film distance must be increased. This distance can be sizable in some areas, such as the maxillary molar projection, where the film may have to be held at the midline of the palate to achieve this parallelism.

The increased object-film distance results in loss of image sharpness; using an increased 16-in focal-film distance (FFD) compensates for these problems (Figure 10-9).

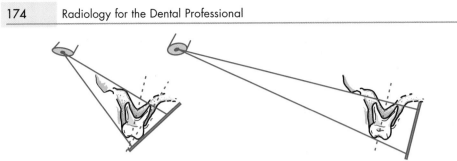

Figure 10-9. Bisecting 8-in focal-film distance technique and paralleling 16-inch extended-cone technique. Note superimposition of zygomatic arch on apices of maxillary molar in bisecting technique. *(Courtesy DENTSPLY Rinn, Elgin, IL.)*

Unfortunately, the paralleling technique has too often been called the *long cone technique*. This terminology emphasizes the length of the position-indicating device (PID) rather than the parallel relationship of the object and the film. Better names for this method are the *extension paralleling technique* or *right-angle technique*, both of which stress the important components of the technique.

Advantages and Disadvantages of the Paralleling Technique Compared with the Bisecting Technique

When the paralleling and bisecting techniques are compared, the consensus is that dental professionals prefer the paralleling method as the technique of choice. The American Academy of Oral and Maxillofacial Radiology through its Parameters of Care Committee states, "The paralleling technique should be used with its appropriate armamentarium, when possible, as it provides the most geometrically accurate image of the dentition." The paralleling technique produces better diagnostic images, less exposure to critical organs such as the thyroid gland and the lens of the eye, a smaller exit dose, and easier standardization and execution than the bisecting technique. This text takes the position that the paralleling technique is the method of choice.

Advantages

The major advantage of the paralleling technique is that when performed correctly it forms an image on the film with both linear and dimensional accuracy to support a more valid diagnosis. The key terms are *dimensional accuracy* and *dimensional distortion*.

The bisecting technique, if used properly, correctly represents the teeth linearly but produces dimensional distortion. The bisecting technique can project the images and surrounding structures on the film in a true linear relationship without elongation or foreshortening. When radiographed with the bisecting technique, performed ideally, a tooth 22 mm in length is shown on the radiograph as 22 mm long. The teeth and bone, however, are three-dimensional objects, and although their overall length may be recorded accurately,

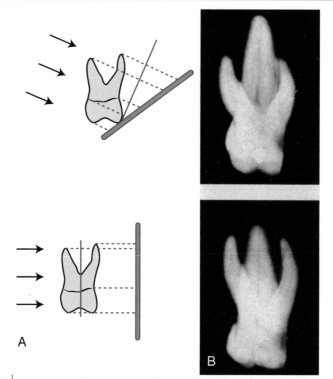

Figure 10-10. Radiographs of maxillary molar taken with **(A)** bisecting technique and the **(B)** paralleling technique *(Courtesy DENTSPLY Rinn, Elgin, IL.)*

the relationship of one part of the tooth to another is distorted dimensionally (Figure 10-10). Those parts of the tooth that lie farthest from the film, such as the buccal plate of bone and buccal roots, are foreshortened, although their lingual linear counterparts are not. A classic clinical example consists of comparing the length of the buccal roots with that of palatal roots in maxillary first molars. Clinicians who have used the bisecting technique for many years may come to believe that the buccal roots are much shorter than they really are because of dimensional distortions. One may argue that this may not be clinically important, except in an initial endodontic measurement, but when this distortion is applied to periodontal evaluation of alveolar bone levels, the clinical importance becomes apparent (Figure 10-11). In the bisecting technique the image of the buccal bone level is figuratively added to the palatal bone height to give a distorted image. A diagnosis and treatment plan could assume the presence of adequate bone for restorations, fixed splinting, and so forth on the basis of distorted radiographic images.

With the paralleling technique, it is possible to diagnose and evaluate caries and alveolar bone height accurately on all radiographs and not rely on the bitewing projections, as users of the bisecting technique do. It is interesting to note that bitewing projections in both techniques are paralleling films.

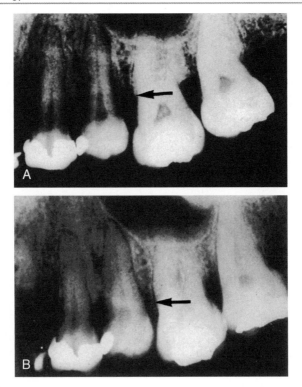

Figure 10-11. | Radiographs of the same area: **A,** taken with the paralleling technique and **B,** the bisecting technique. Note the difference in alveolar bone height as indicated by arrows.

In the bisecting technique the radiopaque image of the zygomatic arch is often superimposed on the apices of the maxillary molars, making diagnosis difficult if not impossible. This superimposition is understandable because the point of entry of the central ray for molar projections is along the zygomatic arch.

The paralleling technique produces no superimposition because the central ray, which is perpendicular to the long axis of the molars, enters below the level of the zygomatic arch. Also, in the paralleling technique the vertical angulation of the primary beam is rarely more than ±10 degrees, compared with vertical angulation of +40 to +50 degrees in the bisecting technique. The lack of extreme vertical angulation reduces the exposure to the thyroid gland and the lens of the eye because they no longer lie in the path of the primary beam. The literature reports thyroid exposure of 25 mR for a full-mouth survey using the paralleling technique, compared with 60 mR for the bisecting technique. In addition, the 16-in FFD used with the paralleling technique reduces the volume of tissue irradiated when compared with the 8-in FFD used in the bisecting technique (see Figure 6-10).

The paralleling technique is easier to standardize than the bisecting technique, and serial comparison radiographs of the same area have greater validity.

This is especially important in evaluating alveolar bone levels of periodontal patients at recall examinations.

If a film-holding device with a localizing ring is used, in the paralleling technique the patient does not have to be positioned so that the occlusal plane of the jaw being radiographed is parallel to the floor. This is especially helpful in contour chairs or when patients are treated in the supine position. In both of these instances, it is difficult to position the patient with the occlusal plane parallel to the floor.

Disadvantages

One of the objections most often raised about the paralleling technique is the difficulty in placement and the degree of discomfort caused by the devices used to hold the film parallel to the long axis of the tooth. This may present some problems for patients with small mouths, children, and patients with low palatal vaults, but the more adept an operator becomes with the technique, the less these problems are a factor. In the pediatric patient, if it is impossible to position the film for the paralleling method, decrease the film size and then, if a backup strategy is needed, use the bisecting method. It is said that paralleling is more difficult to learn and takes clinically longer to do. Experience with novice students has disproved this argument. At least the time element is the same, and learning the paralleling technique is as easy as or easier than learning the bisecting technique, especially when using paralleling instruments.

Objections also focus on the "long, bulky" 16-in PID that is used in the paralleling technique. The claim is that these PIDs are difficult to work with in small operatories. The difference is 8 inches, and in a well-designed office this cannot be a factor. This objection has no validity in the newer x-ray machines with the extended FFD within the tube head as a result of a recessed target (see Figure 3-12).

Another supposed disadvantage of the paralleling technique is that with the 16-in FFD, longer exposure times are necessary, resulting in a greater chance of *patient movement*. With the use of faster film, this is no longer true. This chapter compares exposure times of 1/5 versus 4/5 second (inverse square law), and the difference in possible patient movement within these time frames is not significant. Previously with the use of slower film, the possibility of patient movement with a 4-second exposure was greater than that with a 1-second exposure, and the objection was valid.

EXPOSURE ROUTINE

Regardless of which technique is used, certain basic rules must be followed for barrier technique, infection control preparation of the patient, and radiation hygiene. Operators should develop an *exposure routine* to avoid mistakes that necessitate the retaking of films. Retaking a radiograph because of operator error adds unnecessarily to the patient's radiation burden.

The patient should be seated comfortably in the chair, with the back well supported and the head positioned in such a way that the jaw can be radiographed correctly. Except when localizing rings are used, the occlusal plane of the jaw being radiographed must be parallel to the floor when it is in the open position.

The patient should remove any nonfixed prosthetic appliances from his or her mouth, as well as eyeglasses and facial jewelry such as nose rings. Failure to do this is a common error. Glass and any metallic frame are radiopaque and may be superimposed on any film in which jewelry is worn. The patient should be draped with a lead apron and thyroid collar. This is done routinely for all patients, for a single film and the full-mouth series. Then the operator turns on the x-ray machine and selects the desired kilovoltage and milliamperage. In busy private practices or large clinics, the on/off switches as well as the kVp and mA values may be left unchanged through the working day.

The infection control procedures outlined in Chapter 9 should be followed. Many dental offices have a semiautomatic, lead film dispenser in each operatory, enabling the operator to withdraw one film at a time. The operator should take care not to touch the dispenser with the gloved hand after it has been in the patient's mouth. If a dispenser is to be used, it should be activated with the upper part of the arm or elbow. The exposed films can be placed in a paper cup within a lead receptacle. If there is no lead dispenser, the desired number of films, as well as additional supplies, such as bitewing tabs and *bite blocks*, should be brought near the operatory at this time.

If there are no lead film dispensers and no exposed film receptacles, both the exposed and unexposed films must be kept out of the room where the x-ray machine is used. Many diagnostic dental films are fogged by secondary radiation and thus made unacceptable if left on the bracket table in the dental operatory when other films are being exposed. Again, poor technique on the part of the operator leads to film retakes and unnecessary exposure for the patient.

One of the more important general principles of taking intraoral radiographs is to have the positioned film in the patient's mouth for as short a time as possible. This decreases the likelihood of gagging and patient movement. The desired exposure time on the machine always should be set before the film is placed in the patient's mouth. Many seconds can be wasted in consulting exposure charts and setting the timing dial while the film is in the patient's mouth.

While the exposure is being made from the required 6-ft distance, the operator should watch the patient. If the patient moves, the operator can see the problem and retake the film immediately. A simple command to the patient such as "hold still" can be helpful at this time. A properly designed office permits observation from behind a suitable barrier.

After the exposure has been made, the operator removes the film from the patient's mouth, dries it of saliva, and places it in the exposed film receptacle. Some definite order should be followed for a full-mouth series of radiographs.

Skipping from area to area without a set pattern often results in an omitted film. A good place to start is with the maxillary central incisor film or maxillary central/lateral incisor film; it is probably the easiest to position and the easiest for the patient to tolerate. One should never start with the maxillary molar film because this is the projection most likely to excite the gag reflex; once the reflex is excited, the patient may gag on films that normally could be tolerated. After starting with the maxillary central/lateral incisor, the maxillary canine, premolar, and molar are radiographed in that order. The opposite side of the maxilla is then radiographed. It is poor technique to radiograph left canine, right canine, left premolar, and so forth. This necessitates moving the tube head constantly from one side of the patient to the other and can result in an omitted film.

The bitewing films are taken after maxillary periapicals because the same head position and occlusal plane orientation are used. The mandibular periapical films are taken in the same order as the maxillary films.

Film Holders

The use of film holders is strongly recommended. In the paralleling technique the film packet must be held in its proper position by one of a variety of film-holding devices all serving one purpose: to position the film parallel to the long axis of the tooth. Some examples of devices include *hemostats*, Stabe, XCP, RAPD, Precision, and Intrex holders (Figure 10-12). *Localizing rings* align the PID with the film in both the horizontal and vertical planes and help to reduce the incidence of collimator cutoff ("cone cutting"). The localizing rings are a great aid with some contour dental chairs, which make it difficult to position the patient so that the occlusal plane is parallel to the floor. As long as the open-ended PID can be brought into flat contact with the localizing ring, strict adherence to occlusal plane orientation is not necessary. Also, the relationship between the end of the PID and the ring can alert the operator

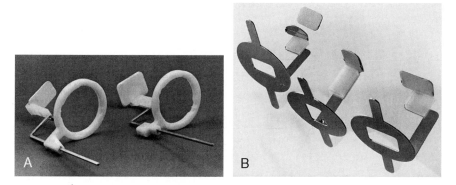

Figure 10-12. | Film-holding (receptor) devices in paralleling technique. **A,** XCP instruments. **B,** Precision paralleling devices.

Continued

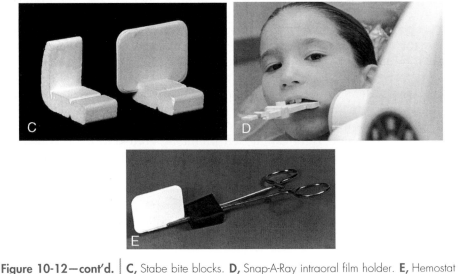

Figure 10-12—cont'd. | **C,** Stabe bite blocks. **D,** Snap-A-Ray intraoral film holder. **E,** Hemostat and rubber bite block. *(From White SC, Pharoah MJ: Oral radiology: principles and interpretation, ed 4, St Louis, 2000, Mosby.* **A and C,** *Courtesy DENTSPLY Rinn, Elgin, IL.)*

to exposure errors before they get a chance to happen. For example, if there is spacing on the right or left of the ring, the operator should correct the horizontal angulation. In addition, if the spacing is on the top or bottom, the operator should correct the vertical angulation. Furthermore, some manufacturers have included notches on circular localizing rings to assist operators with proper placement of a rectangular PID.

Film holders are either disposable (e.g., Styrofoam bite blocks) or nondisposable (e.g., XCP, RAPD). Nondisposable film holders must be sterilized and not just disinfected. As described in Chapter 9, the accepted methods of sterilization include steam autoclaving and dry heat. Some holding devices have plastic or vinyl parts that are not considered autoclavable.

METHOD

The following six factors must be considered in any periapical projection: exposure time, chair position, film position and placement, point of entry of the beam, vertical angulation, and horizontal angulation.

Exposure Time

Exposure time is determined by the area being radiographed, film speed, kilovoltage peak, milliamperage, and FFD. Exposure charts are readily available, and most x-ray film packages contain them. It is customary to post such a chart near the machine so that exposure times need not be committed to memory. In some cases, the time can also be set automatically simply by choosing an icon representing the area of exposure on the control panel (see Figure 2-6). In any event, the timer should be set before the film is placed in the patient's mouth.

Chair Position: Occlusal and Sagittal Plane Orientations

The patient is positioned so that when the mouth is open and the film packet is in position, the occlusal plane of the jaw being radiographed is parallel to the floor. In the maxilla this plane corresponds to the ala-tragus line on the face. When the maxilla is radiographed, the headrest is positioned high on the back of the patient's head, forcing the chin down (Figure 10-13). When the mandible is radiographed, the headrest is placed below the occipital eminence in what would be the normal dental chair position (Figure 10-14). For both upper and lower jaws, the patient's head is positioned so that the *sagittal plane* is perpendicular to the floor (Figure 10-15).

Film Position

The film packet is held with its long dimension vertical for anterior projections and horizontal for posterior periapical and bitewing projections. The edge of the film always should extend evenly either 1/8 in below (maxillary) or 1/8 in above (mandibular) the occlusal plane. This film position ensures

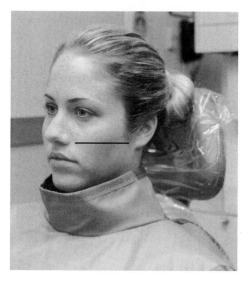

Figure 10-13. | Proper patient position for maxillary periapical radiographs and bitewing films. Note that the occlusal plane of maxillary teeth, or ala-tragus line, is parallel to the floor.

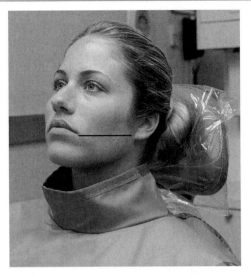

Figure 10-14. Proper patient position for mandibular periapical radiographs. Note that when the mouth is open, the occlusal plane of lower teeth is parallel to the floor.

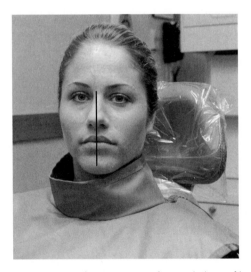

Figure 10-15. Proper patient position for orientation of sagittal plane of head perpendicular to the floor.

that adequate film remains at the apical areas and at the incisal or occlusal surfaces to record the image. The film packet should be placed in the patient's mouth so that the mounting orientation button is toward the occlusal surface (Figure 10-16). This helps in mounting and precludes the possibility of the dots being superimposed over the apex of a tooth. The film is held in position by the patient with a bite block or other film-holding device. One useful way

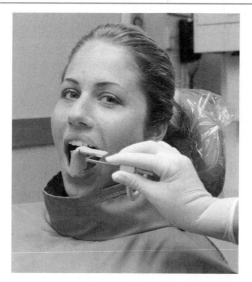

Figure 10-16. Placement of film-holding device in patient's mouth by operator. Note that the correct side of film packet faces the tube head and the mounting dot is toward the occlusal surface.

of remembering the correct positioning of the film packet in the holding device is by use of the slogan "dot in the slot and the white toward me." This will ensure that the operator will prevent having the dot superimposed over the apex of the root, and the incidence of reversed films will be decreased.

Point of Entry

The *point of entry* is the anatomic position on the patient's face at which the central ray of the x-ray beam is aimed. It corresponds to the middle of the film packet in the patient's mouth. The operator should know these anatomic points but also should align the beam with the film as viewed in the patient's mouth. The localizing ring, when used, determines the point of entry by its predetermined relationship to the film packet. The use of rectangular collimation does not change this relationship among the localizing ring, PID, and point of entry.

Vertical Angulation

In the paralleling technique the *vertical angulation* is set to make the central ray perpendicular to the film. In the bisecting technique (see Chapter 11), the vertical angulation is determined by the bisection of the angle. The vertical angulations for the bisecting technique given in this text and elsewhere should be used only as guide angles. These angles can be strictly adhered to if film is positioned accurately; however, not all mouths allow this type of film positioning. Some mouths have crowded arches, misplaced teeth, tight muscle attachments, or other anatomic constraints. In these cases the bisection of the film-tooth angle results in different vertical angulations than those listed. Vertical angulation of the x-ray beam is set according to the dial on the side of the tube head (Figure 10-17).

Horizontal Angulation

To achieve *horizontal angulation*, the central ray is directed so that it is perpendicular to the film in the horizontal plane. The central ray is directed through the interproximal spaces to avoid overlapping of structures. It may be easier for the operator to sight on the horizontal axis of the tube head and make this parallel to the film in the horizontal plane.

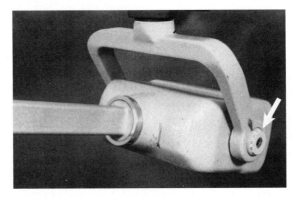

Figure 10-17. | Tube head of x-ray machine, with arrow pointing to setting for vertical angulation.

THE FULL-MOUTH SERIES

Maxillary Central and Lateral Incisors (Figure 10-18)

Chair Position. The maxillary occlusal plane is positioned parallel to the floor, and the sagittal plane of the patient's face is perpendicular to the floor.

Film Position. The film is held vertically and positioned in the palate away from the lingual surfaces of the teeth so that the long axis of the film packet is parallel to the long axis of the teeth. The center of the film packet is positioned between the central and lateral incisors. The film is placed in the palate so that the entire lengths of the teeth are shown. This parallel placement of the film is held in position by one of the devices previously mentioned.

PROCEDURE 10-1

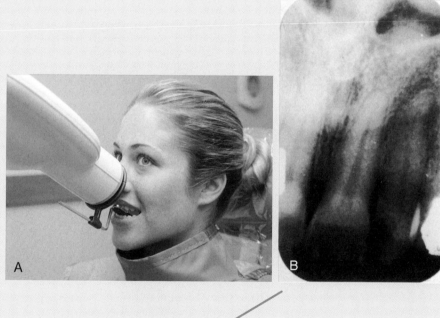

A

B

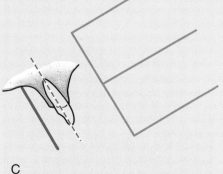

C

Figure 10-18. Maxillary central and lateral incisors. **A,** Film holder and position-indicating device (PID). **B,** Radiograph. **C,** Diagram.

Point of Entry. The central ray is directed at the center of the film. If a localizing ring is used, the open face of the PID contacts the ring; this determines the point of entry and vertical and horizontal angulation of the x-ray beam.

Vertical Angulation. The central ray is perpendicular to the tooth and film packet.

Horizontal Angulation. The central ray is perpendicular to the tooth and film in the horizontal plane.

If one film is to be used for the maxillary right and left central and lateral incisors, the center of the film is placed between the central incisors and the central ray is directed perpendicular to the center of the film packet (Figure 10-19).

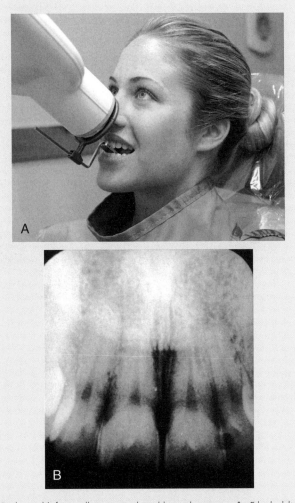

Figure 10-19. | Right and left maxillary central and lateral incisors. **A,** Film-holding device and PID. **B,** Radiograph.

Helpful Hint: When using a localizing device, make sure that it is as close to the patient's face without touching as possible. This prevents the ring position being away from the film, which would result in a thin (light) image because of the application of the inverse square law.

Maxillary Canines (Figure 10-20)

Chair Position. The maxillary occlusal plane is parallel to the floor, and the sagittal plane of the patient's face is perpendicular to the floor.

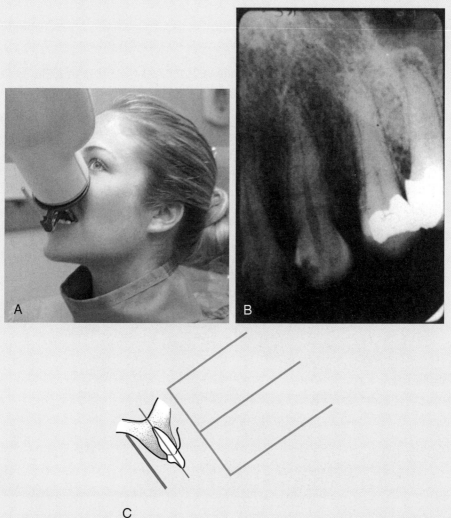

C

Figure 10-20. | Maxillary canine. **A,** Film-holding device and PID. **B,** Radiograph. **C,** Diagram.

PROCEDURE 10-1

Film Position. The film is held vertically, away from the lingual surface of the canine and parallel to its long axis. The center of the film packet is behind the canine and positioned in the palate so that the entire length of the canine is shown. The film packet is held in position by a holding device.

Point of Entry. The central ray is directed at the center of the film packet, or if a localizing ring is used, it is brought into flat contact with the open-ended PID.

Vertical Angulation. The central ray is perpendicular to the film packet.

Horizontal Angulation. The central ray is perpendicular to the film in the horizontal plane.

Helpful Hint: Film placement of the maxillary cuspid may be very difficult. In order to achieve parallelism the film packet may have to be positioned across the arch, resulting in an increased object-film distance. Also, the operator should make sure that the film is curved away from the source of radiation to accommodate the palatal arch. If the film is curved toward the radiation, the lead foil backing will be superimposed over the superior aspect of the film. Furthermore, the operator must make sure that the film doesn't come out of the holder when it contacts the palate so as not to cut off the incisal edge.

Maxillary Premolars (Figure 10-21)
Chair Position. The maxillary occlusal plane is parallel to the floor, and the sagittal plane of the patient's face is perpendicular to the floor.

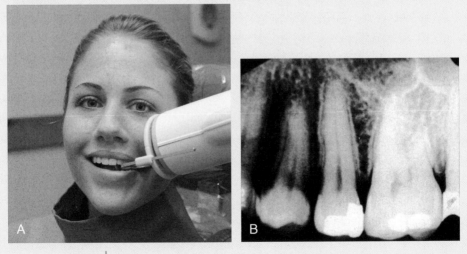

Figure 10-21. | Maxillary premolars. **A,** Film-holding device and PID. **B,** Radiograph.
Continued

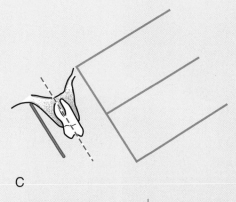

Figure 10-21—cont'd. | **C,** Diagram.

Film Position. The film is held horizontally and positioned away from the lingual surfaces of the premolar so that its long axis is parallel to the long axis of the premolar. In the maxillary premolar and molar region, film position may be in the middle of the palate. The center of the film aligns with the second premolar. The packet is positioned in the palate so that the entire length of the teeth is shown on the film. The packet is held in position by a holding device.

Point of Entry. The central ray is directed at the center of the film, or if a localizing ring is used, it is brought into flat contact with the open-ended PID.

Vertical Angulation. The central ray is perpendicular to the film.

Horizontal Angulation. The central ray is perpendicular to the film in the horizontal plane.

> **Helpful Hint:** If one is having difficulty centering the premolar film packet, it may be helpful to mark the middle of the packet with a vertical line, and this line should always be aligned with the second premolar. Make sure as the arch starts to turn that the film packet remains parallel to the long axis as well as the horizontal axis of the teeth being radiographed.

Maxillary Molars (Figure 10-22)
Chair Position. The maxillary occlusal plane is positioned parallel to the floor, and the sagittal plane of the patient's face is perpendicular to the floor.

Film Position. The film is held horizontally and positioned away from the lingual surfaces of the molars so that the long axis of the film lies parallel to the long axes of the molars. The center of the film packet aligns with the middle of the second

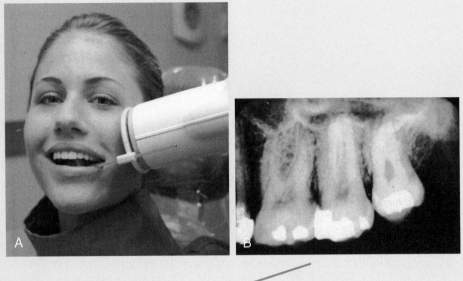

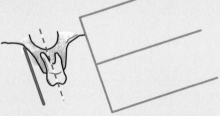

Figure 10-22. | Maxillary molars. **A,** Film-holding device and PID. **B,** Radiograph. **C,** Diagram.

molar, and the packet is positioned in the palate so that the entire length of the teeth is shown. The film packet is held in position by a holding device.

Point of Entry. The central ray is directed at the center of the film, or the localizing ring is brought into flat contact with the open-ended PID.

Vertical Angulation. The central ray is perpendicular to the film.

Horizontal Angulation. The central ray is perpendicular to the film in the horizontal plane.

Helpful Hint: If you are not using a localizing ring, you can offset the film packet by placing the film packet distally in the bite block and have the center of the block be over the first molar.

If the mouth is unusually small or the teeth crowded, it may be necessary to use a smaller film, such as #0 or #1. Remember it is the anatomic variants of the teeth and bone that dictate the film size that should be used.

If the operator is having difficulty placing the packet to include the third molar region, he or she can place the packet on the first molar when the mouth is fully open and ask the patient to close slightly and then place the film on the second molar before finally securing the packet.

Bitewing Films

The technique for bitewing films is the same in the paralleling and bisecting-angle techniques except for the use of the 16-in FFD and thus increased exposure time. Bitewing films are always parallel films, no matter what technique is used for the periapical films. The film is positioned by the bite tab parallel to the crowns of both upper and lower teeth, and the central ray is directed perpendicular to the film.

Premolar and Molar Bitewing Projections (Figure 10-23)

Chair Position. The maxillary occlusal plane is positioned parallel to the floor, and the sagittal plane of the patient's face is perpendicular to the floor.

Film Position. When the premolars are radiographed, the bite tab is placed on the occlusal surface of the second mandibular premolar. This depresses the film packet into the floor of the mouth. While the operator holds the tab down with thumb and forefinger, the patient is instructed to bite on the tab. The operator

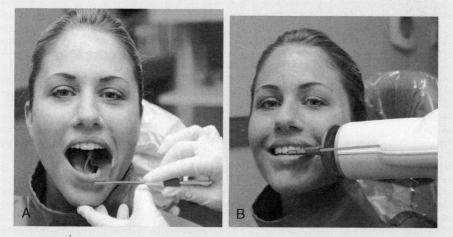

Figure 10-23. Bitewing projection. **A,** Film-holding device being placed on occlusal surfaces of lower teeth. **B,** Patient bites on bite block.

PROCEDURE 10-1

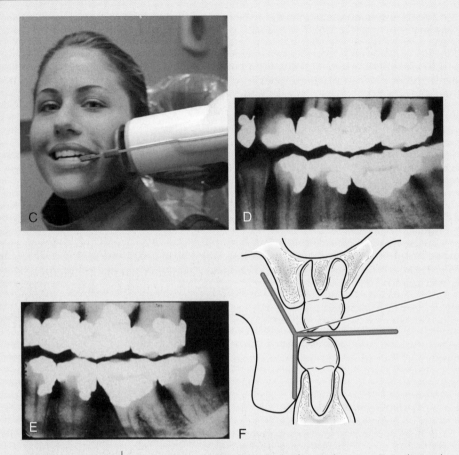

Figure 10-23—cont'd. **C,** PID positioned, **D,** Radiograph of premolar area. **E,** Radiograph of molar area. **F,** Diagram.

should be sure that the patient is biting on the back teeth and not just bringing the incisors together. If the back teeth are not moved to centric occlusion, the film packet is not secure; it may move and not be oriented correctly. The procedure for radiographing the molars is the same as that previously mentioned, except that the bite tab is centered over the occlusal surface of the second molar.

Point of Entry. The central ray is directed at the bitewing tab, which is held in position by the patient's teeth. If a localizing ring and film holder are used, the open end of the PID is placed against the ring.

Vertical Angulation. The central ray is perpendicular to the film.

Horizontal Angulation. Horizontal angulation is a critical factor in the bitewing film, and utmost attention should be paid to horizontal positioning. An overlapping image on the bitewing film is useless. The central ray should be perpendicular to the film packet in the horizontal plane and should go through the contact points of the premolars or molars.

Helpful Hint: When taking bitewings without the use of a localizing ring, it helps to align the beam by having your index finger touching the bitewing tab in the buccal sulcus of the patient's mouth in an effort to use your finger as an extension of the PID. You can also ask the patient to smile so that the tab is revealed.

Vertical Bitewings (Figure 10-24)

Vertical bitewings are used when the desired area would not be seen on the film with normal bitewing placement; this could be the case in advanced bone loss, root caries, or tooth eruption. The film is placed in the patient's mouth with the longer side vertically positioned. All other exposure factors remain the same. It is necessary to use the paste-on tabs and not the loops or the preformed bitewing packets in this technique. The vertical bitewing can be used in a posterior or anterior region. There are paralleling instruments available in the contemporary market that now include vertical bitewing attachments.

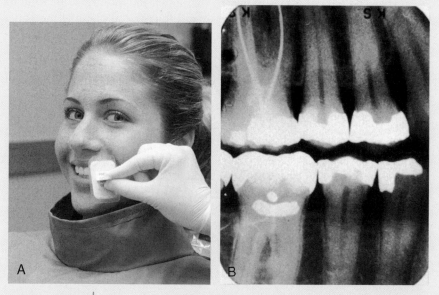

Figure 10-24. | Vertical bitewing. **A,** Posterior film position. **B,** Posterior radiograph.

PROCEDURE 10-1

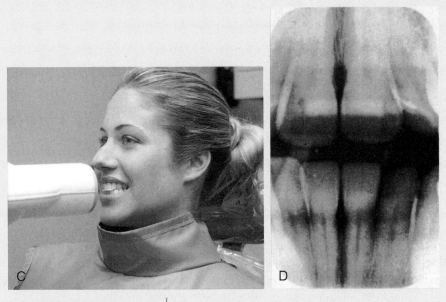

Figure 10-24—cont'd. │ **C,** Anterior film position. **D,** Anterior radiograph.

Mandibular Incisors (Figure 10-25)

Chair Position. The patient is positioned so that when the mouth is open the mandibular occlusal plane is parallel to the floor and the sagittal plane of the patient's face is perpendicular to the floor.

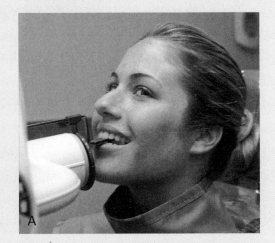

Figure 10-25. │ Mandibular incisors. **A,** Film-holding device and PID.

Continued

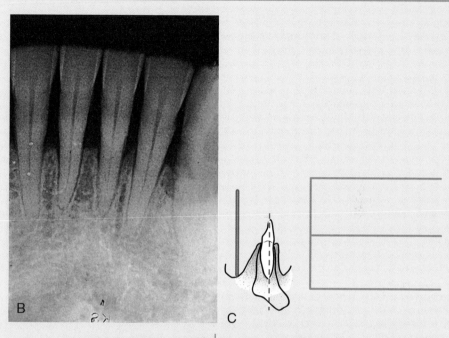

PROCEDURE 10-1

B

C

Figure 10-25—cont'd. | **B,** Radiograph. **C,** Diagram.

Film Position. The film is held vertically and positioned away from the lingual surfaces of the incisors so that the long axis of the film is parallel to the long axes of the incisors. The center of the packet is positioned at the midline so that all four incisors appear on the film. The film is depressed into the floor of the mouth so that the entire length of the teeth is shown. It may be necessary to displace the tongue distally and to depress the floor of the mouth to achieve this. The film packet is held in position by a holding device.

Point of Entry. The central ray is directed at the center of the film, or the localizing ring is brought into flat contact with the open-ended PID.

Vertical Angulation. The central ray is perpendicular to the film.

Horizontal Angulation. The central ray is perpendicular to the film in the horizontal plane.

Helpful Hint: When taking this projection, remember that in order to achieve parallelism between the teeth and the film packet in some cases it may be necessary to position the packet far back in the floor of the mouth at the level of the molars. You may also start out with the film on an angle and then bring the film into a parallel

> position slowly with the closure of the mandible. The operator may also place a gauze pad under the film to prevent it from irritating the floor of the mouth.

Mandibular Canines (Figure 10-26)

Chair Position. The patient is positioned so that when the mouth is open the mandibular occlusal plane is parallel to the floor and the sagittal plane of the patient's face is perpendicular to the floor.

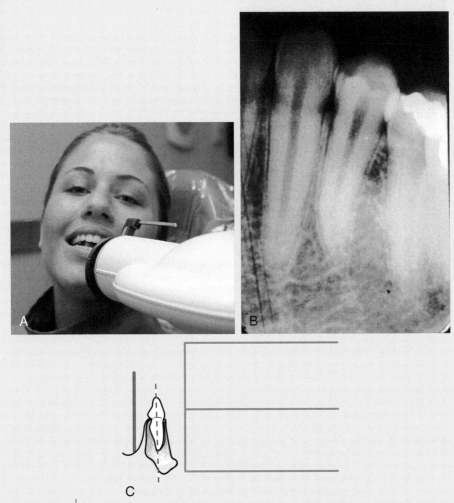

Figure 10-26. Mandibular canine. **A,** Film-holding device and PID. **B,** Radiograph. **C,** Diagram.

Film Position. The film is held vertically and positioned away from the lingual surface of the canine so that its long axis is parallel to that of the canine. The packet is positioned so that the canine is in the center of the film. The packet is depressed into the floor of the mouth so that the entire length of the tooth is shown on the film. The packet is held in position by a holding device.

Point of Entry. The central ray is directed at the center of the film, or the localizing ring is brought into flat contact with the open-ended PID.

Vertical Angulation. The central ray is perpendicular to the film.

Horizontal Angulation. The central ray is perpendicular to the film in the horizontal plane.

> **Helpful Hint:** Be sure that the film packet is placed below and not above the tongue, as it is skeletal muscle and very difficult to displace. As it is said, "in a war with the tongue, the tongue always wins."

Mandibular Premolars (Figure 10-27)

Chair Position. The patient is positioned so that when the mouth is open the mandibular occlusal plane is parallel to the floor and the sagittal plane of the patient's face is perpendicular to the floor.

Film Position. The film is held horizontally and positioned so that it is parallel to the long axis of the premolar. The object-film distance in both the mandibular

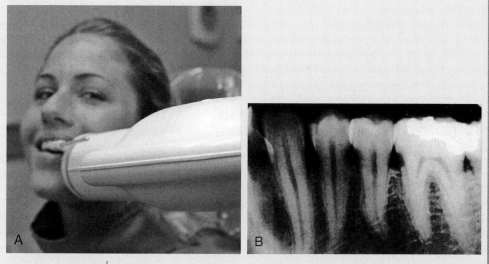

Figure 10-27. │ Mandibular premolar. **A,** Film-holding device and PID. **B,** Radiograph.

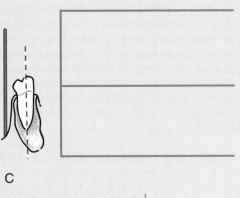

C

Figure 10-27—cont'd. | **C,** Diagram.

premolar and molar regions is almost minimal because the anatomy allows the film to be positioned very close to the tooth and still be parallel. The second premolar is centered behind the center of the film packet. The packet is depressed into the floor of the mouth so that the entire length of the teeth shows on the film. The film is held in position by a holding device.

Point of Entry. The central ray is directed at the center of the film, or if a localizing ring is used, it is brought into flat contact with the open-ended PID.

Vertical Angulation. The central ray is directed perpendicular to the film.

Horizontal Angulation. The central ray is perpendicular to the film in the horizontal plane.

> **Helpful Hint:** In a small mouth, it may be helpful to roll (not bend) the lower anterior corner of the film packet to ensure the patient's comfort.

Mandibular Molars (Figure 10-28)

Chair Position. The patient is positioned so that when the mouth is open the mandibular occlusal plane is parallel to the floor and the sagittal plane of the patient's face is perpendicular to the floor.

Film Position. The film is held horizontally and positioned lingually to the molar so that the long axis of the film is parallel to the long axes of the molars. The film is centered behind the second molar and depressed into the floor of the mouth so that the entire length of the teeth appears on the film. The packet is held in position by a holding device.

Point of Entry. The central ray is directed at the center of the film, or if a localizing ring is used, it is brought into flat contact with the open-ended PID.

PROCEDURE 10-1

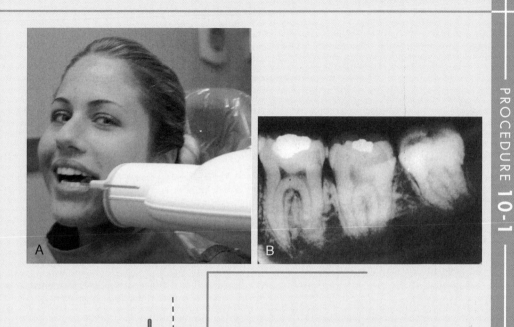

Figure 10-28. | Mandibular molars. **A,** Film-holding device and PID. **B,** Radiograph. **C,** Diagram.

Vertical Angulation. The central ray is directed perpendicular to the film.

Horizontal Angulation. The central ray is perpendicular to the film in the horizontal plane.

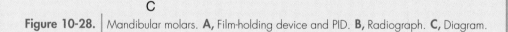

Helpful Hint: When positioning the film packet, make sure that the middle of the packet, which may be marked, is aligned with the middle of the second molar.

COMMON ERROR 10-1

THE PARALLELING METHOD (also see the Appendix)

All of the errors mentioned and illustrated in this chapter also are possible in the bisecting technique, but the incidence differs. Although elongation and foreshortening are the most common bisecting errors, they are not as common in the paralleling technique. The most common error in the paralleling technique, even with the use of positioning devices, is in film placement. If the film packet and film holder are not placed correctly in the patient's mouth, the paralleling technique does not work. The most common error is not to place the film packet deep enough in the floor of the mouth or high enough in the palate, thus cutting off the apices of the teeth as a result of inadequate closure.

With the use of the localizing ring, which is aligned with the center of the film packet, collimator cutoff ("cone cutting") can be practically eliminated.

Occlusal plane and sagittal plane orientation of the patient's head is not important if the localizing ring on the film-holding device is used, as long as the open end of the PID is brought into flat contact with the localizing ring.

Horizontal overlapping of the images also is eliminated with the proper use of the positioning device and localizing ring.

The rest of the errors mentioned in this chapter (i.e., film reversal, overbending, crescent marks, overexposing and underexposing, double exposure, and failure to remove dental appliances) are all possible with the bisecting technique, and their remedies are the same.

Collimator cutoff (cone cutting) (Figure 10-29). An unexposed area on the radiograph occurs when the x-ray beam is not centered on the film packet. This is called *collimator cutoff* and is caused by improper alignment of the x-ray beam and film.

Remedy. The central ray of the x-ray beam should be aligned carefully with the center of the film packet. With circular collimation the aperture of the diaphragm

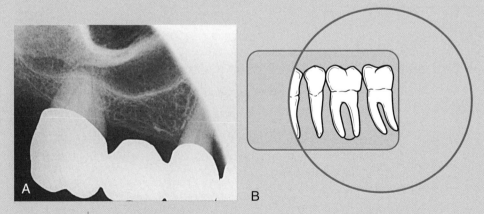

Figure 10-29. | **A,** Collimator cutoff ("cone cutting"). Central ray positioned too far distal.
B, Diagram of cone cutting. Central ray positioned too far mesial.

Continued

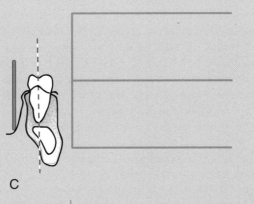

C

Figure 10-29—cont'd. | **C,** Cone cutting with rectangular collimation.

allows for a beam diameter, measured at the face, of $2^3/_4$ in. Size #2 adult film is $1^1/_4 \times 1^5/_8$ in, which leaves almost $^1/_2$-in leeway for error in all directions. It is not sufficient to identify collimator cutoff; it should be analyzed to pinpoint the error. If it is always the distal part of a radiograph in a projection that is cut off, then the point of entry must be moved mesially. A localizing ring, with a film-holding device, aligns the beam and the film and eliminates collimator cutoff with both circular and rectangular collimation.

Film reversal (Figure 10-30). *Film reversal* is sometimes referred to as the "herringbone effect" because the herringbone pattern that is embossed on the lead foil backing is transferred to the processed reversed radiograph. The herringbone, light (thin) image results from placing the film packet backward in the patient's mouth. The x-rays are attenuated in a pattern by the lead foil before striking the film. The geometric pattern embossed by the lead foil backing distinguishes this light radiograph from other *underexposure* errors. The original geometric pattern

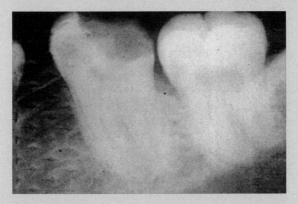

Figure 10-30. | Film reversal. Film packet placed in mouth with the wrong side toward the tube.

was that of a herringbone, and the name has survived even though the present pattern now resembles tiny adjacent boxes, a checkerboard, or even tire tracks.

Remedy. The front and the back of the film packet should be identified. Some manufacturers color-code or change the texture of the back of the film packet. Operators should develop the habit of looking for these aids.

Poor film placement (Figure 10-31). The film has been poorly positioned if the whole tooth does not show on the film and the image is not elongated; there is no film behind the apex of the tooth to record the image or the tooth that should be centered is not.

Remedy. Only $^1/_8$ in of film should project above or below the occlusal or incisal edges of the teeth. If a bite block is used, the teeth being radiographed must bite firmly on the block.

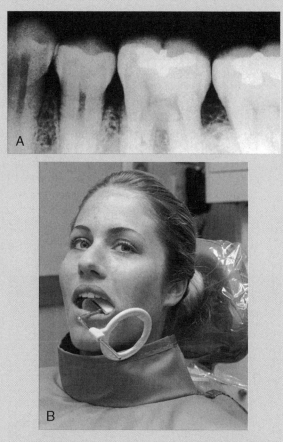

Figure 10-31. | **A,** Nondiagnostic image caused by poor film packet placement. Note that apices of teeth are not seen. **B,** Poor film placement. Note how much film is visible above occlusal plane of tooth.

Overlapping (Figures 10-32 and 10-33). *Overlapping* of the images of the teeth will result if the central ray is not perpendicular to the film and teeth in the horizontal plane.

Remedy. The film should be aligned with some part of the tube head that is perpendicular to the central ray. In some cases, there is a horizontal bar with the manufacturer's name on it that can be used for this purpose. Standing in front of the patient, the operator should retract the patient's cheek and check the horizontal alignment. As in collimator cutoff, a positioning device with a localizing ring can be used to prevent overlapping. If the film is placed parallel to the teeth, the localizing ring aligns the beam perpendicular to the film.

Crescent marks and bent films (Figures 10-34 and 10-35). Black crescent-shaped marks can be caused by excessive bending of the film packet, which cracks the emulsion. The crescent marks show when the film is developed. A film may be overbent to such a degree that the x-rays cannot strike it at all.

Remedy. Films can be made more pliable by rolling them slightly against one's index finger, which also may allow them to fit better in the patient's mouth. Films

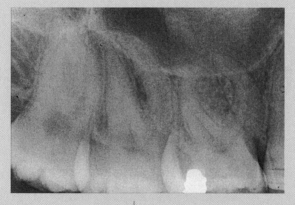

Figure 10-32. Overlapped images.

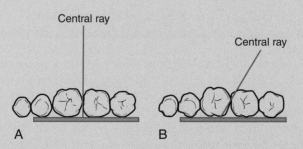

A   B

Figure 10-33. Proper **(A)** and improper **(B)** horizontal angulation of x-ray beam.

COMMON ERROR 10-1

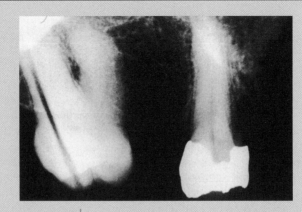

Figure 10-34. Black line caused by cracking of film emulsion.

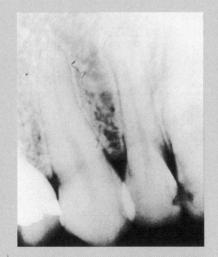

Figure 10-35. Result of overbending film packet. Note upper-right corner.

should not be bent to adapt to anatomic surfaces; they should be gently shaped to conform to the arch. X-rays travel in straight lines; they do not turn corners to expose bent films.

Light films (Figure 10-36). Light (thin) films without adequate density can result from underexposure or underdevelopment, assuming that the proper kVp has been used. If not enough kVp has been used, the dental structures are not adequately penetrated, and the film does not differentiate structures of different density. The operator should avoid removing his or her finger from the exposure button prematurely because this can cause an underexposed film as well.

Remedy. For preventing underexposure, all settings on the machine should be checked before an exposure is made (mA, time, kVp).

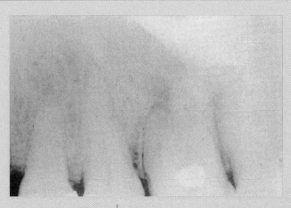

Figure 10-36. | Underexposed radiograph.

A very common error that leads to underexposure is unwittingly increasing the FFD by failing to bring the open end of the PID close to the patient's face. The exposure times are calculated for an FFD that assumes a PID placement close to the face. If the PID is carelessly positioned away from the face, the inverse square law intensifies the error, not just by the increased distance but by the square of that distance (Figure 10-37). For a discussion of underdevelopment, see Chapter 8.

Dark films (Figure 10-38). Dark (dense) films are the result of overexposure or overdevelopment, the opposites of the causes of light films. The length of the PID prevents the possibility of decreased FFD. If a film is overpenetrated, it is black and none of the dental structures show or they are difficult to differentiate.

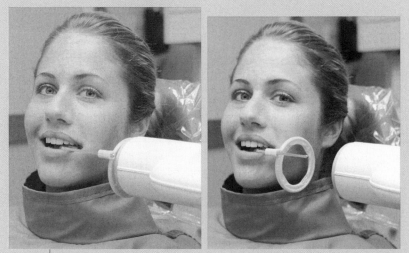

Figure 10-37. | Light film can be caused by increased focal-film distance without compensatory increase in exposure time. Note distance between the patient's face and PID.

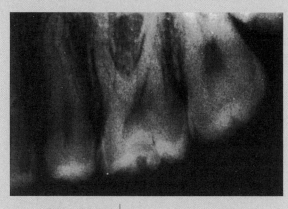

Figure 10-38. | Overexposed radiograph.

Remedy. To avoid overexposure, operators should check all settings on the control panel before making an exposure. For a discussion of overdevelopment, see Chapter 8.

Double exposure (Figure 10-39). A *double exposure* results from using the same film packet twice. This is an inexcusable error and indicates lack of attention to detail.

Remedy. After the film packet has been exposed, it should be placed in a lead receptacle. Exposed films and unexposed films should never be kept on the same shelf. When barrier envelopes are used, they can be removed between exposures to easily distinguish exposed films from unexposed films.

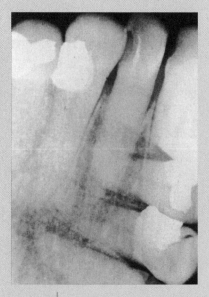

Figure 10-39. | Double exposure on a radiograph.

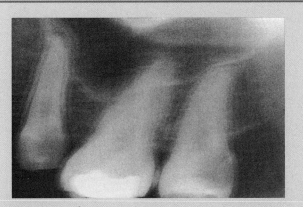

Figure 10-40. | Blurred image caused by patient movement.

Blurred images (Figure 10-40). Blurred images are the result of patient, film, or tube head movement during the exposure.

Remedy. Tube heads and arms should be adjusted to prevent vibration and drifting. In most states, drifting is a serious health code violation. Good chairside technique prevents film and patient movement.

Failure to remove dental appliances or facial jewelry (Figures 10-41 and 10-42). If dental appliances or pieces of facial jewelry are not removed, the metallic portions will be superimposed on the tooth structure.

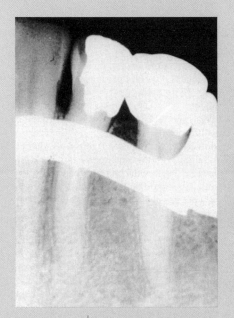

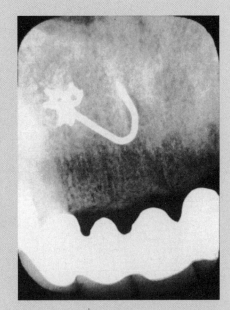

Figure 10-41. | Patient's metal-based partial denture was not removed.

Figure 10-42. | Facial jewelry (nose ring) was not removed.

Remedy. It should be a part of the work routine to have patients remove all dentures, nose and lip jewelry, and eyeglasses. For panoramic and extraoral projections, patients also must remove earrings, hearing aids, and hair clips.

Poor bitewings (Figure 10-43). The three most common errors seen on bitewing radiographs are overlapping, collimator cutoff, and poor film placement.

Overlapping (see Figure 10-43, *A*). Overlapping results from improper horizontal beam alignment.

Remedy. The beam should be aligned in the horizontal plane so that it is at right angles to the film packet.

Collimator cutoff (cone cutting) (see Figure 10-43, *B*). Collimator cutoff is failure to align the central ray with the center of the film packet. It occurs most often because the operator loses sight of the bite tab when the patient closes the mouth.

Remedy. The bite tab should be kept visible by asking the patient to smile while biting. If this is not possible, the operator can touch the tab with one hand while aligning the beam with the other. The central ray is directed at the tab. A localizing ring also can be used to help center the x-ray beam.

Poor film placement (see Figure 10-43, *C*). Poor film placement occurs in bitewing films when the patient is allowed to bite the film into position after the operator has let go of the tab or when the patient bites in protrusive instead of centric relation, allowing the film to float free and be repositioned by the tongue.

Remedy. The operator should not let go of the film tab until the patient is biting on it in centric occlusion.

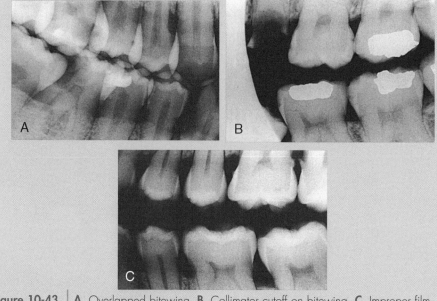

Figure 10-43. | **A,** Overlapped bitewing. **B,** Collimator cutoff on bitewing. **C,** Improper film placement.

SUGGESTED READINGS

American Academy of Oral and Maxillofacial Radiology: Standards of care, intraoral imaging, AAOMR Newslett 25, 1998.

American Dental Association Council on Scientific Affairs: An update on radiographic practices: information and recommendations, J Am Dent Assoc 132:234-238, 2001.

National Center for Health Care Technology: Dental radiology: a summary of recommendations from the Technology Assessment Forum, J Am Dent Assoc 103:423-425, 1981.

Stabulas JJ: Vertical bitewings, the other option, J Prac Hyg 11(3):46-47, 2002.

U.S. Department of Health and Human Services, Public Health Service FDA: The selection of patients for dental radiographic examinations, HHS/PHS/FDA, 88-827310-21, 1987.

White SC, Pharoah MJ: Oral radiology: principles and interpretation, ed 5, St Louis, Mosby, 2004.

CHAPTER 11

Accessory Radiographic Techniques: Bisecting Technique and Occlusal Projections

EDUCATIONAL OBJECTIVES

1. Understand the geometry of film placement and beam alignment in the bisecting technique.
2. Be able to apply this understanding in the clinical setting and take a full-mouth survey for dentulous and edentulous patients using the bisecting technique.
3. Understand the indications for occlusal radiographs and be able to take these films.

KEY TERMS

bisecting the angle
film plane
headrest position
imaginary bisecting line

occlusal film
occlusal projection
right-angle occlusal
  projection

topographic occlusal
  projection

BISECTING TECHNIQUE

Another method for taking intraoral periapical radiographs is the bisecting technique. In the bisecting technique the film packet is placed as close to the tooth as possible without bending the film. Because of the anatomy of the mouth, the long axis of the tooth is not parallel in most areas to the plane of the film with this placement. The vertical angulation of the tube head is directed so that the central ray is perpendicular to an imaginary line that bisects the angle formed by the long axis of the tooth and the plane of the dental film (see Figure 3-14). With this film placement, the object-film distance is minimal. No compensation for image enlargement is necessary, and therefore the technique usually calls for an 8-inch focal-film distance (FFD). Although a "short cone" is used, this is not the determining factor in the technique. Bite blocks should be used in this method.

Before listing the supposed advantages of the bisecting technique, we must note again that the consensus of opinion now among dental professionals and the standard of care for intraoral imaging of the American Academy of Oral and Maxillofacial Radiology call for the paralleling technique as the technique of choice for periapical radiography. The bisecting technique should be considered an ancillary method that can be used in special circumstances when it is not possible to use the paralleling technique. It is in this context that the bisecting technique is presented in this textbook.

Advantages

The bisecting technique is said to be easier to perform and is still used by some dentists in practice at this time. The use of the patient's finger or simple bite blocks for holding the film packets in position precludes the need for the paralleling instruments. For patients with small mouths, children, and patients with low palatal vaults, paralleling devices may be extremely difficult to use.

Because the film is held close to the tooth, it is possible to use an 8-in FFD (focal-film distance), and the objectionable, bulky, extension cylinder necessary in the paralleling technique can be avoided. This objection to the 16-in FFD is not valid in the newer machines with a recessed target within the tube head. Another argument is that a well-designed office should have room for the extra 8 in of the position-indicating device (PID).

Shorter exposure times can be used in the bisecting technique because of the shorter FFD; hence there is less chance for patient movement. In reality, this may not be a valid objection; with the use of faster film, we are comparing exposure times of $\frac{1}{10}$ versus $\frac{1}{10}$ second (inverse square law). Previously, with the use of slower films, the possibility of movement with a 4-second exposure compared with a 1-second exposure was greater, and the advantage was clear.

Disadvantages

The major disadvantage of the bisecting technique is that the image projected on the film is dimensionally distorted (see Chapter 10).

The bisecting technique is difficult to perform with the patient in a contour chair or in the supine position, as used in four-handed dentistry. With the newer dental chairs, it is very hard to place the patient in the correct position so that the occlusal plane of the jaw being radiographed is parallel to the floor. All vertical angulations used in the bisecting technique are measured from this line. Other disadvantages of the bisecting technique are related to the use of an 8-in FFD. The 8-in FFD when compared with the extended 16-in FFD causes greater image enlargement and distortion (see Figure 3-8). There is also more tissue volume exposed with an 8-in FFD than with a 16-in FFD (see Chapter 6). If the patient's finger is used to support the film, as is common in this method, then the patient's finger and hand are exposed unnecessarily to primary radiation. A bite block always should be used instead of the patient's finger.

Method

In this periapical technique the film is held as close to the tooth as possible without bending the film. The long axis of the film therefore is not parallel to the long axis of the tooth. An *imaginary bisecting line* is drawn to bisect the angle formed by the long axis of the tooth and the plane of the film. The central ray of the x-ray beam is directed perpendicular to this bisecting line; this determines the vertical angulation of the x-ray beam (see Figure 3-14). For the maxillary teeth, positive angulation (PID pointing down) is used, and for mandibular teeth, negative angulation (PID pointing up) is used. At zero-degree angulations, the PID is parallel to the floor; this becomes the reference point from which vertical angulations are measured. Therefore it is crucial to have the occlusal plane of the jaw being radiographed positioned parallel to the floor for predetermined angulations to be valid.

THE FULL-MOUTH SERIES

PROCEDURE 11-1

Maxillary Central and Lateral Incisors (Left or Right) (Figure 11-1)

Chair Position. The maxillary occlusal plane is positioned parallel to the floor, and the sagittal plane of the patient's face is perpendicular to the floor.

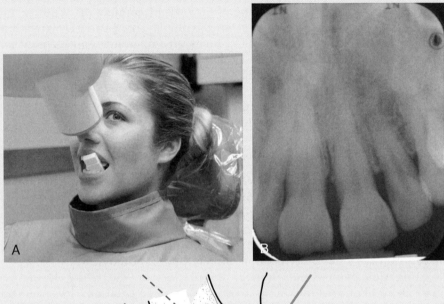

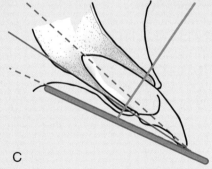

Figure 11-1. | Maxillary central and lateral incisors. **A,** Film packet and position-indicating device (PID). **B,** Radiograph. **C,** Diagram.

Film Position. The film packet is held vertically so that it extends evenly ⅛-in below the incisal edge of the incisors. The midpoint of this ⅛-in border should be between the lateral and central incisors. The film packet is positioned as close to the lingual surface of the incisors as possible without bending it.

Point of Entry. The central ray is directed just below the midpoint of the nares, aimed at the center of the film packet.

Vertical Angulation. +50 degrees.

Horizontal Angulation. The central ray is perpendicular to the film packet in the horizontal plane.

If only one film is to be used for the right and left maxillary central and lateral incisors, the center of the film packet is placed between the central incisors and the central ray is directed just below the tip of the nose (Figure 11-2).

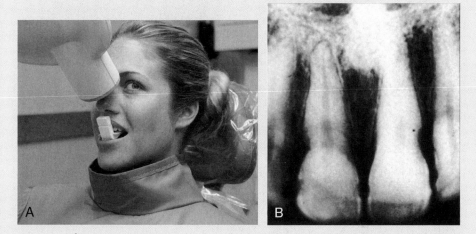

Figure 11-2. | Right and left central and lateral incisors. **A,** Film packet and PID. **B,** Radiograph.

> **Helpful Hint:** Make sure that the occlusal plane is kept parallel to the floor, because patients tend to change positions in the chair.

Maxillary Canines (Figure 11-3)

Chair Position. The maxillary occlusal plane is positioned parallel to the floor, and the sagittal plane of the patient's face is perpendicular to the floor.

Film Position. The film packet is held vertically and extends ⅛-in below the tip of the canine. The canine is in the center of the film packet, which is held firmly against the lingual surface of the canine.

Point of Entry. The central ray is directed at the base of the lateral nasal groove, aimed at the center of the film packet.

Vertical Angulation. +50 degrees.

Horizontal Angulation. The central ray is perpendicular to the film packet in the horizontal plane.

> **Helpful Hint:** Try to avoid bending the film packet in a small mouth to prevent crescent-shaped marks. New fast speed films are more sensitive to the consequences of excessive manipulation.

PROCEDURE 11-1

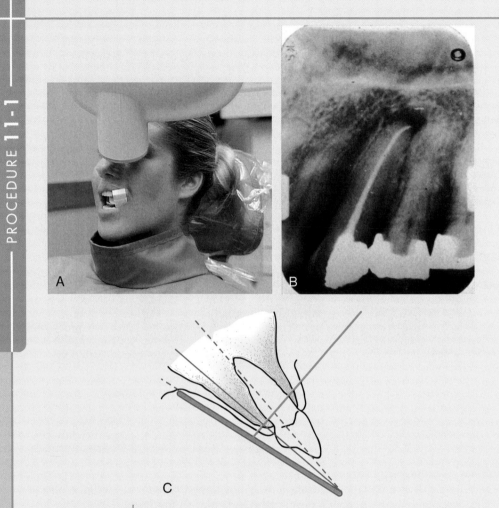

Figure 11-3. │ Maxillary canines. **A,** Film packet and PID. **B,** Radiograph. **C,** Diagram.

Maxillary Premolars (Figure 11-4)

Chair Position. The maxillary occlusal plane is positioned parallel to the floor, and the sagittal plane of the patient's face is perpendicular to the floor.

Film Position. The film packet is held horizontally and extends ⅛-in below the occlusal surfaces of the teeth. The second premolar is in the center of the film packet. The packet is held in position against the lingual surfaces. The operator should avoid shaping the packet to the arch.

Point of Entry. The central ray is directed at the most anterior part of the cheekbone, aimed at the center of the film packet.

Vertical Angulation. +40 degrees.

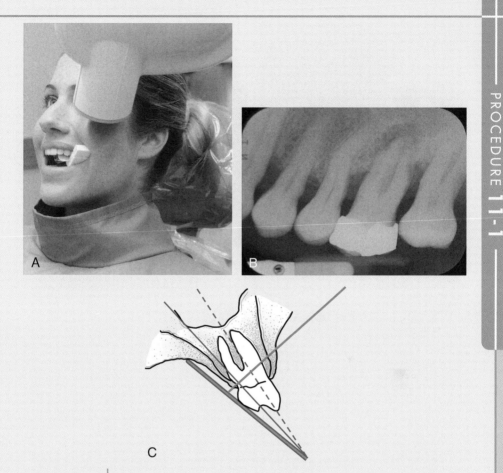

Figure 11-4. | Maxillary premolars. **A,** Film packet and PID. **B,** Radiograph. **C,** Diagram.

Horizontal Angulation. The central ray is perpendicular to the film packet in the horizontal plane and is directed through the interproximal spaces.

Helpful Hint: Make sure that the anterior part of the film packet is positioned behind the center of the cuspid.

Maxillary Molars (Figure 11-5)

Chair Position. The maxillary occlusal plane is positioned parallel to the floor, and the sagittal plane of the patient's face is perpendicular to the floor.

Film Position. The film is held horizontally and extends ⅛-in evenly below the occlusal surfaces of the teeth. The second molar is in the center of the film packet. The film packet is held against the lingual surfaces of the teeth.

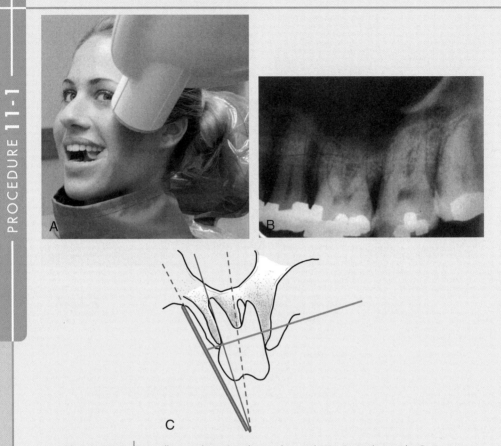

Figure 11-5. | Maxillary molars. **A,** Film packet and PID. **B,** Radiograph. **C,** Diagram.

Point of Entry. The central ray is directed through the zygomatic arch at the center of the film. The distal curvature of the open-ended "cone" should not be distal to the outer canthus (corner) of the eye.

Vertical Angulation. +30 degrees.

Horizontal Angulation. The central ray is perpendicular to the film packet in the horizontal plane and is directed through the interproximal spaces.

Helpful Hint: Make sure that the middle of the film packet, in the horizontal position, is at the center of the second molar.

Mandibular Incisors (Figure 11-6)
Chair Position. The patient is positioned so that when the mouth is open, the mandibular occlusal plane is parallel to the floor and the sagittal plane of the patient's face is perpendicular to the floor.

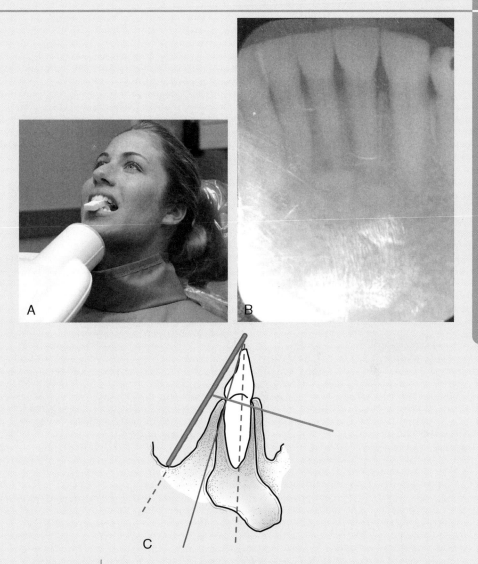

Figure 11-6. Mandibular incisors. **A,** Film packet and PID. **B,** Radiograph. **C,** Diagram.

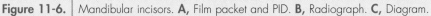

Film Position. The film packet is held vertically so that it extends ⅛-in above the incisal edges of the incisors. The midpoint of this ⅛-in border should be between the central incisors. All four lower incisors are shown on one film. The film is held against the lingual surfaces of the incisors.

Point of Entry. The central ray is directed at the depression in the face just above the chin (mental groove), aimed at the center of the film.

Vertical Angulation. −20 degrees.

Horizontal Angulation. The central ray is perpendicular to the film in the horizontal plane.

> **Helpful Hint:** In some small and crowded arch shapes, it may be necessary to use size #1 film for a lower anterior film.

Mandibular Canines (Figure 11-7)

Chair Position. The patient is positioned so that when the mouth is open, the mandibular occlusal plane is parallel to the floor and the sagittal plane of the patient's face is perpendicular to the floor.

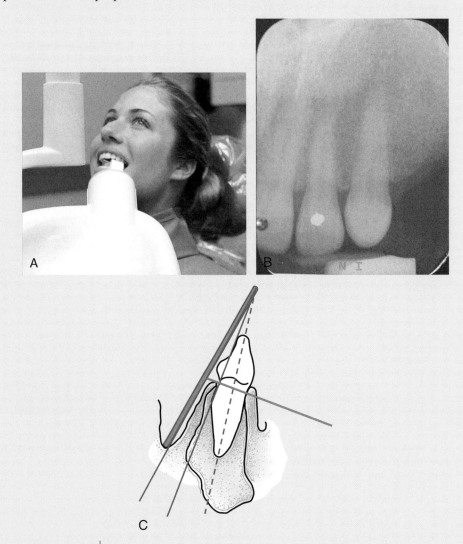

Figure 11-7. | Mandibular canines. **A,** Film packet and PID. **B,** Radiograph. **C,** Diagram.

Film Position. The film packet is held vertically and extends ⅛ inch above the tip of the canine, which is in the center of the film packet. The film packet is held against the lingual surface of the canine.

Point of Entry. The central ray is directed at the root of the canine, aimed at the middle of the film packet.

Vertical Angulation. −20 degrees.

Horizontal Angulation. The central ray is perpendicular to the film in the horizontal plane.

Helpful Hint: In the cuspid area, it may be necessary to use one or two extra size #1 films to cover the cuspid area completely.

Mandibular Premolars (Figure 11-8)

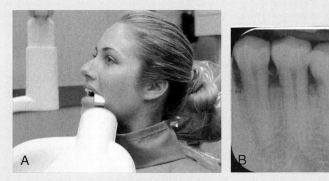

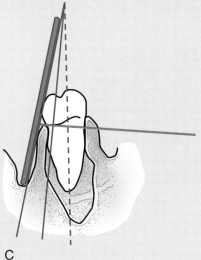

Figure 11-8. │ Mandibular premolars. **A,** Film packet and PID. **B,** Radiograph. **C,** Diagram.

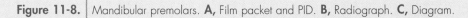

Chair Position. The patient is positioned so that when the mouth is open, the mandibular occlusal plane is parallel to the floor and the sagittal plane of the patient's face is perpendicular to the floor.

Film Position. The film packet is held horizontally and extends ⅛ in above the occlusal surfaces of the teeth. The second premolar is in the center of the film. The film packet is held against the lingual surfaces of the teeth.

Point of Entry. The central ray is directed at the mental foramen, aimed at the center of the film packet.

Vertical Angulation. −15 degrees.

Horizontal Angulation. The central ray is perpendicular to the film in the horizontal plane.

> **Helpful Hint:** It may be necessary to bend the inferior anterior corner of the film packet to follow the curve of the arch.

Mandibular Molars (Figure 11-9)

Chair Position. The patient is positioned so that when the mouth is open, the mandibular occlusal plane is parallel to the floor and the sagittal plane of the patient's face is perpendicular to the floor.

Film Position. The film packet is held horizontally and extends ⅛ in above the occlusal surfaces of the molars. The second molar is in the middle of the film. The film is held against the lingual surface of the molars. Because of the anatomy of the area, the film packet is almost parallel to the long axis of the tooth, and most molar periapical films done in the bisecting technique are really parallel films.

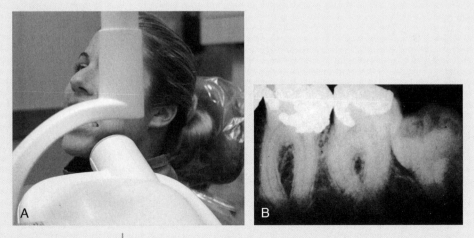

Figure 11-9. | Mandibular molars. **A,** Film packet and PID. **B,** Radiograph.

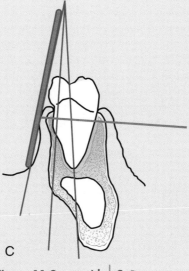

Figure 11-9—cont'd. │ **C,** Diagram.

Point of Entry. The central ray is directed at the roots of the molars, aimed at the center of the film packet.

Vertical Angulation. −5 degrees.

Horizontal Angulation. The central ray is perpendicular to the film packet in the horizontal plane.

> **Helpful Hint:** When inserting the film packet, use a finger from your other hand to depress the floor of the mouth.

Bitewings

The technique for the bitewing projection is the same as in the paralleling method as both call for the film and the teeth to be parallel and the x-ray beam to be at right angles to both.

> **Helpful Hint:** Make sure that the patient closes in centric and not protrusive relation when biting on the bitewing tab.

BISECTING TECHNIQUE (see also the Appendix)

The following text presents the most common errors seen in the bisecting technique. Recognition and correction of occasional errors in technique are important. Not all patients are cooperative or have mouths that are anatomically easy to radiograph. Remember that films retaken because of poor technique add unnecessarily to the patient's radiation burden (see Chapter 10 for a discussion of other chairside errors).

Elongation (Figure 11-10). Elongation, or lengthening of the image on the film, can be caused by inadequate vertical angulation, improper occlusal plane orientation because of patient position, or poor film placement.

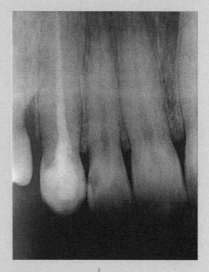

Figure 11-10. Elongated image.

Remedy. The film and the central ray must be in the correct relationship. In the bisecting-angle technique the vertical angulation should be increased to correct elongation. The occlusal plane of the jaw being radiographed should be parallel to the floor. Patients tend to move after a few exposures or lift their heads to watch the operator. Their movements disorient the occlusal plane. Check the patient's head position before making each exposure.

Foreshortening (Figure 11-11). Foreshortening (the shortening of the image on the film) is not as common an error as elongation. It can be caused by excessive vertical angulation or poor occlusal plane orientation.

Remedy. In the bisecting-angle technique, the vertical angulation should be decreased to overcome errors of foreshortening.

Sagittal plane orientation (Figure 11-12). When the periapical radiographs show the occlusal surfaces of the teeth, the patient's head has tipped away from the proper sagittal plane. This is accompanied by elongation of the image.

Remedy. The operator should make sure the patient does not tip his or her head away from the tube head as it is brought into approximation with the skin.

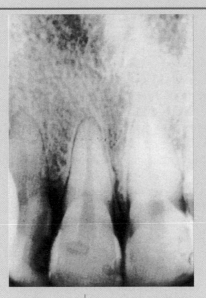

Figure 11-11. | Foreshortened image.

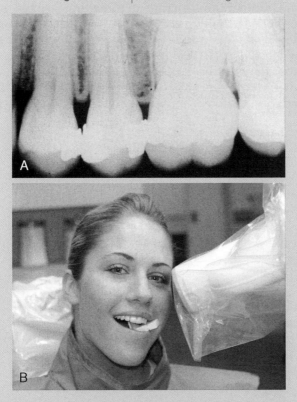

Figure 11-12. | **A,** Elongated and distorted radiograph caused by poor sagittal plane orientation of the patient's head. **B,** Poor sagittal plane orientation.

OCCLUSAL FILM PROJECTIONS

Occlusal film packets should be part of every dental office's radiographic armamentarium. The film packets are relatively inexpensive, come in small quantities, and can be obtained either as single or double films and at speeds corresponding to those of other intraoral films. In some cases the occlusal projection is the one of choice, whereas in others it may be used when extraoral or panoramic views are not available.

Occlusal projections are used to localize objects and pathologic conditions in the buccolingual dimension and to visualize areas that would not be seen on periapical films because of the insufficient field size. The right-angle occlusal technique is used for localizing in the buccolingual dimension; the topographic occlusal technique is used for the large pathologic areas. *Occlusal films* also are used when proper placement of periapical films is not possible in children or handicapped patients (Box 11-1; see Chapter 18).

Right-Angle Projections

In *right-angle occlusal projections* the central ray is directed at an angle of 90 degrees to the film. For example, this technique would be used to locate an object such as an impacted tooth in the third dimension. It has been mentioned that dental radiographs picture a three-dimensional subject in a two-dimensional plane, usually vertical and horizontal. The radiographs do not indicate depth. In the example of the impacted tooth, one might know from a conventional radiograph the impaction's mesiodistal location and its vertical height from the crest of the alveolar ridge, but we would not know its depth in the bone in a buccolingual dimension. One way to determine whether an impacted mandibular molar lies buccal or lingual to the alveolar

---

BOX 11-1   USE OF OCCLUSAL PROJECTIONS

Clinical examples of the use of occlusal projections include the following:
- To locate retained roots of extracted teeth
- To locate supernumerary (extra) unerupted or impacted teeth
- To locate foreign bodies in the maxilla or the mandible
- To locate salivary stones in the floor of the mouth and in the submandibular duct and gland
- To locate and evaluate the extent of intraosseous lesions (e.g., cysts, tumors, malignancies) in the maxilla or mandible
- To evaluate the boundaries of the maxillary sinus
- To evaluate fractures of the maxilla or mandible
- To aid in the examination of patients who cannot open their mouths more than a few millimeters
- To examine the area of a cleft palate
- To evaluate changes in the size and shape of the maxilla or mandible

ridge is to take a radiograph from another direction. In this example, it would be an occlusal radiograph, with the central ray coming from underneath the mandible, directed at a right angle to a film placed on the occlusal surface of the mandibular teeth.

Topographic Projections

The angulation of the *topographic occlusal projection* may vary from 45 to 75 degrees, depending on the anatomic area. Because the occlusal packet is approximately four times the size of the intraoral packet, it can record areas that would not be seen on the smaller film. The extreme vertical angulations are necessary to compensate for the lack of parallelism between the object and the film. This is a modification of the bisecting-angle technique.

Film Packet

The occlusal film packet (size #4) is 2½ × 3 in and is supplied in either single or double films (Figure 11-13), available in film speed D, E, or F. These films are sometimes called "sandwich films" because they are positioned in the patient's mouth with the teeth closed on the film packet, resembling the biting of a sandwich. Occlusal films are processed in the darkroom in the same way as other intraoral films. The exposure time is greater than that of intraoral periapical films because the FFD is greater.

Mandibular Occlusal Technique

In the mandibular occlusal technique, the film packet is placed in the patient's mouth on the occlusal surfaces of the lower teeth. The back of the film packet faces the palate, with the front (white side) of the packet facing the tongue on the occlusal surfaces of the lower teeth. In patients with small mouths, it is possible to get both right and left sides of the mandible on one film if it is inserted with the longer side extending across the patient's mouth. In patients with larger mouths, it may be necessary to take a separate film of each half of the mandible. In this instance, the longest dimension of the film packet will run anteroposteriorly. The film is placed as far posterior on the mandible as possible so that

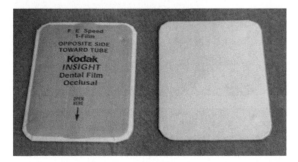

Figure 11-13. │ Front and back of occlusal film packet.

the edge of the packet touches the ascending ramus of the mandible. The patient is directed to bite gently on the film packet. For the right-angle projection, the central ray of the x-ray beam is directed from under the mandible, so that it is perpendicular to the center of the film packet (Figures 11-14 and 11-15). For the topographic view of the mandible, the central ray is directed at a point just above the mental eminence at a vertical angulation of 65 degrees. To accomplish these angulations the operator must tip the headrest position of the chair back and have the patient extend his or her head and neck posteriorly (Figures 11-16 and 11-17).

Maxillary Occlusal Technique

In an anterior topographic occlusal view of the maxilla, the film packet is placed in the patient's mouth with the front of the film packet facing the

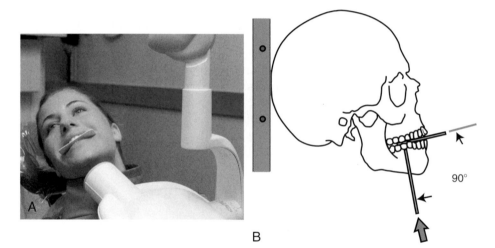

Figure 11-14. | **A,** Film placement and PID position for mandibular right-angle occlusal film. Note that the central ray is directed at 90 degrees to center of film packet. **B,** Diagram.

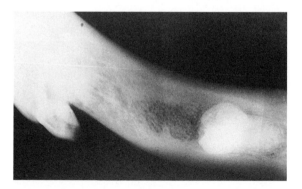

Figure 11-15. | Right-angle occlusal radiograph of patient's mandibular posterior area. Note buccal and lingual cortex of bone and central position of the impaction.

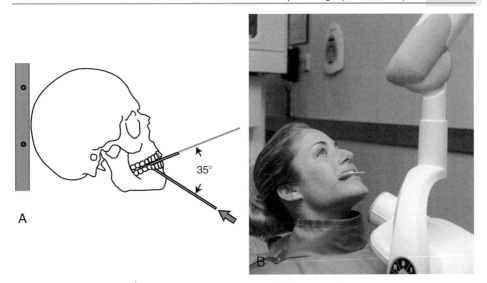

Figure 11-16. | **A,** Topographic mandibular occlusal projection. **B,** Diagram.

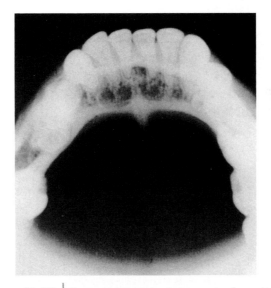

Figure 11-17. | Topographic occlusal projection of mandible.

palate and the long dimension of the packet running across the mouth. The packet is positioned as far posterior as possible so that the posterior edge of the film packet touches the ascending ramus of the mandible. With the patient's head positioned so that the *film plane* is parallel to the floor, the central ray is directed at a 50- to 65-degree vertical angulation through the bridge of the nose (Figures 11-18 and 11-19). In the right-angle occlusal view of the maxilla, the film is placed in the same position in the patient's mouth, but

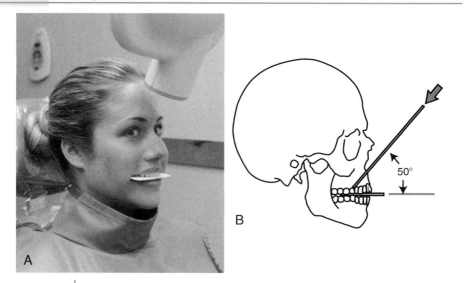

Figure 11-18. | **A,** Film placement and PID position for topographic occlusal view of maxilla. Note that the central ray is directed at 50 to 65 degrees to bridge of nose. **B,** Diagram.

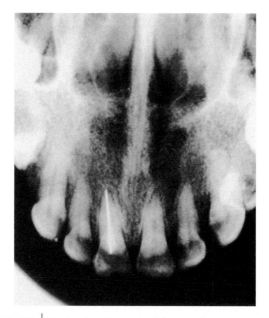

Figure 11-19. | Occlusal radiograph of the maxilla, topographic view.

the central ray is directed perpendicular to the center of the film packet. To do this the PID must be positioned above the patient's head at about the hairline. The vertical angulation is 90 degrees. Because there is an increased FFD when compared with the maxillary topographic view, this projection requires a longer exposure time (Figures 11-20 and 11-21).

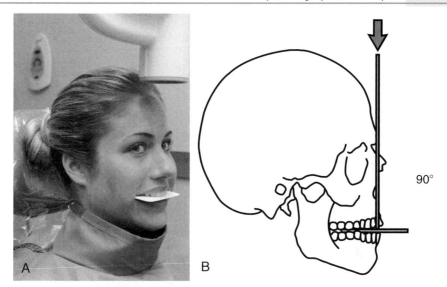

Figure 11-20. **A,** Film placement and PID position for a right-angle occlusal view of maxilla. Note that the central ray is directed at 90 degrees to film packet. **B,** Diagram.

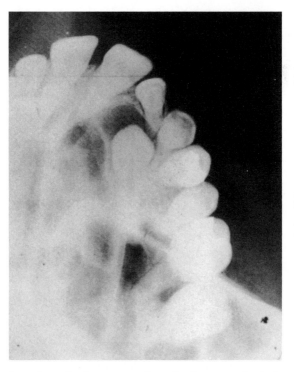

Figure 11-21. Right-angle occlusal projection of maxilla showing palatal relationship of impacted canine.

The posterior occlusal topographic view can be considered a topographic view of the maxillary sinus and surrounding structures. The film packet is positioned on either the left or the right side of the patient's mouth, from the midline, laterally with the long side running anteroposteriorly. The central ray is directed to a point just above the apices of the premolars at a vertical angulation of 55 degrees (Figures 11-22 and 11-23).

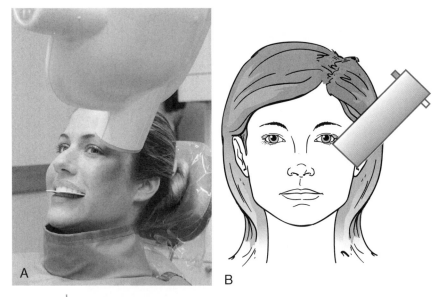

Figure 11-22. | **A,** Posterior topographic occlusal projection. **B,** Diagram. The point of entry corresponds to the apices of the premolars, and vertical angulation is approximately 55 degrees.

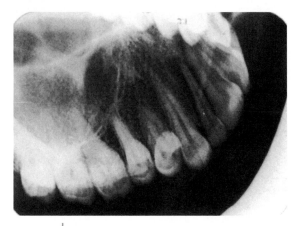

Figure 11-23. | Topographic occlusal radiograph of maxillary sinus.

CHAPTER 12

Panoramic Radiography

CHAPTER OUTLINE

EDUCATIONAL OBJECTIVES

1. Understand the principles of tomography and how they apply to dental panoramic x-ray units.
2. Be able to learn to use any of the panoramic units available today.

KEY TERMS

ala-tragus line
centers of rotation
flexible cassette
focal trough
Frankfort plane
ghost image
image layer
laminogram
midsagittal plane
panoramic film
"Panorex"
pantomogram
point of rotation
slit beam
tomogram
tomography

Panoramic dental x-ray units have become commonplace in dental offices, and the panoramic radiograph is considered today by some to be an essential element in radiographic diagnosis. Therefore dental professionals should be familiar with panoramic x-ray machines, technique, and interpretation. As shown in this chapter, the panoramic radiograph is not meant to replace intraoral periapical and bitewing films, but rather to complement them in the diagnostic process.

The term *panorama* means "an unobstructed view of a region in any direction"; thus a *panoramic film* shows the mandible and maxilla on one radiograph from condyle to condyle.

Panoramic radiography is a relatively new technique that was introduced into the U.S. dental market in 1959 by the S.S. White Corp. as their "Panorex" unit. The design of this unit was based mainly on the work of Dr. Y.V. Paatero, a Finnish dentist, and was published in 1949.

Two techniques are currently available that produce panoramic films. The first of these involves the use of an intraoral x-ray source in which the x-ray tube is placed in the patient's mouth and emits a 180-degree x-ray beam that hits a film wrapped externally around the patient's jaws. This technique, although theoretically interesting and innovative, is not commonly used because no commercial units are currently available. The radiographs produced in this method show a great deal of distortion; however, the radiation exposure is significantly decreased. The second technique, by far the more extensively used, makes use of a slit beam and curved or flat-surface rotational tomography.

The term *slit beam* refers to the width, usually 1 to 2 mm, of the beam that is produced by the collimator (Figure 12-1). Compare the size and shape of this x-ray beam with the standard intraoral x-ray beam that is $2^{3}/_{4}$ in in diameter.

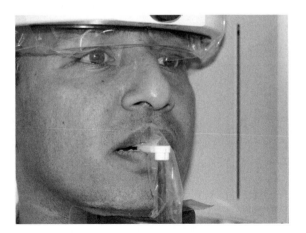

Figure 12-1. Slit beam collimator. Only the part of the film that is in back of the narrow beam is exposed.

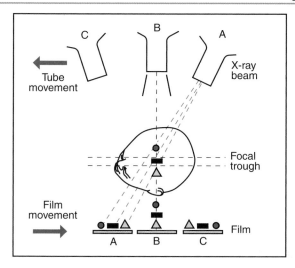

Figure 12-2. Principles of tomography. Note that only objects in the focal trough (square) project onto the same area of the film and are not blurred out.

Tomography is a radiographic technique that allows radiographing in one plane of an object while blurring or eliminating images from structures in other planes. *Tomo* is the Greek word for "section," and sections or radiographic slices of the object are seen. These projections also could be but are not often called *laminograms*, from the word *lamina* (layer), as this is a layered radiographic technique. Tomography is used extensively in medicine and is the basis for computed tomography (CT) and magnetic resonance imaging (MRI), both of which are discussed in Chapter 16.

A tomogram is made by moving the x-ray source and the film in opposite directions in a fixed relationship through one or a series of rotation points while the patient remains stationary (Figure 12-2). The plane of the object that is not blurred on the radiograph is called the "plane of acceptable detail" or *focal trough*. It is also called the *image layer* (Figure 12-3). The image layer is an invisible area that is located in the space between the source of radiation and the image receptor. The shape of the image layer varies. Clinically this concept is very important because many of the errors in technique that are discussed later in the chapter are caused by improper patient positioning, the result of which is not having the desired area in the image layer. The *points of rotation* around which the tube head travels can be either inside or outside of the focal trough. The width or thickness of the focal trough is governed by many factors, including the angle of movement of the x-ray beam, the width of the x-ray beam, and the size of the focal spot. Any object that lies in the focal plane is shown clearly, and objects above and below it appear blurred. By varying the focal-object distance—the distance between the tube head and the patient—on a tomographic series, different focal troughs or "cuts" can be achieved. A tomographic series is usually composed of multiple cuts, 0.5 cm apart, with the number of cuts varying according to the thickness of the object (Figure 12-4).

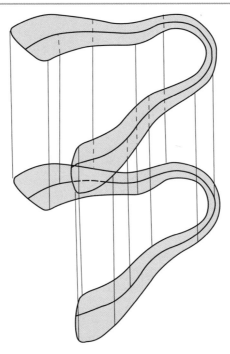

Figure 12-3. Image layer, or focal trough. *(Courtesy Eastman Kodak Co., Rochester, NY.)*

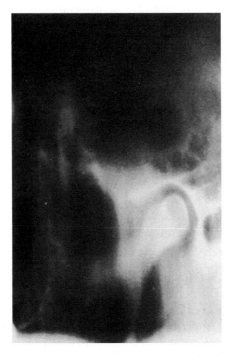

Figure 12-4. Tomogram of the temporomandibular joint. Note the clarity of the condyle and the blurring of the rest of the image.

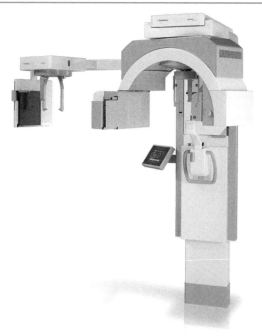

Figure 12-5. Soredex's CRANEX TOME tomographic unit. The unit can also be used to take panoramic and cephalometric radiographs. *(Courtesy Soredex, Helsinki, Finland.)*

Some tomographic units are made combined with a panoramic unit specifically for use in the head and neck region. These units enable dentists to do tomography in their own offices. Indications for dental office tomography include implant planning, temporomandibular joint (TMJ) tomography, and diagnosis of pathologic lesions. The majority of these tomographic units are computer-driven (Figure 12-5). This means that the computer controls the motion of the tube head and film and other exposure parameters based on choices and information entered by the operator. This use of the computer should not be confused with digital imaging which is described in Chapter 15. In the computer-directed units, the imaging system is still a film screen combination, not the electronic sensor to be described later. In these systems the computer does not produce or store images as in digital imaging; it simply directs the patient exposure, after which the film is processed to produce the diagnostic image.

PANTOMOGRAM

A panoramic radiograph of the maxilla and the mandible produced by using tomography is properly called a *pantomogram*. The pantomogram is a curved-surface tomogram (Figure 12-6), in contrast to the plane surface or straight-line tomogram illustrated in Figure 12-2. In common usage the term *panoramic*

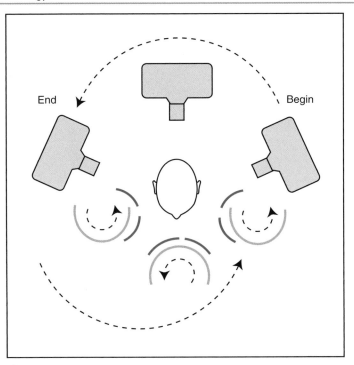

Figure 12-6. Rotational tomography. Note the slit opening in the film carrier and that the film and the tube travel around the patient in opposite directions.

radiograph is usually substituted for *pantomogram*. The term *panorex* should never be used as a substitute for a *panoramic radiograph* unless the Panorex unit is being used. It is not a generic term, but the manufacturer's name for the first panoramic unit introduced in the dental market.

Many pantomographic units are available on the market today. They differ primarily in the number and locations of the *centers of rotation*, the choice of a fixed or adjustable focal trough, and the type and shape of the film transport mechanism. All units use intensifying screens, with a film size of either 5½ or 6½ in. Design differences include head-positioning devices, manual or automatic setting controls, bite blocks, kVp and mA range, standing or sitting patient position, and wall-mounted or freestanding units. Some more advanced units offer the option of being able to do other extraoral projections, cross-sectional tomography, or digital imaging. Individual manufacturers use trade names for their own panoramic units. Examples include Orthophos Plus, PM 2002 CC Proline, and the GX-PAN. Each manufacturer's machine has its own technique for operation, which can be learned easily from the instruction manual (Figures 12-7 and 12-8). However, there are certain positioning requirements that are common to all units, and these are discussed in Procedure 12-1.

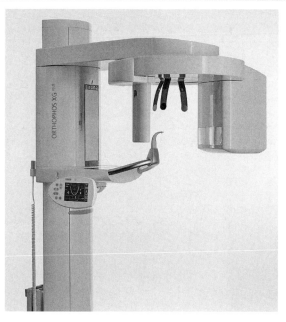

Figure 12-7. Orthophos Plus panoramic unit (also available with or without cephalometer and direct digital sensor technology). *(Courtesy Sirona Dental Systems, Bensheim, Germany.)*

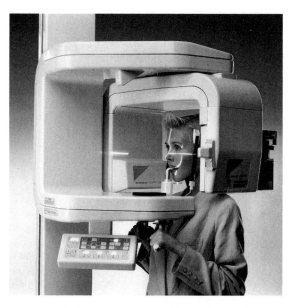

Figure 12-8. PM 2002 CC Proline panoramic machine. *(Courtesy Planmeca, Inc., Roselle, IL.)*

PROCEDURE 12.1

COMMON POSITIONING REQUIREMENTS FOR PANORAMIC UNITS

1. Midsagittal plane: This plane should be perpendicular to the floor (Figure 12-9).

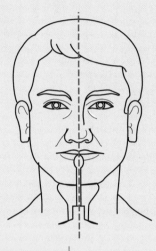

Figure 12-9. | Midsagittal plane.

2. Frankfort plane: This is the imaginary line connecting the floor of the orbit and the external auditory meatus. In most units this plane should be parallel to the floor (Figure 12-10). Some units may use the ala-tragus line for patient positioning.
3. Bite block position: The anterior teeth should be positioned in the proper groove in the bite block (Figure 12-11) and not forward or posterior to the groove (Figures 12-12 and 12-13). If the patient is edentulous, then some other type of extraoral positioner should be used (Figure 12-14).

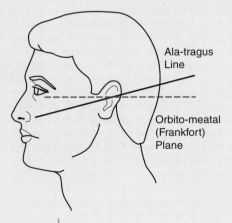

Figure 12-10. | Anatomic horizontal positioning planes.

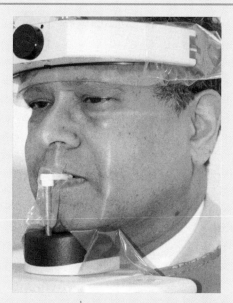

Figure 12-11. | Patient positioned with anterior teeth in placement groove.

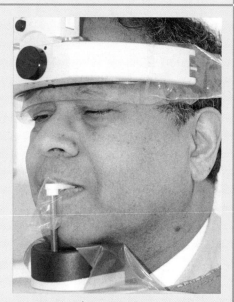

Figure 12-12. | Patient positioned with anterior teeth forward of the groove.

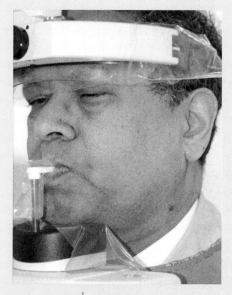

Figure 12-13. | Patient positioned with anterior teeth posterior to the groove.

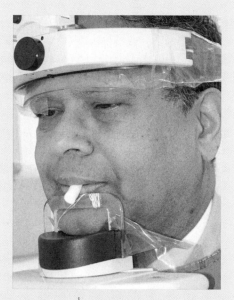

Figure 12-14. | Positioning of the edentulous patient.

PROCEDURE **12.1**

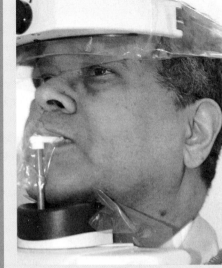

Figure 12-15. | Patient positioned incorrectly with the chin up.

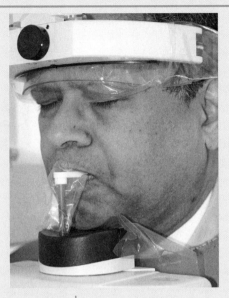

Figure 12-16. | Patient positioned incorrectly with the chin down.

4. Chin position: The chin should not be angled up or down (Figures 12-15 and 12-16).
5. Head tilted: The head-positioning devices should be firm to prevent tipping or rotating during the exposure and loss of proper midsagittal orientation (Figure 12-17).
6. Patient movement: The patient must not move during the exposure or a blurred image will result.
7. Tongue position: The patient should place and maintain his or her tongue against the roof of the mouth.
8. Posture: The patient should not slump but should keep the spine erect.
9. Lead apron: If a lead apron is used, as it should be, it should not have a thyroid collar because such a collar will block the primary beam (Figure 12-18).

Helpful Hint: Patient posture is very important. Without correct positioning of the posture, the structure to be radiographed may not be in or remain in the plane of focus and will appear blurred on the radiograph.

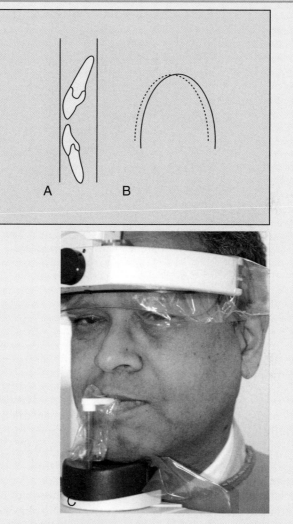

Figure 12-17. | **A,** Anterior teeth positioned correctly. **B,** Broken line is focal plane, and unbroken line is mandibular arch, showing that neither side is in the focal plane. **C,** Patient positioned with head rotated.

PROCEDURE 12.1

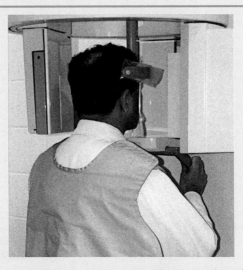

Figure 12-18. | Patient with lead apron in place. Note there is no thyroid collar used.

Pantomographic Image

The image on a panoramic film shows the entire dentition and supporting bone from condyle to condyle on one film. However, the image does not have the same definition seen on an intraoral periapical or bitewing film. This factor is inherent in the pantomographic process and the use of intensifying screens. These images also have a significant amount of horizontal distortion but less vertical distortion.

All objects in the field of the x-ray beam, even those out of the plane of focus, are projected onto the film, but most are not seen. The objects that have the greatest density (e.g., bone or metal objects) and are out of the plane of acceptable detail (focal trough) are shown in two places on the panoramic film. One place is the intended image or the usable image, and the other is referred to as the *ghost image* (Figure 12-19). The ghost image always has less sharpness and is seen at a point higher on the film than the desired image. The ghost image is always reversed; that is, the left appears on the right and vice versa. This can be best illustrated by a film in which the patient did not remove large earrings (Figure 12-20.).

Some panoramic units can be used to take tomograms of the TMJ (Figure 12-21). To accomplish this, the unit must have an adjustable focal plane. The plane is set for the position of the condyle instead of the usual focal plane, which is through the body of the mandible. By stopping the rotation and rewinding the film carrier, an open view and a closed view can be taken on each side with one piece of film.

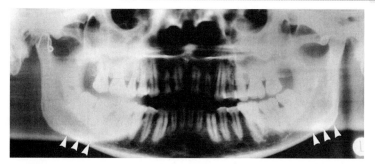

Figure 12-19. | Ghost images of the opposite sides of the mandible, outlined by the arrows.

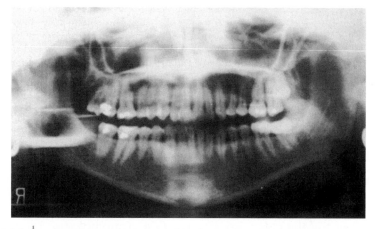

Figure 12-20. | Radiopaque markings caused by the patient's earring. Note the ghost image and the sharp image.

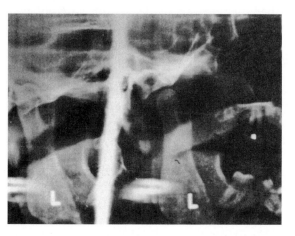

Figure 12-21. | Pantomography of the temporomandibular joint done using a panoramic unit with an adjustable focal trough. The focal trough is set for the plane of the condyles instead of the body of the mandible.

Digital Radiography

With the wide use of digital imaging for intraoral periapical and bitewing projections, it should come as no surprise that digital imaging is now available for panoramic units. Digital radiography is discussed in detail in Chapter 15, where the basic principles of intraoral digital imaging are shown to apply to panoramic digital radiography. Basically a digital sensor approximately the size of the slit beam collimating device is placed in the carrier instead of a film screen combination. As the carrier moves around the patient, the electronic impulses are sent back to the computer and an image is generated.

ADVANTAGES AND DISADVANTAGES: PANORAMIC TOMOGRAPHY

Like any technique, panoramic tomography has its advantages and disadvantages when compared with conventional intraoral techniques. The pantomographic unit is expensive (approximately four times the cost of a regular x-ray tube head). The standard x-ray unit is still necessary even in an office with a panoramic unit. The full-mouth series, composed of periapical and bitewing films, has been and still is the gold standard for dental radiography, and any other technique should be judged in comparison.

Advantages

Size of the Field

Field size is one of the major advantages of the pantomogram. The full-mouth series is not composed of radiographs of the entire mouth but only of the teeth, alveolar ridges, and part of the supporting bone. The pantomogram covers an area that includes all of the mandible from condyle to condyle and the maxillary regions extending superiorly to the maxillary sinus and nasal cavity (Figures 12-22 and 12-23). Areas of the mandible, such as the condyles, inferior border, angle, ascending ramus, and coronoid process, as well as the entire maxillary arch, which are not visualized on intraoral surveys, are seen routinely on pantomograms. Lesions that might be undetected on intraoral surveys may be seen in the field of pantomograms.

A new indication for the use of panoramic films has recently been reported. Some patients who are at risk for cerebrovascular accidents because of the presence of atherosclerotic plaque in their carotid arteries can be identified in the dental office by appropriate evaluation of their panoramic films for calcifications. Most pantomograms will show the area adjacent to or below the intervertebral space between C3 and C4, which is the location of the carotid arteries that might show evidence of calcifications (Figure 12-24). Pantograms should not be taken solely to screen for carotid artery atherosclerotic plaque. However, their presence should be evaluated on every patient who has a pantomogram. It is your professional

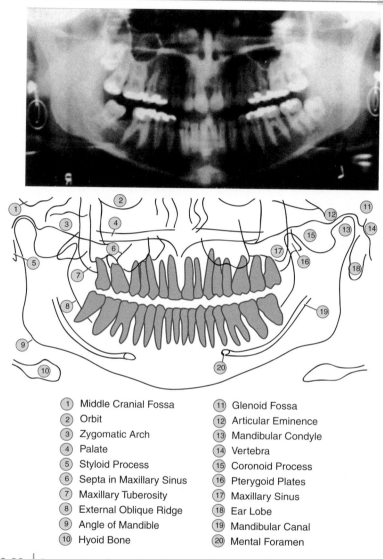

①	Middle Cranial Fossa	⑪	Glenoid Fossa
②	Orbit	⑫	Articular Eminence
③	Zygomatic Arch	⑬	Mandibular Condyle
④	Palate	⑭	Vertebra
⑤	Styloid Process	⑮	Coronoid Process
⑥	Septa in Maxillary Sinus	⑯	Pterygoid Plates
⑦	Maxillary Tuberosity	⑰	Maxillary Sinus
⑧	External Oblique Ridge	⑱	Ear Lobe
⑨	Angle of Mandible	⑲	Mandibular Canal
⑩	Hyoid Bone	⑳	Mental Foramen

Figure 12-22. Panoramic radiograph and tracing showing numbered anatomic landmarks. (Courtesy KaVo Dental/GENDEX Imaging, Lake Zurich, IL.)

obligation to do this, and patients should be referred to a physician regardless of their symptoms.

Quality Control

In maintaining quality control, good chairside technique is essential so that the undistorted complete image is seen. Full visualization of all the teeth and surrounding bone, including the third molar area, is of prime importance. This is more easily done with a pantomographic unit than an intraoral

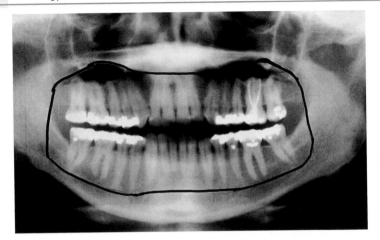

Figure 12-23. | Panoramic radiograph with tracing of the area seen on a full-mouth survey outlined.

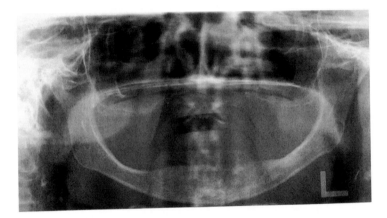

Figure 12-24. | Panoramic radiograph showing calcifications in the left carotid arteries distal and inferior to the angle of the mandible. *(Courtesy Dr. Laurie Carter.)*

full-mouth series because the technique, although not simple, is not as demanding as intraoral radiography. There are fewer retakes, and quality control is easier to maintain. Quality control for processing of pantomograms is discussed in Chapter 8.

Simplicity
Pantomographic procedures, as mentioned, are relatively simple to perform. With minimal training and strict attention to detail, any member of the dental team can become proficient in taking these films.

Patient Cooperation
Because pantomography is an extraoral procedure, it requires a minimum of patient cooperation in comparison with intraoral techniques. No film packet

is placed in the patient's mouth. The patient is asked to bite on a rod and is only required to sit or stand still for 12 to 22 seconds of exposure. When applicable, most units can be operated without radiation to demonstrate to an apprehensive patient what the procedure will be like.

Pantomography practically eliminates problems with intractable gaggers, patients with trismus, and fearful or uncooperative children.

Time
Less time is required for a pantomographic examination than an intraoral survey. The most skilled operator requires at least 15 to 20 minutes to do an intraoral survey; pantomograms can be taken in less than 5 minutes.

Dose
There seems to be general agreement that the radiation dose to the patient is less than or at most equal to that in intraoral radiography, depending on technique and on how and where measurements are made. The panoramic radiograph delivers a bone marrow dose that is 20% less than that received from a full-mouth conventional intraoral series. The panoramic dose is about equivalent to that received from four bitewing films. This dose can be reduced even further by using rare earth intensifying screens in the panoramic cassettes. The patient dose is relatively higher in the regions of the centers of rotation. Significant thyroid dose during the panoramic procedure also has been reported.

Disadvantages

Image Quality
Tomograms inherently show magnification, geometric distortion, and poor definition. Compared with an intraoral radiograph, the pantomogram does not give comparable definition. Besides the tomographic process, other factors that tend to degrade the images as compared with intraoral films are (1) external placement of the film with resulting increased object-film distance, (2) the use of intensifying screens, and (3) faster film with large grain size.

Many diagnostic problems in dentistry require a high degree of radiographic definition. Early detection of such conditions as interproximal caries, disruption of the lamina dura, loss of crestal alveolar bone, and a thickened periodontal membrane all require the maximum of radiographic definition. Because of these factors, pantomographs have very limited value in the diagnosis of periodontal disease and the detection of caries and early periapical lesions. These are common diagnostic problems for practitioners, and the pantomographic technique is lacking in these areas. If a pantomogram is used instead of a full-mouth series, it must be augmented with bitewings and selected periapical films where indicated.

Focal Trough (Image Layer)
Areas that lie outside (either in front of or behind) the focal trough may be seen poorly or not at all. The focal trough or plane of acceptable detail is not as wide as either the mandible or maxilla, and only structures or changes that

lie within the trough are visualized clearly. Pantomographic units that have adjustable focal troughs have far greater diagnostic capabilities than those that do not, but the cost is greater.

Overlap
Pantomographic units have a tendency to produce overlapping images, particularly in the premolar area.

Superimposition
Often superimposition of the spinal column shows up on the anterior portion of the pantomogram. If the patient is positioned properly, this should not happen. However, not all patients are perfect, and some have physical problems that make proper positioning difficult. The anterior teeth and periapical bone are the most difficult to interpret on pantomograms.

Distortion
The amount of vertical and horizontal distortion varies from one part of the film to another, resulting in an uneven magnification of the image; therefore structures, spaces, and distances may appear larger than they actually are. This is a critical factor because some dentists use panoramic radiographs for bone evaluation and case planning involving implant patients.

Overuse
Overuse is one of the prime concerns regarding patient exposure. The ease and convenience in obtaining the pantomograph might lead to careless substitution for other projections that would yield better results. The pantomogram might be taken instead of a periapical film of an area.

Cost
Panoramic units are not inexpensive, but they are a great aid to a practice. Costs vary from about $9000 to $26,000 depending on manufacture and design. It is very desirable to have a pantomographic unit in a dental office and, if not, to have a pathway for referrals.

INDICATIONS

The main indication for panoramic radiography is attaining a larger field size than is possible with periapical and bitewing radiography. Clinical situations in which a panoramic unit is useful and helpful include detecting large areas of pathologic conditions; visualizing impacted teeth; jaw fractures; patients who cannot or will not open their mouths; evaluating tooth development and eruption patterns and timing for both the permanent and deciduous dentition; TMJ problems; foreign bodies; and implant evaluation.

INTERPRETATION

Because there is a larger field size, it follows that it will be necessary to be able to identify more anatomic structures not seen on an intraoral survey. There will be some structures that will be seen on both. The new structures are (see Figure 12-22) the middle cranial fossa, orbit, styloid process septa in the maxillary sinus, angle of the mandible, hyoid bone, TMJ, vertebra, coronoid process, pterygoid plate, the entire maxillary sinus, tonsillar tissue, ear lobe, and mandibular canal.

TECHNIQUE

Procedure 12-2 presents the general rules of technique for preparing and positioning the patient for panoramic radiography. These rules are valid for all units, but some slight technique changes may be necessary for individual units, depending on the manufacturer's specific instructions.

> **Helpful Hint:** Always follow the manufacturer's manual regarding which anatomic line is to be used for positioning the patient. For example, the ala-tragus line is tilted slightly down, about 5 degrees, from a parallel line to the floor, or the Frankfort plane is parallel to the floor.

PROCESSING

Panoramic films are processed with regular dental solutions either by hand-processing or automatically if the processor can accommodate the panoramic size film. The time-temperature method is used with the same fixation and washing times as with intraoral films. The film used in panoramic radiography, as in other extraoral projections, is especially sensitive to excessive safelighting or exposure to cell phone light and may not be merely fogged but ruined. One should make sure that the film-screen combination used is compatible with the intensity and type of safelight used.

One of the most common artifacts seen on panoramic films is caused in the darkroom by static electricity. Multiple black linear streaks resembling tree branches without leaves appear on the radiograph (Figure 12-25). This artifact can be caused by pulling a piece of film quickly and forcefully out of a tightly packed full box of film or when loading or unloading film between the intensifying screens of a flexible cassette. Static electricity is produced most often on cold, dry days.

RULES AND TECHNIQUE FOR PREPARING AND POSITIONING THE PATIENT FOR PANORAMIC RADIOGRAPHY

PROCEDURE 12.2

1. Explain the procedure to the patient, pointing out the importance of not moving during the procedure. Point out the movement of the film cassette and tube around the patient's head and the possibility that the film cassette may touch the shoulder or ear gently during the exposure rotation.
2. Have the patient remove a jacket or any other bulky piece of clothing that might interfere with movement of the cassette holder.
3. Ask the patient to remove any dentures, eyeglasses, earrings, nose rings, hearing aids, and hairpins to avoid their appearance on the film.
4. Seat or stand the patient in the most erect position possible so that the spinal column is straight. Instruct the patient to hold the support handles on the unit, take one step forward, and keep the feet together.
5. Align the patient's head so that the midsagittal plane is perpendicular to the floor.
6. Place the patient's chin on the chin rest. Secure the head-positioning devices to prevent head movement.
7. Drape the front and back of the patient with the lead apron. Do not use a thyroid collar or a bib chain because it would be superimposed on the image.
8. Place a cotton roll or a bite stick, if the unit has one, between the patient's upper and lower incisors.
9. Have the patient close the lips and place the tongue against the roof of the mouth. In addition, instruct the patient to swallow and hold this position. These instructions help to prevent the formation of an airspace that is represented as a radiolucent area above the apices of the upper teeth.
10. Take any readings or measurements called for and set exposure factors if required.
11. Make the exposure. Because the exposure can be as long as 22 seconds as the tube and film cassette travel around the patient, the operator should, despite being positioned outside of the room, talk to the patient, reminding him or her not to move.

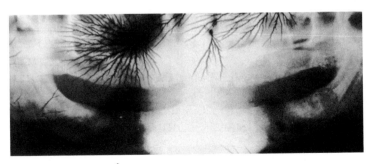

Figure 12-25. Panoramic radiograph showing static marks.

PANORAMIC FILMS

Patient positioned too far forward (Figure 12-26). If the patient is positioned in front of the focal plane, the upper and lower anterior teeth appear blurred and narrow. The spinal column is superimposed on the ramus, and the premolars are overlapped.

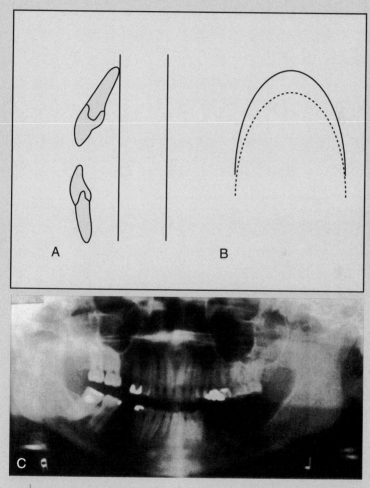

Figure 12-26. Patient positioned too far forward. Anterior teeth appear blurred and narrow. Spinal column is superimposed on the ramus, and premolars are overlapped. **A,** Anterior teeth forward of the focal plane. **B,** Dental arch (*solid line*) anterior to focal plane (*broken line*). **C,** Radiograph.

Remedy. The patient's teeth or edentulous ridges must be in the proper position in the anterior-posterior plane. Check the position of the teeth on the bite block or bite stick and the position of the patient's chin on the rest. Make sure the distance setting is correct.

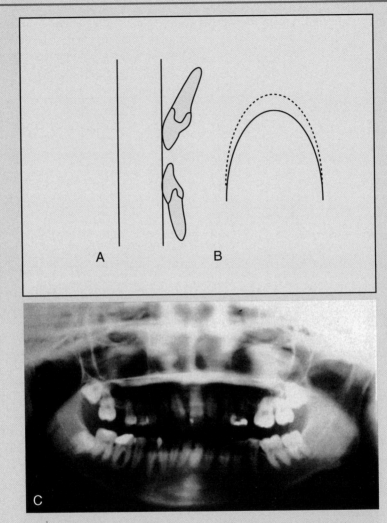

Figure 12-27. Patient positioned too far back. Upper and lower anterior teeth appear blurred and widened. **A,** Anterior teeth positioned behind the focal plane. **B,** Dental arch (*solid line*) posterior to focal plane (*broken line*). **C,** Radiograph.

Patient positioned too far back (Figure 12-27). If the patient is positioned in back of the focal plane, the upper and lower anterior teeth appear blurred and widened. Increased ghosting of the mandible also appears.

Remedy. The patient's teeth or ridges must be in the proper position on the bite block or bite stick. Check the position of the chin rest and the chin for the correct distance in the posterior-anterior plane.

Patient's head tilted up (Figure 12-28). If the patient's head is tilted up, the forehead is too far back and the chin too far forward. This position causes the

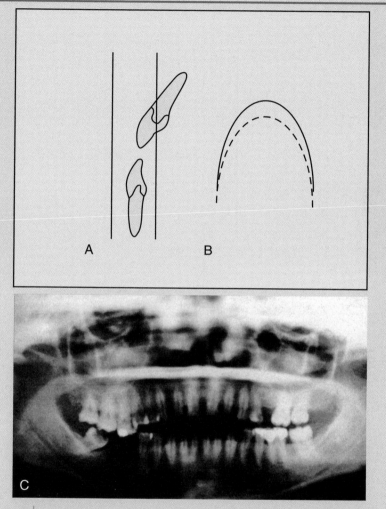

Figure 12-28. Patient's head tilted up. Hard palate (radiopaque band) is superimposed on apices of upper teeth. **A,** Roots of maxillary incisors outside of focal plane. **B,** Mandibular arch (*unbroken line*) in focal trough. Maxillary arch (*broken line*) positioned in back of focal plane. **C,** Radiograph.

upper incisors to be out of focus, and the radiopaque hard palate is superimposed over the apices of the upper teeth. The condyles may be off the film.

Remedy. The reference lines on the patient's face, the Frankfort plane or the ala-tragus line, should be aligned parallel to the floor.

Patient's head tilted down (Figure 12-29). If the patient's head is tilted down, then the chin is back and the forehead is forward. This position causes the lower incisors to be blurred. The radiopaque image of the hyoid bone is superimposed

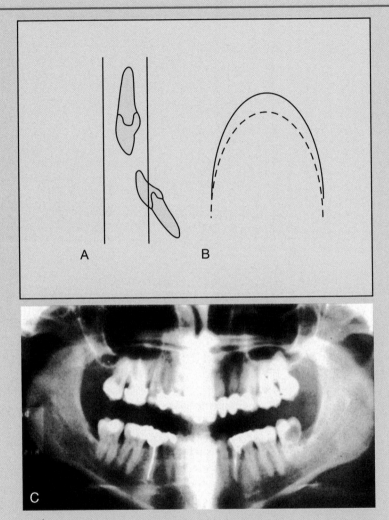

Figure 12-29. | Patient's head is tilted down. Lower incisors are blurred, and image of the hyoid bone is superimposed on the mandible. **A,** Roots of mandibular teeth outside of focal plane. **B,** Maxillary arch (*unbroken line*) positioned in focal plane. Mandibular arch (*broken line*) positioned in back of focal plane. **C,** Radiograph.

on the anterior part of the mandible. The superior portions of the condyles may be cut off the film, and the premolars are overlapped.

Remedy. The reference lines on the patient's face, the Frankfort plane or the ala-tragus line, should be aligned parallel to the floor.

Patient moved during exposure (Figure 12-30). If the patient moves anytime during the exposure, the part of the film that was being exposed at that time will appear blurred. This effect differs from that in intraoral radiography, in which patient movement blurs the entire film.

COMMON ERRORS 12-1

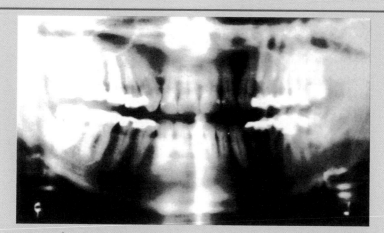

Figure 12-30. | Patient movement during exposure. Note the blurred and sharp areas.

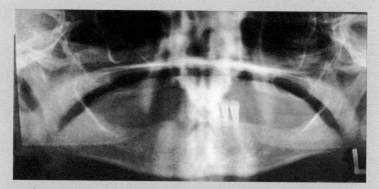

Figure 12-31. | Tongue not against roof of the patient's mouth. Note the large radiolucent band superimposed over apices of the maxillary teeth.

Remedy. Talk to the patient during the exposure, reminding him or her not to move.

Large radiolucent area below the palate (Figure 12-31). If the patient does not hold the tongue against the roof of the mouth, a pharyngeal air space is created that produces a black shadow on the radiograph.

Remedy. Remind patients during the exposure to keep the tongue against the roof of the mouth.

Patient does not sit or stand erect (Figure 12-32). If the patient slumps while standing or sitting, the spinal column causes a triangular radiopacity to be superimposed on the anterior teeth.

Remedy. When positioning a patient, keep his or her spine erect. If the patient is seated, the operator can place a cushion or support in the small of the patient's back to help him or her sit upright.

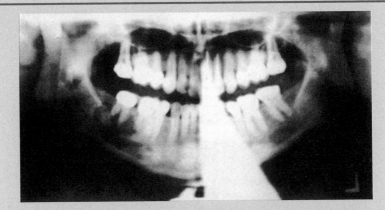

Figure 12-32. Patient slouching. Note superimposition of triangular radiopacity representing the spinal column and not a lead apron.

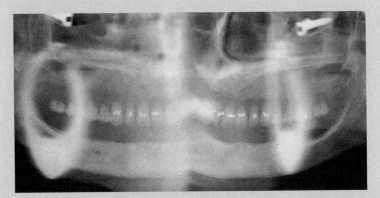

Figure 12-33. Failure to remove metal earrings, maxillary denture, and eyeglasses from patient's face. Note ghosting effect of the metal.

Failure to remove metal objects such as dentures, jewelry, and eyeglasses from the face, head, and mouth (Figure 12-33). These metal objects, if not removed, cause radiopaque ghosting on the opposite side of the film and may obscure structures, making the film undiagnostic.

Remedy. Remove all dentures from the patient's mouth as done in intraoral radiography. All objects must be removed from the face as well.

Lead apron placed too high on the patient (Figure 12-34). The lead apron cannot be placed on the patient above the level of the clavicles because it will create a large radiopacity on the film.

Remedy. Keep the lead apron low on the patient and never use a thyroid collar when taking a panoramic radiograph.

Film cassette slowing down because of patient contact (Figure 10-35). If the film cassette is slowed down or stopped for an instant during the exposure travel

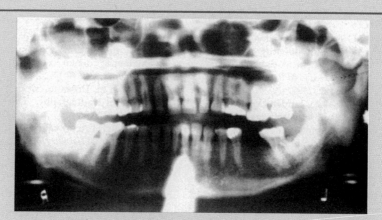

Figure 12-34. Placement of the lead apron too high on the patient's neck.

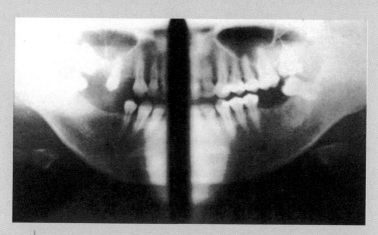

Figure 12-35. Film cassette slowed because of patient contact. Note radiolucent band where the overexposure took place.

around the patient, black vertical bands will appear on the film as a result of the localized overexposure.

Remedy. Position the patient carefully. With large-framed patients, the operator should run the machine first without radiation to acquaint the patient with the procedure and to check on the patient's position.

CONTEMPORARY PANORAMIC IMAGING ARTIFACTS

There have been new findings evident in dental panoramic imaging that reflect changes in society over time. Although we may interpret these findings as "artifacts," they could simply be images that we cannot readily identify.

One of these artifacts that accurately reflects today's lifestyle is cell-phone fogging on panoramic images. Panoramic film is much more sensitive to light than intraoral film, and it takes longer for the entire panoramic film to be fed into an automatic film processor. Although it may seem unlikely, when the operator exposes the panoramic film to the light emitted from a cell phone, the film becomes fogged and is, therefore, not acceptable for diagnostic use (Figure 12-36).

There are several fashion trends not seen in the past that are common today and, therefore, they are visible more often on panoramic dental films. Common among these are facial jewelry. These items should be removed before dental radiographic exposure when possible. If they are metallic in composition, they could be superimposed over images that are wished to be observed and/or they could cause ghosting on panoramic radiographs that interferes with the diagnostic capability of the image. In some instances the patient is unable to remove the piercings because, in keeping with contemporary body piercing procedures, they were soldered into place permanently. The artifacts will be visible, along with the ghosting caused by these objects, which appear more superior, reversed, and with less definition than the actual images (Figure 12-37).

Figure 12-36. | Panoramic film-fogging because of exposure from cell-phone light.

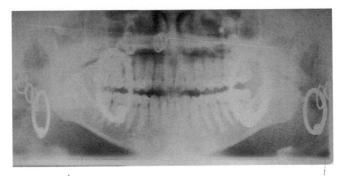

Figure 12-37. | Ghosting of various piercings on a panoramic radiograph.

Images that involve medical consideration and surgical intervention can also be seen on panoramic radiographs. These images may include carotid stents, aneurysm clamps, and hearing aids (Figures 12-38, 12-39, and 12-40).

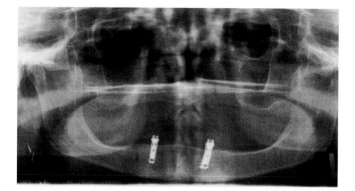

Figure 12-38. | Carotid artery stents on patient's right side on a panoramic radiograph.

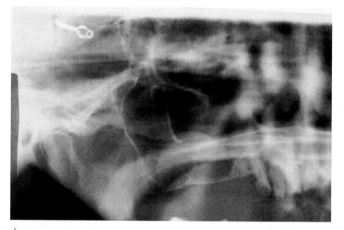

Figure 12-39. | Aneurysm clamp seen on upper border of panoramic radiograph, on patient's right side.

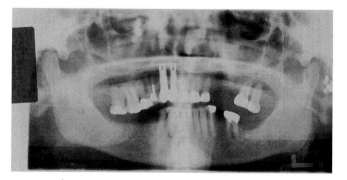

Figure 12-40. | Hearing aid in patient's left ear on a panoramic radiograph.

SUGGESTED READING

Carter LC, et al: Use of panoramic radiography among an ambulatory dental population to detect patients at risk of stroke, J Am Dent Assoc 28:977-984, 1997.

Friedlander AH, et al: The prevalence of calcified carotid artery atheromas on the panoramic radiographs of patients with have type 2 diabetes mellitus, J Am Dent Assoc 133:1516-1523, 2002.

Frommer HIT, Stabulas-Savage JJ: A sign of the times: contemporary dental imaging artifacts, N Y State Dent J 74:37-39, 2008.

White SC, Pharoah MJ: Oral radiology: principles and interpretation, ed 5, St Louis, Mosby, 2004.

CHAPTER 13

Extraoral Techniques

EDUCATIONAL OBJECTIVES

1. Understand the indications for extraoral projections, and apply them in clinical practice.
2. Understand the use of intensifying screens and grids and their clinical importance.
3. Be able to expose the extraoral projections discussed in the chapter.

KEY TERMS

anteroposterior
    projection
cassette
cephalometric
    radiography
cephalostat

extraoral films
grid
lateral oblique projection
lateral skull projection
posteroanterior
    projection

submentovertex
    projection
Waters' view

The scope of dental radiology is constantly expanding; it is not limited to pantomography and the intraoral periapical, bitewing, and occlusal films that have been previously described. There is an ever-increasing use of the term *maxillofacial radiology*. There are many accessory techniques, intraoral and extraoral, using different imaging systems and film-screen combinations, different projections, and computers. If a person is going to be responsible for the maxillofacial area, then he or she must be able to image that area in any way possible. All of the extraoral techniques that are described in this chapter can be performed with the conventional dental x-ray unit in the dental office, because their kilovoltage and milliamperage requirements are within the capability of the dental unit.

As is the case with intraoral radiographs, dental professionals should be knowledgeable and skilled in these accessory techniques. However, some states have statutes that prohibit or limit the dental professional from performing certain extraoral techniques. Information about these restrictions is readily available from the appropriate agencies in individual states.

Newer imaging techniques such as tomography, computed tomography (CT), and magnetic resonance imaging (MRI) also are used by dentists to make complicated diagnoses and treatment planning. They are discussed in Chapter 16.

INDICATIONS

There are two main categories of indications for the use of *extraoral films*. The first is a situation in which a patient cannot or will not open his or her mouth to allow the film packet to be placed intraorally. Handicapped patients may be unable to open their mouths for film placement, and uncooperative patients may simply refuse (see Chapter 18). Patients with trismus or temporomandibular joint (TMJ) ankylosis cannot open their mouths. These indications are very similar to those listed for pantomography, but they require no additional expensive equipment.

The second indication is when the area being radiographed is larger than or cannot be seen on intraoral films. Many areas of the mandible and maxilla cannot be seen on intraoral films. The scope of dental treatment, as mentioned previously, is not limited to the teeth and alveolar bone; it may be necessary to radiograph such areas as the angle and ramus of the mandible to visualize impactions or the skull for orthodontic *cephalometric radiography* analysis. Extraoral radiographs can be used to image the TMJ, maxillary sinus, or lesions that grow so large that they cannot be captured completely on periapical films. Through a combination of extraoral radiographs, it is also possible to locate objects in the third plane, which is necessary for implant evaluation and with occlusal radiography (see Chapter 11).

EQUIPMENT

The radiographic equipment needed to do standard extraoral projections is minimal because extraoral radiographs can be taken with a standard dental x-ray unit and dental chair. Extraoral techniques require a regular dental x-ray unit, film cassettes, 8 × 10-in or 5 × 7-in film, intensifying screens, and cassette holders or angling boards. The darkroom must have the capacity to process the larger film size. The use of grids, although optional, results in better image definition.

X-ray Unit

For extraoral radiographs the x-ray machine must be positioned in the operatory so that a focal-film distance (FFD) of 36 in can be achieved. This distance is necessary to get a sufficiently large divergent beam size at the patient's face so the complete area of interest can be seen. The kilovoltage and milliamperage of the dental x-ray machine are in the suitable range for extraoral radiography.

Cassettes

The films are contained in a carrier called a *cassette*. Cassettes can be rigid or flexible and are available in varying sizes corresponding to the size of the film used (Figure 13-1). The rigid cassette may be cardboard, metal, plastic, or a combination of these materials. A cassette must be light-tight but allow the passage of x-rays to affect the x-ray film and intensifying screen contained in the cassette. The film packet wrapping in intraoral film also can be considered a cassette—a paper cassette—although it is never referred to as such.

Cassettes must be marked with lead letters to identify the left or the right side of the film, or it will not be possible to orient the finished radiograph. Extraoral films have no raised dot to signify which side of the film should face the x-ray tube. Lead strips are available to imprint the patient's name and the date on the film.

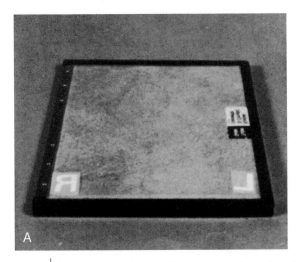

Figure 13-1. **A,** Front view of 8 × 10-in cassette with marking letters.

Continued

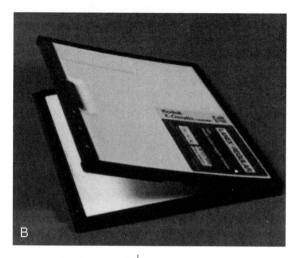

Figure 13-1—cont'd. | **B,** Cassette partially open.

FILM-SCREEN COMBINATION

The imaging system used in extraoral radiography is a film-screen system (see Chapter 4). To reduce radiation exposure to the patient, the film is used in combination with intensifying screens. Previously in dentistry, to obtain better detail, some extraoral projections were taken with film alone in the so-called nonscreen technique. Today with the improved film quality and concern for radiation safety, all extraoral films should be taken using intensifying screens. The screen film used is more sensitive to the light emitted by the intensifying screens than it is to radiation. However, the film used must be sensitive to the type of light emitted by the particular screen (e.g., blue light or green light).

As mentioned in Chapter 4, extraoral film is available in 5 × 7-in or 8 × 10-in sizes and in the panoramic 5 × 12-in and 6 × 12-in sizes.

Holding Devices

Extraoral cassette holders are available that can be wall-mounted or used on a tabletop. If no positioning device is available, the patient can hold the cassette on his or her shoulder. Holding devices have the advantage of standardizing techniques for comparison of films and preventing patient and film movement (Figure 13-2).

Grids

The use of *grids* for extraoral radiography is not common in dental practice and is mostly confined to cephalometric and TMJ radiographs. The function of the grid is to decrease the amount of scatter radiation originating in the

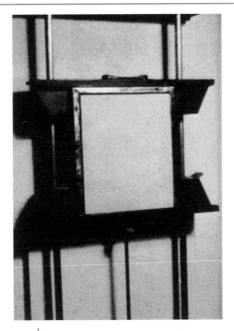

Figure 13-2. | Cassette in a wall-mounted, film-holding device.

object (Figure 13-3). This scatter degrades the image by decreasing the contrast. The grid is a thin plate composed of radiotransparent and radioabsorptive strips that is placed in front of the cassette. The grid absorbs all radiation leaving the object that is not at right angles to the film. In doing so it decreases the effect of scatter on the diagnostic image. Grids are not used in intraoral

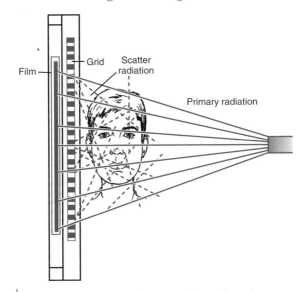

Figure 13-3. | Grid. Note absorption of scatter radiation by radioresistant strips of grid.

radiography because the secondary radiation does not greatly degrade the image as a result of the small field size. The panoramic units, with their narrow exposure field size, also do not need grids. Medical x-ray units use grids routinely. Extraoral radiographs taken with a medical x-ray machine have better-quality density and contrast than similar films taken with a dental x-ray unit because of the use of a grid.

FILM SENSITIVITY AND PROCESSING

Extraoral screen films are more sensitive to light than are intraoral films. Therefore what would be acceptable safelight conditions in the darkroom for processing intraoral films might fog the extraoral films. The films used in panoramic radiography are also especially sensitive to excessive safelighting and may not be merely fogged but ruined. Safelighting always should be checked by the coin test before processing extraoral films.

Extraoral films are processed in the same manner as intraoral films, either manually or by automatic processors that can accommodate large-size film. For manual processing the time-temperature method is used with the same fixation and washing time as with intraoral films. The only difference is that special sizes of film hangers are used (Figure 13-4). Operators should take special care when processing the large films because they are easier to scratch when more than one film is processed at a time.

PROJECTIONS

As in intraoral radiography, certain factors must be known for every projection made, such as (1) the relationship of the film to the patient, (2) the relationship of the central ray of the x-ray beam to the patient and the film, (3) the FFD, (4) the point of entry of the x-ray beam, (5) the kVp, and (6) the mAs.

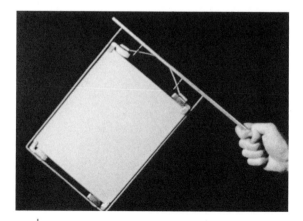

Figure 13-4. | Piece of 8 × 10-in film mounted on a processing film hanger.

EXTRAORAL RADIOGRAPHIC TECHNIQUE

1. Load the extraoral cassette in the darkroom under the proper safelight procedures for the film being used.
2. Set the kVp, mA, and time for the desired values.
3. Place the cassette in the holding device.
4. Have the patient remove all nonfixed prostheses, jewelry, eyeglasses, and so forth that might be seen on the radiograph.
5. Cover or disinfect ear rods, chin positioner, headrest, biteblock, or edentulous positioner.
6. Explain the exposure procedure to the patient.
7. Seat the patient and place the lead apron without a thyroid collar on the patient.
8. Position the patient's head according to the projection, align the x-ray beam, and make the exposure.

Helpful Hint: Remember that extraoral film is more sensitive to light than intraoral film. Be sure to double check that acceptable safelight conditions are being used before beginning to process the film.

PROCEDURE 13-1

Suggested exposure times and mA and kVp settings are given, but these may vary, depending on the film speed, intensifying screen used, and size of the patient. The suggested exposure times that follow assume the use of rare earth intensifying screens.

Lateral Oblique Projection of the Mandible

The *lateral oblique projection* of the mandible is used for surveying one side of the mandible entirely from the distal of the canine to the angle of the ramus, the ramus, condyle, and coronoid process. This projection is ideal for visualizing impactions, fractures, and large areas of pathologic conditions that would not be seen on periapical films. It is not diagnostic anterior to the canine because of the superimposition caused by the anterior curve of the mandible. Before the advent of pantomography, it was the most commonly used extraoral technique for mandibular pathologic conditions and impactions. Today the left and right lateral oblique projections have been replaced in many offices by a pantomograph.

An 8 × 10-in or a 5 × 7-in cassette may be used for this projection. The cassette is supported by the patient's shoulder or a holding device on the side of the mandible to be radiographed. The cassette is in contact with the cheekbone and mandible. The patient's head is inclined about 15 degrees away from the x-ray tube. The central ray is directed from under the opposite side of the mandible at right angles to the cassette. The FFD is 14 in. An average exposure time at 65 kVp and 10 mA would be 5 to 10 impulses (Figure 13-5). This technique can be used

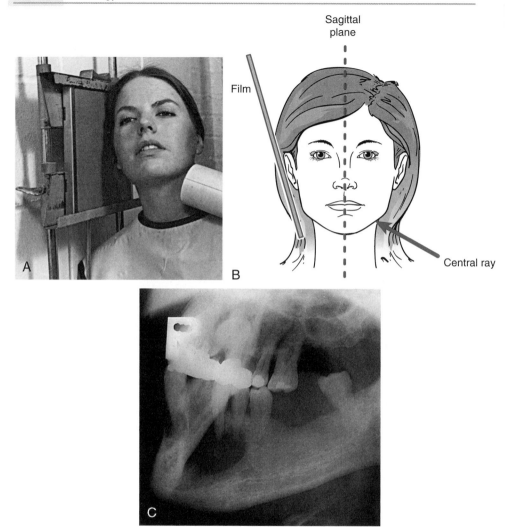

Figure 13-5. | Lateral oblique projection. **A,** Central ray is directed at cassette from beneath opposite side of mandible. **B,** Drawing. **C,** Radiograph.

with an occlusal film packet or in the reverse bitewing technique but with increased exposure times (see Chapter 18).

Clinical indication: viewing mandibular third molar impactions and pathologic conditions.

Lateral Skull Projection

The *lateral skull projection* is used to survey the whole skull in the sagittal plane. The right and left sides of the skull are superimposed on each other, with the side nearer the tube magnified slightly more than the side nearer the film.

Clinical example: It is used in dentistry to detect fractures and systemic pathologic conditions that are also manifested in the jaws, such as Paget's disease. It is the radiographic projection used by orthodontists to obtain lateral cephalometric radiographs.

An 8 × 10-in cassette is used with intensifying screens. The cassette is held in position by the patient, supported on the patient's shoulder or by some supportive device. The cassette is positioned parallel to the sagittal plane of the skull. The central ray is directed at the external auditory meatus at an FFD of 36 in. The vertical angulation is zero degrees. An average exposure time for an adult at 65 kVp and 10 mA would be 8 to 15 impulses (Figure 13-6).

Clinical indication: detection of skull pathologic conditions and cephalometrics.

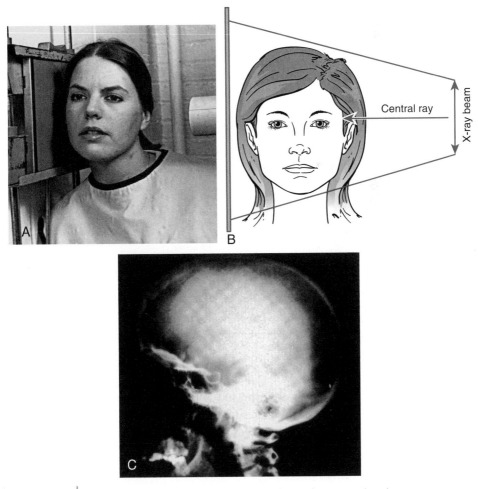

Figure 13-6. | Lateral skull projection. **A,** Central ray is directed at external auditory meatus at a minimum focal-film distance of 36 in. **B,** Drawing. **C,** Radiograph.

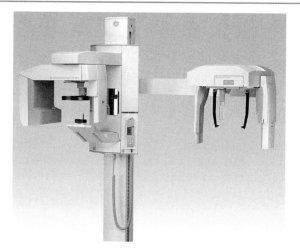

Figure 13-7. Orthoceph OC100 D direct digital cephalometric imaging unit. Note the cephalostat (head holder). The unit can also be used for panoramic digital imaging. *(Courtesy GE Healthcare, Dental Imaging, Milwaukee, WI).*

If the lateral skull projection is to be used for cephalometric measurement, then a head-positioning device *(cephalostat)* must be used (Figure 13-7). The cephalostat ensures that the patient's head is accurately aligned with the sagittal plane and allows reproducibility of patient position so that films taken during and after treatment are valid for comparison.

Posteroanterior Projection

The *posteroanterior projection* is the companion projection to the lateral skull, is used to survey the skull in the anteroposterior plane (coronal, frontal), and provides a means of localizing changes in a mediolateral direction. The left and right sides of the facial structures are not superimposed on each other as in the lateral skull projection.

Clinical indication: In dentistry this projection is used to detect fractures and their displacements, tumors, and large areas of disease. It is not effective for studying the maxillary sinus because of the superimposition of other cranial structures on the sinuses. Although the anteroposterior projection will show the same area, the posteroanterior is preferred in dental radiography because the structures that are of greatest interest are closer to the film in a posteroanterior than an *anteroposterior projection* and hence show less enlargement.

An 8 × 10-in cassette is used with intensifying screens. The cassette can be held in position by the patient, but some type of cassette-holding device is preferable. The patient is positioned with the nose and forehead touching the cassette. The central ray is directed at a zero-degree vertical angulation, aimed at the external occipital protuberance (the prominent bump near the base of the skull). The FFD is 36 in. An average exposure time at 65 kVp and 10 mA would be 8 to 15 impulses (Figure 13-8).

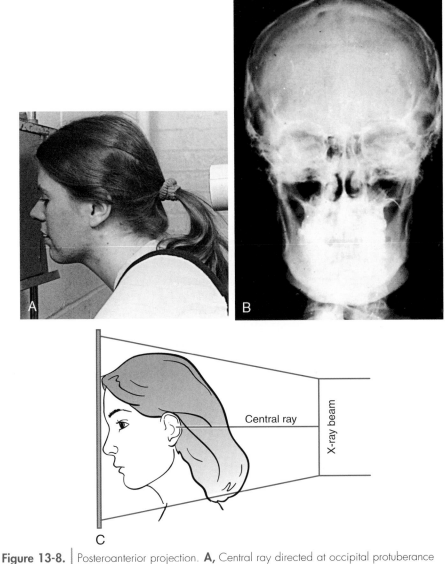

Figure 13-8. | Posteroanterior projection. **A,** Central ray directed at occipital protuberance at minimum focal-film distance of 36 in. **B,** Radiograph. **C,** Drawing.

Posteroanterior (Waters') View of the Sinuses

The *Waters' view* is a variation of the posteroanterior projection that enlarges the middle third of the face and is useful in the diagnosis of maxillary sinus and other pathologic conditions occurring in the middle third of the face. It differs from the posteroanterior projection positioning in that the patient's mouth is kept open while the nose and chin are touching the cassette. The central ray is again directed at the external occipital protuberance, and an FFD of 36 in is used. An average exposure time at 65 kVp and 10 mA would be 15 to 20 impulses (Figure 13-9).

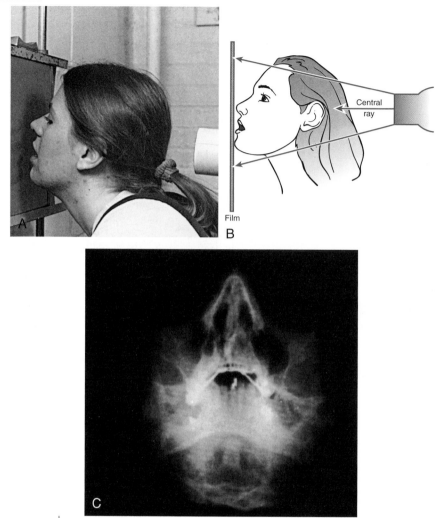

Figure 13-9. Posteroanterior projection of the sinuses (Waters' view). **A,** Central ray is directed perpendicular to cassette at occipital protuberance using 36 in focal-film distance. **B,** Drawing. **C,** Radiograph.

Clinical indication: maxillary sinus pathologic condition, facial fractures of the middle third of the face.

Submentovertex Projection

The *submentovertex projection* is used to detect fractures of the zygomatic arch and visualize the sphenoid and ethmoid sinuses, as well as the lateral wall of the maxillary sinus. It is also used in tomography as a scout film to determine the positions of the condyles.

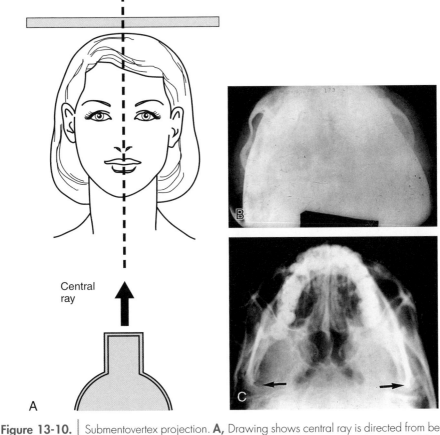

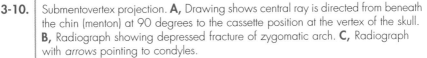

Figure 13-10. | Submentovertex projection. **A,** Drawing shows central ray is directed from beneath the chin (menton) at 90 degrees to the cassette position at the vertex of the skull. **B,** Radiograph showing depressed fracture of zygomatic arch. **C,** Radiograph with *arrows* pointing to condyles.

The cassette is positioned on the vertex of the patient's skull, and the central ray is directed from underneath the patient's chin (menton) perpendicular to the cassette. An average exposure time at 65 kVp and 10 mA would be 8 to 10 impulses (Figure 13-10).

SUGGESTED READINGS

Brooks SL, et al: Imaging of the temporomandibular joint: a position paper of the American Academy of Oral and Maxillofacial Radiology, Oral Surg Oral Med Oral Pathol Oral Radiol Endod 83:609-618, 1997.

White SC, Pharoah MJ: Oral radiology: principles and interpretation, ed 5, St Louis, Mosby, 2004.

CHAPTER 14

Radiography of the Temporomandibular Joint

EDUCATIONAL OBJECTIVES

1. Understand the radiographic anatomy of the temporomandibular joint.
2. Know how to produce various diagnostic images of the joint and surrounding structures.

KEY TERMS

arthrography

temporomandibular joint
   (TMJ)

transcranial projection

Patients with symptoms relating to the *temporomandibular joint* (TMJ) are not uncommon in dental practice. Patients may be referred by other dentists or physicians. They may bring with them previous radiographs, or they may need new or additional radiographs. Some TMJ imaging can be done in the dental office, and some may have to be referred to advanced imaging centers. In either case, dental professionals should feel comfortable in dealing with these images.

ANATOMY OF THE TEMPOROMANDIBULAR JOINT

By understanding the hard and soft tissue anatomy of the TMJ, the problems in imaging the TMJ can be appreciated. The joint is bounded laterally by the zygomatic arch and medially by the petrous ridge of the temporal bone. Structures that the dental professional should be able to identify on radiographs are the external meatus of the ear, the mastoid air cells, the mandibular condyle, the articular fossa, the neck of the condyle, and the articular eminence. The internal and external pterygoid muscles and the articular disc (meniscus) are not seen with routine radiographic imaging (Figures 14-1 and 14-2). Some of the structures are radiolucent and some are radiopaque. The articular disc, which is the major source of TMJ disorders, is not seen on conventional radiographic images because it is fibrocartilaginous and thus radiolucent.

The TMJ pathologic lesions seen on radiographs include fractures, benign and malignant tumors, arthritic changes, ankylosis, disc displacement, fibrous adhesions, and congenital absence of structures. Because the condyle is a movable structure, it is beneficial to image it in various positions (e.g., open, rest, and closed).

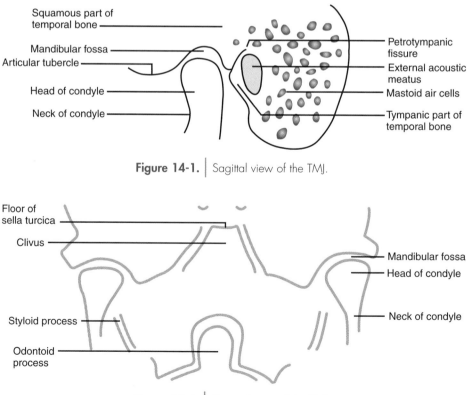

Squamous part of temporal bone
Mandibular fossa
Articular tubercle
Head of condyle
Neck of condyle

Petrotympanic fissure
External acoustic meatus
Mastoid air cells
Tympanic part of temporal bone

Figure 14-1. | Sagittal view of the TMJ.

Floor of sella turcica
Clivus
Styloid process
Odontoid process

Mandibular fossa
Head of condyle
Neck of condyle

Figure 14-2. | Coronal view of the TMJ

TRANSCRANIAL TEMPOROMANDIBULAR JOINT PROJECTION

Next to the panoramic view the *transcranial projection* is the one that is most commonly used in the dental office for TMJ radiography. A 5 × 7-in cassette can be used if there is to be only one exposure. Usually radiographs are taken of both the left and right condyles in both the open and closed position. Because the diagnostic area is relatively small, the four views can be placed on an 8 × 10-in film if appropriate lead shielding is used on the cassette. The patient's head is positioned parallel to the cassette, with the side to be imaged closest to the cassette. The cassette can be supported on the patient's shoulder or on a positioning device in either the upright or horizontal position. The point of entry for the central ray of the x-ray beam is on the opposite side of the head from the condyle being radiographed, approximately 2½ in above and ½ in in front of the external auditory meatus. The x-ray beam is directed at a vertical angulation of 20 to 25 degrees. The open surface of the position-indicating device approximates the skin. An average exposure time at 65 kVp and 10 mA using a fast film and intensifying screens would be 7 to 15 impulses (Figure 14-3). Positioning boards (angling boards) are available to use with the transcranial technique. These boards also incorporate means to hold the patient in a fixed position while allowing movement of the cassette to give up to three exposures for each condyle (open, closed, and rest) on an 8 × 10-in film (Figure 14-4).

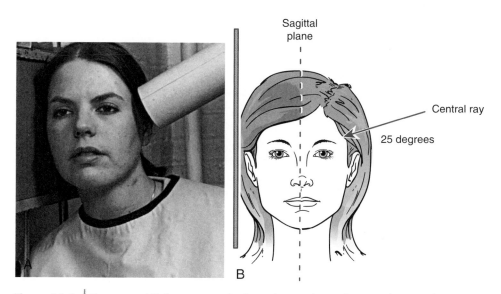

Figure 14-3. Transcranial TMJ projection. **A,** Central ray is directed 2½ in above and ½ in forward of external auditory meatus, with vertical angulation of 20 to 25 degrees. **B,** Drawing.

Continued

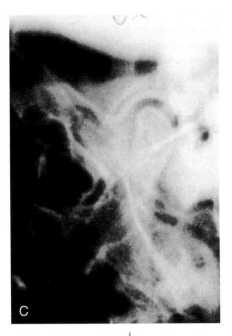

Figure 14-3—cont'd. | **C,** Radiograph.

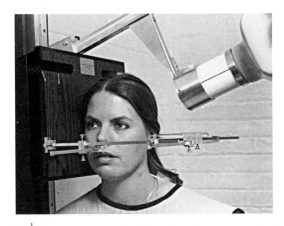

Figure 14-4. | A positioning (angling) board used for transcranial projection.

SUBMENTOVERTEX (BASILAR) PROJECTION

Besides the clinical indications noted in Chapter 14, submental or basilar views can also be used to view the TMJ from the axial plane (Figure 14-5), allowing visualization of the medial and lateral aspects of the condyle. The submentovertex (SMV) projection is also used as a scout film for

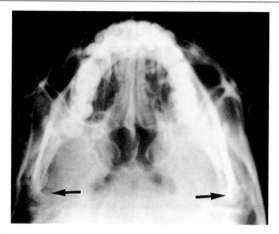

Figure 14-5. Submentovertex projection. Radiograph with *arrows* pointing to condyles.

tomograms of the TMJ, because the projection will relate to the position of the long axis of the condyles with the midsagittal plane.

PANORAMIC PROJECTION

A conventional panoramic projection shows both left and right joints in the lateral plane as well as an overall view of the mandible and maxilla. These views can be used for screening or as a scout film to detect any other existing condition that might be the cause of TMJ pathologic processes (Figure 14-6). If the panoramic film shows a pathologic process, a more advanced projection can be used to make the diagnosis. Some panoramic units have specific programs for the TMJ that will also allow one to take views in the open and

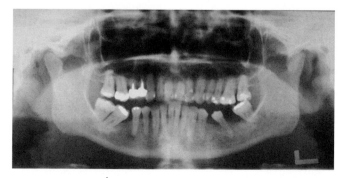

Figure 14-6. Conventional panoramic view of the TMJ.

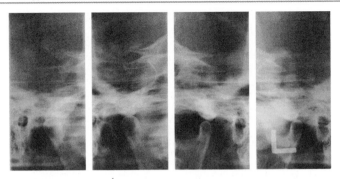

Figure 14-7. | Modified panoramic view of the TMJ.

closed positions. The glenoid fossa and the condyle will be seen, but the articular disc will not (Figure 14-7).

CONVENTIONAL TOMOGRAPHY

Before the wide use of computed tomography (CT) scanning, conventional tomography was one of the better ways to examine the condyle radiographically. Dedicated dental tomographic units are available (Figure 14-8) that produce tomographic images of the TMJ (Figure 14-9). The images are better than panoramic projections and in some ways equivalent to a CT scan. Again, however, the articular disc is not seen, but the fossa, neck, and head of the condyle are seen.

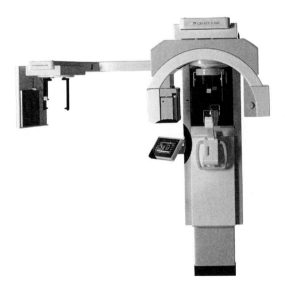

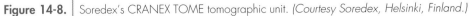

Figure 14-8. | Soredex's CRANEX TOME tomographic unit. *(Courtesy Soredex, Helsinki, Finland.)*

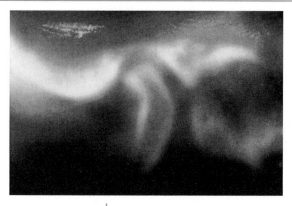

Figure 14-9. | Tomographic view of the TMJ.

COMPUTED TOMOGRAPHY

As discussed in Chapter 16, CT facilitates viewing of an area in three planes and is an excellent means for examining the bones of the TMJ. However, the scans do not include diagnostic images of the articular disc (Figures 14-10 to 14-12).

MAGNETIC RESONANCE IMAGING

Magnetic resonance imaging (MRI) is a very effective means for viewing soft tissue and thus for viewing the articular disc of the TMJ. Because the disc is an important factor in TMJ pathologic processes, the use of MRI should be considered. If one remembers the basic anatomy of the TMJ, the images are not

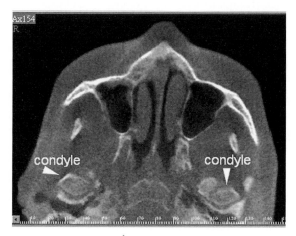

Figure 14-10. | CT axial view of the TMJ.

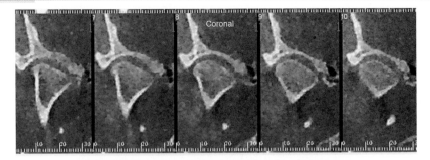

Figure 14-11. │ CT coronal view of the TMJ.

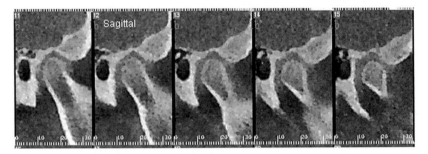

Figure 14-12. │ CT sagittal view of the TMJ.

difficult to read. What is radiolucent on a CT scan or radiograph will be opaque on a magnetic resonance image, indicating high soft tissue density or a strong signal. What is radiopaque on a CT scan will appear lucent on a magnetic resonance image, indicating low soft tissue density or a weak signal (Figure 14-13).

ARTHROGRAPHY

One of the means of radiographing soft tissue is to outline it with a radiographic opaque contrast medium (see Chapter 18). In the case of the articular disc, a contrast medium is injected into both the upper and lower joint space, thus outlining the disc (Figure 14-14). *Arthrography* is an invasive procedure that may have complications if the contrast medium is not placed in the correct space. After considering the options, MRI is the system of choice when imaging the disc and other soft tissues of the TMJ.

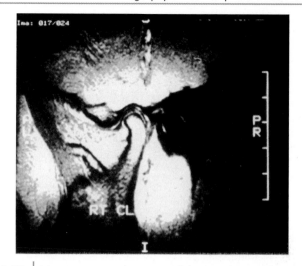

Figure 14-13. | Magnetic resonance image of the TMJ showing the articular disc.

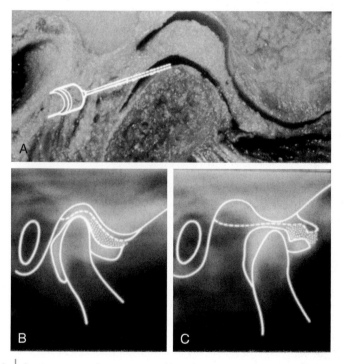

Figure 14-14. | **A,** Contrast medium is injected into the joint space. **B** and **C,** Arthrogram images of the TMJ.

Digital Imaging

EDUCATIONAL OBJECTIVES

1. Understand the principles of digital imaging and how they can be used in the dental office.
2. Be able to make images using digital radiography.

KEY TERMS

analogue
charged coupling device (CCD)
complementary metal oxide semiconductor (CMOS)
detector
digital image
digitize

direct digital radiography
gray level
hard copy
image manipulation
imaging plate
indirect digital radiography
line pairs per millimeter
monitor

optically scanned digital radiography
paperless office
photostimulable phosphor plate (PSP)
pixels
RVG system
sensor
storage phosphor

One of the newest and most exciting technologies introduced in dentistry in recent years is digital imaging. Instead of film or a film-screen combination, this new imaging system uses electronic sensors to record the penetration of the x-ray photons and sends this information to a computer that *digitizes* (converts to numbers) these electronic impulses. This allows the computer to produce a diagnostic image on a monitor almost instantaneously. Digital imaging was introduced into dentistry in 1987 by Dr. Francois Mugnon with his *RVG system* (RadioVisioGraphy). Since that time the market has exploded with numerous companies making competing products. This chapter does not focus on a particular digital unit, but it attempts to explain the basic principles of digital imaging, as well as the technique, advantages, and disadvantages of the system.

DIGITAL IMAGE

A *digital image* is an image formed by the use of an electronic sensor that is connected in some manner to a computer. Early in the development of digital imaging it was often referred to as "filmless radiography," but that name is no longer completely accurate. The basic elements necessary to acquire a digital image are (1) an x-ray machine; (2) an electronic sensor or *detector;* (3) an analogue-to-digital converter; (4) a computer, which can be a laptop version; and (5) a *monitor* (Figure 15-1).

Presently there are three basic types of digital imaging systems (Figure 15-2):

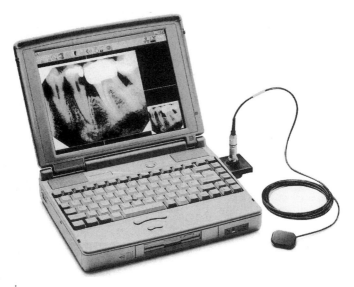

Figure 15-1. | A laptop can be used for digital imaging. Note the attached sensor. *(Courtesy DEXIS LLC, Atlanta, GA.)*

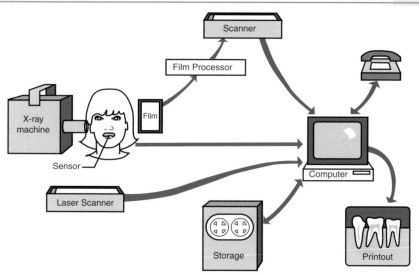

Figure 15-2. | Different digital imaging systems.

1. *Direct digital radiography.* This system uses a sensor wired directly to the computer with the sensor either a charged coupling device (CCD) or a complementary metal oxide semiconductor (CMOS).
2. *Indirect digital radiography (storage phosphor).* This wireless system employs a *photostimulable phosphor plate (PSP)* and laser beam scanning to produce the image.
3. *Optically scanned digital radiography.* In this system a finished processed radiograph is scanned and digitized in much the same way a document is scanned. The new digitalized image can be manipulated in the same manner that direct and indirect images are.

X-ray Unit

The standard dental intraoral x-ray machine can be used for digital radiography, so it is not necessary to purchase a digital-specific unit. Digital panoramic units are now available that combine the advantages of digital imaging with those of pantomography. Some existing panoramic units can be retrofitted for digital radiography. During the early development of these digital systems, because the sensors were so sensitive to radiation, some units needed their own dedicated x-ray units capable of delivering exposures of less than one impulse.

SENSORS

The most critical part of a digital radiography system is the sensor that is placed in the patient's mouth. Presently sensors are available that are equal in size to #0, #1, #2, and panoramic films (Figure 15-3). Earlier

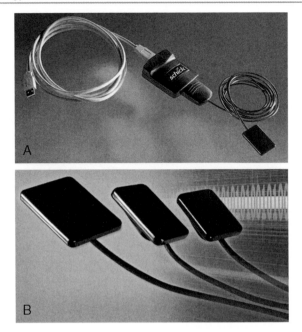

Figure 15-3. **A,** A digital sensor. **B,** Sensors are available in different sizes. *(Courtesy Schick Technologies, Inc., Long Island, NY.)*

sensors had field sizes smaller than standard intraoral film, which thus limited their diagnostic ability. This problem no longer exists, because both film and digital sensors have the same field size. Direct sensors have wires leading to the image processor and solid-state electronic devices. The most common sensor in use is the CCD, which is a chip of pure silicon that is divided into a two-dimensional display called *pixels*. When either x-ray or light photons interact with a CCD, depending on the system used, an electric charge is created and stored. After the exposure is completed, the charges on the CCD are sequentially removed electrically creating a continuous *analogue* output signal. An analogue signal represents data in a continuous mode, just like a wristwatch with hour, minute, and second hands. This information must be converted to digital units that can be assigned numbers. An analogue-to-digital converter is used to convert the analogue output signal to a digital signal that is then sent to the computer. The CMOS sensors are also wired directly to the computer and produce an instantaneous image. CMOS sensors have less power and are less expensive. CMOS sensors have more noise (lesser image definition) than the CCD and hold less diagnostic information. However, they are less fragile and sensor replacement is less common.

The direct CMOS sensor is also wired to the computer to produce an instantaneous image. There is presently debate on which type of wired sensor produces the best results.

A storage phosphor sensor (or PSP) produces images in a two-step process by using a reusable plastic *imaging plate* that is not wired to the computer and is thinner, less expensive, and less rigid and fragile than the CCD and CMOS sensors. The phosphor material in the sensor stores the x-ray energy until it is scanned by a laser. Acquiring the image from the laser can take between 1½ and 5 minutes, depending on the number of images being scanned. The light released by the laser is captured as an electronic signal and is converted to a digital image that is seen on the monitor.

The sensors are reusable after sterilization, and the processing of the image and recharging of the PSP sensor do not necessitate that the room be completely dark as the use of standard film does.

NATURE OF THE IMAGE

A digital image is composed of structurally ordered areas called *pixels*. A pixel would be the digital equivalent of a silver halide crystal on conventional film, with the difference being that silver halide crystals are randomly positioned in the emulsion, whereas the pixel has a definite location that can be assigned a number (digit). The pixel is a single dot in a digital image, and the image is made up of all the pixels or dots on the image. An analogy would be a photograph in a newspaper. In looking carefully at the image, one will see that it is composed of multiple dots with varying degrees of black and white. When looking at the picture, however, one does not see the dots but rather the whole picture. Besides each pixel having a location, it also has a *gray level* that represents the photon penetration of the object (tooth) in that area. The pixel is represented in the computer by a number that indicates its location and photon penetration, and the total image is a table of numbers that can be manipulated (e.g., added or subtracted).

The pixels can be considered containers for numbers, and the numbers vary from 0 to 256 (black to white). Hence there are usually 256 gray levels in an image. However, the human eye can only discern 32 gray levels. Diagnosis relies more on contrast discrimination (gray levels) than on spatial relations and definition. The fact that digital images have only 9 to 10 *line pairs per millimeter* discrimination as compared with 15 line pairs per millimeter for film is not that important as a disadvantage of digital imaging.

Advantages & Disadvantages

Digital Radiography

Before discussing the technique for each type of unit, first look at the advantages and disadvantages of digital radiography. Any new imaging system should be compared with the existing standard of care, which in this instance is the traditional cellulose acetate film base with the double-coated silver halide emulsion.

Advantages

Faster image acquisition. In clinical practice this is by far the advantage that is most appealing to dentists because processing time is practically eliminated. Depending on the system used, as seen later, the range of time needed before one can view the diagnostic image can vary from instantaneous for one image to about 5 minutes for a full series.

Processing time reduced. Because there is no need for a darkroom, the darkroom-associated errors are eliminated and with them the need for retakes. There is also the time saved in not having to open the film packets and place the film on hangers or feed into an automatic processor. The time spent in processing and drying is eliminated, as is the mounting time, because the images are placed on a predesignated mounting template.

Reduction in radiation dose. A great deal of attention has been given in the press, on television, and in the scientific literature to the fact that digital imaging requires much less radiation than film or film-screen combinations. The reduction is about 90% when compared with the dose from D-speed film and about 60% when compared with E-speed film. Although these reductions in dose are remarkable and desirable, bear in mind that the dental dose using film and a film-screen combination is very small to begin with, and these reductions take place in the fourth decimal place. For example, consider the reduction of gonadal dose from a full-mouth survey. An acceptable gonadal dose range with E-speed film is 0.0003 rem. If one uses a digital system, then the 0.0003 rem is reduced by 60% to 0.00018 rem. The 60% reduction in this context is not as dramatic as expressing the reduction in percentage.

Image adjustment and manipulation (Figure 15-4). Once the image is acquired, the computer can change it in many ways. The image can be enlarged, darkened, or lightened (varying the density and contrast) or have selected areas magnified, colorized, and reversed. Unlike computed tomography, the viewing plane cannot be changed (sagittal to cross-sectional), and if the image is elongated or the apices are not seen, the computer cannot compensate for these technique errors.

Image storage. Because the images are stored in digital form on a disk, the space required is minimal compared with a mounted full-mouth survey kept in a chart. In all the available digital systems, stored images can be called up almost instantaneously. Images taken at different times can be placed on the monitor side by side for comparison.

Remote consultation. The digital images can be transmitted to other dental offices or insurance companies if the intended receiver has the hardware to receive the images. Instead of duplication of radiographs and reliance on the mail, the images are sent immediately to another practitioner, thereby saving valuable time and labor.

Hard copies. If teletransmission of the image is not possible, printouts, or *hard copies*, can be produced immediately, thus eliminating the need for duplication while preserving the integrity of the office records.

Patient education. Patients seem to relate better to a digital image on a monitor than a radiograph or a series of mounted radiographs on a viewbox when the dentist is using them as a visual aid for case presentation. The reason may be that this is a

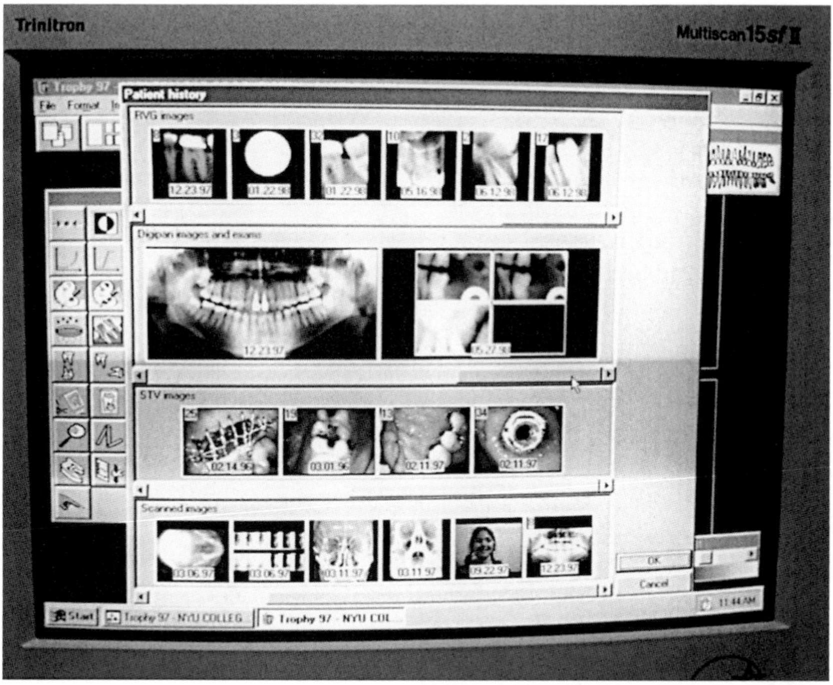

Figure 15-4. | Computer screen showing some of the image-adjustment capabilities.

television age, so patients may be used to the "screen" and close-up views. The ability to look at clinical images or radiographs on the same screen at the same time also helps in case presentation.

Environmentally friendly. Because the silver salts found in film emulsion and processing chemicals are not used in digital imaging, there are no environmental and waste disposal issues. As discussed in Chapter 8, many states now have laws governing the disposal of processing chemicals. This environmental issue is very important and appealing to both patients and dentists. In addition, no lead foil is used in digital radiography.

Paperless office. Most dental offices and clinics are now using computers for record keeping. Software that started out as a means of billing has been expanded to include treatment records, insurance forms, recall systems, birthday and thank-you notes, and so on. The final piece in the puzzle to make the use of the conventional dental chart obsolete is the digital image. With its addition, every type of information about the patient is now available for immediate viewing by just using the tips of one's fingers on the computer keyboard. Lost charts and the tedious storage and retrieval of records can now be a thing of the past because electronic records are copyable and storable. These records should be backed up by a duplicate disk that is stored at another location.

Cross-contamination. Computerized images are clean and sterile because they are not touched by the operator's contaminated gloves when mounting or removing them from the chart or viewbox during an operative procedure.

Disadvantages

Sensor placement. The main disadvantage or difficulty in digital radiography is sensor placement in the patient's mouth (Figure 15-5, A). The sensors are the same size as standard #0, #1, and #2 dental film, but they are thicker and more rigid. Even though manufacturers have tried to make the sensors more user-friendly, it may be difficult or impossible to obtain parallelism between the tooth and sensor in small or crowded mouths to follow the right angle/paralleling technique. However, paralleling instruments are now available for use with direct digital sensors (Figure 15-5, B). If one has to use the bisecting technique, this is a distinct disadvantage, as discussed in Chapter 11. It should be noted that the storage phosphor systems use a thinner and slightly more adaptable

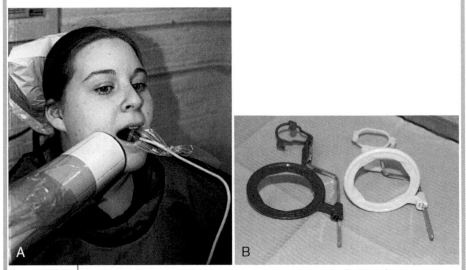

Figure 15-5. | **A,** Charged coupling device sensor in patient's mouth. **B,** Digital imaging paralleling instruments.

sensor than do the direct digital systems (Figure 15-6), and some feel that this gives the system a distinct advantage over the CCD-based system.

Definition. As mentioned, film provides better detail (12 to 15 line pairs per millimeter) than do digital images (6 to 10 line pairs per millimeter). Although this may be the case, the human eye cannot usually make this distinction in clinical situations.

Infection control. Some concern has been expressed about cross-contamination because the sensors cannot be autoclaved. With the use of plastic covers that extend outside the mouth (Figure 15-7) or a self-sealing cover that comes with some units, satisfactory infection control can be obtained.

Cost. The initial cost of a digital system can range from $10,000 to $15,000. Although this may seem like a large expense at first, over time the savings in space,

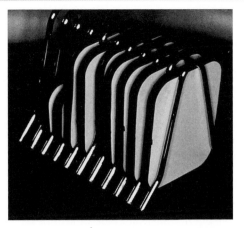

Figure 15-6. │ Storage phosphor sensors.

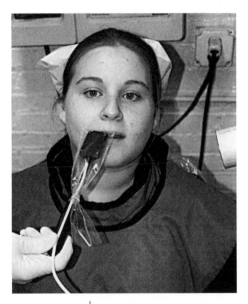

Figure 15-7. │ Sensor with plastic covering.

labor, storage, and so on will justify and amortize the start-up costs. Digital panoramic units can cost about $25,000.

Fragility of sensors. The intraoral sensors are really large silicon chips, and if dropped or abused, their replacement is costly. The cost of the sensor alone is $2000 to $3000. If one drops a piece of film, 10 to 15 cents is wasted. Care in handling should not be the reason for not using digital radiography, but rather it should be a reminder to pay attention to detail.

THE DIGITAL IMAGING TECHNIQUE

The actual exposure technique for digital imaging at chairside is very similar to that of conventional radiography, with the exception of processing and the inclusion of the computer (Figure 15-8).

The main difference between direct and indirect radiography is that the direct digital sensors have wires that are directly connected to the computer and they are less similar to the film packet used in conventional radiography. The sensors used for both techniques are available in different sizes to accommodate varying patients. The operator should still maintain quality assurance in infection control, patient/operator protection, and chairside technique with digital exposures.

The operator is expected to protect himself or herself and the patient against unnecessary radiation exposure. Each patient should be draped with a lead apron and thyroid collar (Figure 15-9). Operators are expected to use sensor-holding devices and not use the patient's finger to stabilize the sensor when exposing images. Digital sensors should be covered with an infection control barrier and handled with extreme caution and care because they are very sensitive devices. The operator's position is maintained at 6 ft from the source of radiation and behind an acceptable barrier.

Optimal chairside technique is extremely important in producing quality films and preventing overexposure to the patient. The operator must avoid retakes as much as possible. The spontaneous image of an error causes retakes to be less time-consuming than conventional radiography, but it still adds to the radiation burden of the patient. Some of the errors previously mentioned do not apply to digital radiography (i.e., reversed film, overbending of the film packet, static electricity artifacts, processing errors) but most exposure errors (i.e., collimator cutoff, foreshortening, elongation, overlap, improper film placement) are still possible.

The Digital Full-Mouth Series

The digital full-mouth series is generally exposed using the paralleling technique with paralleling instruments in use. All principles of the paralleling technique are followed (refer to Chapter 11) with the exception of conventional film being replaced by the digital sensor.

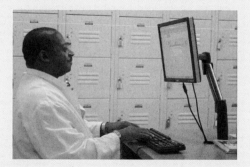

Figure 15-8. Operator accessing digital images.

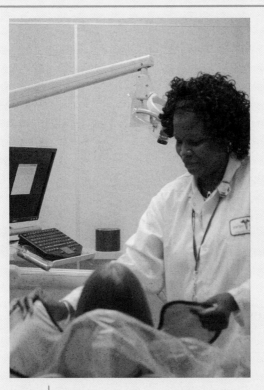

Figure 15-9. │ Operator placing lead apron/collar on patient.

The following account includes the sensor, paralleling instrument, and position-indicating device (PID) position for each projection constituent of a full-mouth series. The combination of the digital sensor, paralleling instruments and collimation contribute to a decrease in radiation exposure to the patient.

Maxillary Central Incisors (Figure 15-10)

The sensor is placed parallel to the teeth in both the vertical and horizontal planes and as close to the teeth as possible. The sensor is placed in the holder in the vertical position. The sensor placement in the patient's mouth may be difficult as a result of the rigidity of the digital sensors. However, the difficulty in placement may be remedied by increasing the distance of the sensor from the central incisors. The center of the sensor is aligned with the junction of both central incisors. The central ray is aimed at the center of the sensor. The PID is placed perpendicular to both the sensor and the tooth in the vertical and horizontal planes. When a localizing device is being used, make sure that the ring is placed as close to the

PROCEDURE 15-1

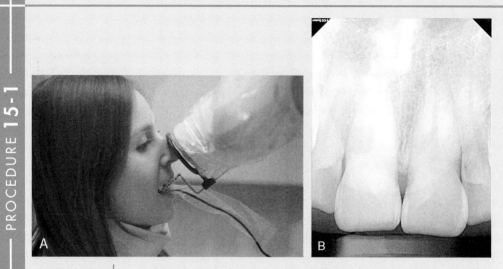

Figure 15-10. | Maxillary central incisors. **A,** Sensor-holding device and PID. **B,** Digital image.

patient's face as possible so as to obtain proper contrast and density of the digital image.

Maxillary Canines (Figure 15-11)
The sensor is placed parallel to the tooth in both the vertical and horizontal planes and as close to the tooth as possible. The sensor is placed in the holder in the vertical position for the anterior projections. The placement of the sensor in the

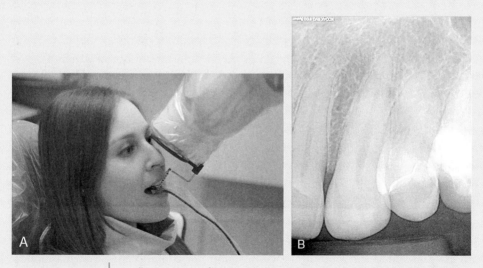

Figure 15-11. | Maxillary canines. **A,** Sensor-holding device and PID. **B,** Digital image.

patient's mouth may be difficult as a result of the rigidity of the digital sensors. However, the difficulty in placement may be remedied by increasing the distance of the sensor from the canine and holding the sensor holder directly on the maxillary canine before asking the patient to bite on the sensor holder. The center of the sensor is aligned with the center of the canine. The central ray is aimed at the center of the sensor. The PID is placed perpendicular to both the sensor and the tooth in the vertical and horizontal planes. When a localizing device is being used, make sure that the ring is placed as close to the patient's face as possible so as to obtain proper contrast and density of the digital image.

Maxillary Premolars (Figure 15-12)
The sensor is placed parallel to the teeth in both the vertical and horizontal planes and as close to the tooth as possible. The sensor is placed in the holder in the horizontal position for the posterior projections. The placement of the sensor in the patient's mouth may be difficult as a result of the rigidity of the digital sensors. However, the difficulty in placement may be remedied by increasing the distance

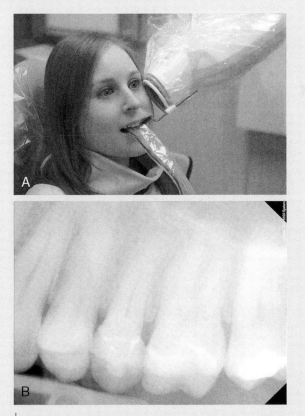

Figure 15-12. | Maxillary premolars. **A,** Sensor-holding device and PID. **B,** Digital image.

PROCEDURE 15-1

of the sensor from the premolars so that the sensor position may be in the middle of the palate. The center of the sensor is aligned with the center of the second premolar. The central ray is aimed at the center of the sensor. The PID is placed perpendicular to both the sensor and the tooth in the vertical and horizontal planes. When a localizing device is being used, make sure that the ring is placed as close to the patient's face as possible so as to obtain proper contrast and density of the digital image.

Maxillary Molars (Figure 15-13)

The sensor is placed parallel to the teeth in both the vertical and horizontal planes and as close to the teeth as possible. The sensor is placed in the holder in the horizontal position for the posterior projections. The placement of the sensor in the patient's mouth may be difficult as a result of the rigidity of the digital sensors. However, the difficulty in placement may be remedied by increasing the distance of the sensor from the molars so that the sensor position may be in the middle of the palate. The center of the sensor is aligned with the center of the second molar.

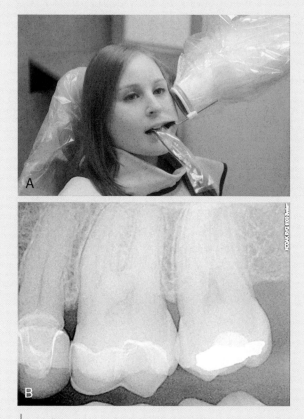

Figure 15-13. | Maxillary molars. **A,** Sensor-holding device and PID. **B,** Digital image.

The central ray is aimed at the center of the sensor. The PID is placed perpendicular to both the film and the tooth in the vertical and horizontal planes. When a localizing device is being used, make sure that the ring is placed as close to the patient's face as possible so as to obtain proper contrast and density of the digital image.

Bitewing Projections (Figure 15-14)

When the premolar bitewings are being radiographed, the center of the sensor is aligned with the center of the mandibular second premolar and the biting surface of the sensor holder is held on the mandibular arch. While the operator holds the sensor in position, the patient is instructed to bite on the film-holding device. The operator should be sure that the patient is biting on the posterior teeth in centric occlusion. The central ray is aimed at the center of the sensor. The PID is placed perpendicular to both the film and the tooth in the vertical and horizontal planes. When a localizing device is being used, make sure that the ring is placed as close to the patient's face as possible. The procedure for radiographing the molars is the same as that mentioned earlier, except that the biting surface of the sensor holder is centered and held on the mandibular second molar. It should also be noted that there are sensor-holding devices available for use with digital vertical bitewing projections as well.

Mandibular Incisors (Figure 15-15)

The sensor is placed parallel to the teeth in both the vertical and horizontal planes and as close to the teeth as possible. The sensor is placed in the holder in the vertical position. The sensor placement in the patient's mouth may be difficult as a result of the rigidity of the digital sensors. However, the difficulty in placement may be remedied by increasing the distance of the sensor from the central incisors. In some cases it may be necessary to position the sensor far back in the floor of the mouth at the level of the molars. The operator may also start out with the sensor on an angle and then bring the sensor into a parallel position slowly with the closure of the mandible. The operator may also place a gauze pad under the sensor to prevent it from irritating the floor of the mouth. The center of the sensor is aligned with the junction of both central incisors. The central ray is aimed at the center of the sensor. The PID is placed perpendicular to both the sensor and the tooth in the vertical and horizontal planes. When a localizing device is being used, make sure that the ring is placed as close to the patient's face as possible so as to obtain proper contrast and density of the digital image.

Mandibular Canines (Figure 15-16)

The sensor is placed parallel to the tooth in both the vertical and horizontal planes and as close to the tooth as possible. The sensor is placed in the holder in the vertical position for the anterior projections. The placement of the sensor in the patient's mouth may be difficult as a result of the rigidity of the digital sensors. However, the difficulty in placement may be remedied by increasing the distance

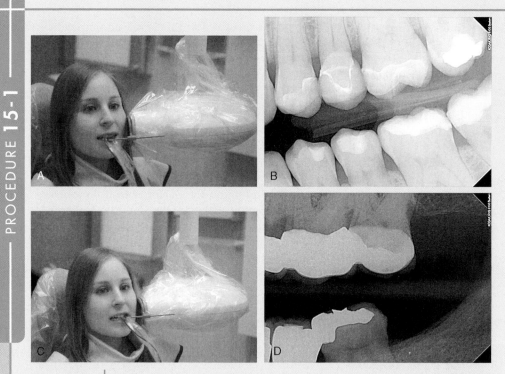

Figure 15-14. Bitewing projections. **A,** Sensor-holding device and PID for premolar bitewing. **B,** Digital image of premolar bitewing. **C,** Sensor-holding device and PID for molar bitewing. **D,** Digital image of molar bitewing.

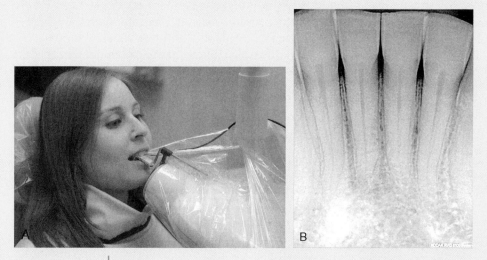

Figure 15-15. Mandibular incisors. **A,** Sensor-holding device and PID. **B,** Digital image.

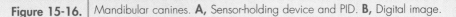

Figure 15-16. | Mandibular canines. **A,** Sensor-holding device and PID. **B,** Digital image.

of the sensor from the canine and holding the sensor holder directly on the mandibular canine before asking the patient to bite on the sensor holder. Be sure that the sensor is placed below and not above the tongue. The center of the sensor is aligned with the center of the canine. The central ray is aimed at the center of the sensor. The PID is placed perpendicular to both the sensor and the tooth in the vertical and horizontal planes. When a localizing device is being used, make sure that the ring is placed as close to the patient's face as possible so as to obtain proper contrast and density of the digital image.

Mandibular Premolars (Figure 15-17)

The sensor is placed parallel to the teeth in both the vertical and horizontal planes and as close to the tooth as possible. The sensor is placed in the holder in the horizontal position for the posterior projections. The placement of the sensor in the patient's mouth may be difficult as a result of the rigidity of the digital sensors. However, the difficulty in placement may be remedied by increasing the distance of the sensor from the premolars so that the sensor position may be in the middle of the floor of the mouth. The anterior corner of the sensor will not curve to accommodate the arch; therefore care must be taken to include the mesial of the first premolar on the image without causing unnecessary discomfort to the patient. The center of the sensor is aligned with the center of the second premolar. The central ray is aimed at the center of the sensor. The PID is placed perpendicular to both the sensor and the tooth in the vertical and horizontal planes. When a localizing device is being used, make sure that the ring is placed as close to the patient's face as possible so as to obtain proper contrast and density of the digital image.

PROCEDURE 15-1

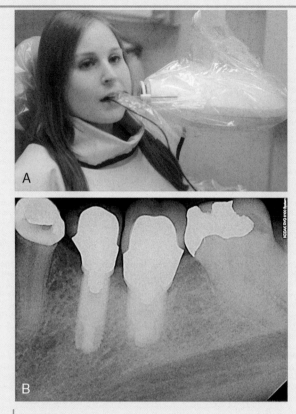

Figure 15-17. | Mandibular premolars. **A,** Sensor-holding device and PID. **B,** Digital image.

Mandibular Molars (Figure 15-18)

The sensor is placed parallel to the teeth in both the vertical and horizontal planes and as close to the teeth as possible. The sensor is placed in the holder in the horizontal position for the posterior projections. The placement of the sensor in the patient's mouth may be difficult as a result of the rigidity of the digital sensors. However, the difficulty in placement may be remedied by increasing the distance of the sensor from the molars so that the sensor position may be in the middle of the floor of the mouth. The center of the sensor is aligned with the center of the second molar. The central ray is aimed at the center of the sensor. The PID is placed perpendicular to both the film and the tooth in the vertical and horizontal planes. When a localizing device is being used, make sure that the ring is placed as close to the patient's face as possible so as to obtain proper contrast and density of the digital image.

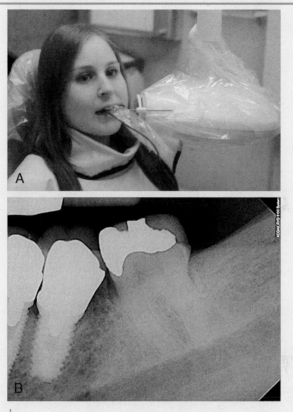

Figure 15-18. | Mandibular molars. **A,** Sensor-holding device and PID. **B,** Digital image.

TYPES OF DIGITAL SYSTEMS

All of the systems mentioned differ in how they acquire the digital image and in what size of receptor plates are available (e.g., panoramic). Once acquired, the systems do not vary greatly in how they display, adjust, store, or transmit the image.

Direct Digital Radiography

In direct digital radiography systems, the sensor, which is placed in the patient's mouth, is connected by a wire to the computer that is visible to the patient, and there is instantaneous image production on the monitor when the exposure is made. Systems vary regarding the type of sensor used to capture the x-ray photons to affect the CCD. Some acquire the photons directly, whereas others use a fiberoptically coupled sensor that operates like a film-screen system, sending light photons to affect the CCD.

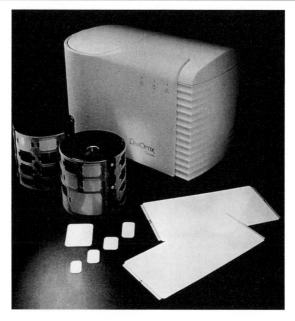

Figure 15-19. | Storage phosphor unit. *(Courtesy KaVo Dental/GENDEX Imaging, Lake Zurich, IL.)*

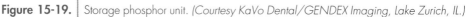

Indirect Digital Radiography (Storage Phosphor)

In indirect digital radiography (storage phosphor), a slightly flexible sensor, which is not connected by wire to the computer, is placed in the patient's mouth and an exposure is made (Figure 15-19). The sensor is then exposed, removed from the mouth, and processed by a laser beam with electronic data sent to the computer, which generates a digital image in 1½ to 5 minutes, depending on the number and types of sensor plates being processed. The plates can then be recharged and used again. Some types of digital scanners have a built-in heat sealer and bag cutter to maintain the sterility of the imaging plates.

Optically Scanned Digital Radiography

In optically scanned digital radiography systems, regular dental film is used to acquire the image with the usual intraoral techniques. The film is then processed in the darkroom, the finished dry film is scanned, and the digital image is produced (Figure 15-20). This digitized image can be used in the same way as those that have been directly acquired. With this method, it takes a great deal of time to acquire a digitized image because complete film processing must be done before the image can be scanned and digitized. The greatest use of optically scanned digital imaging is in filing and storage of images.

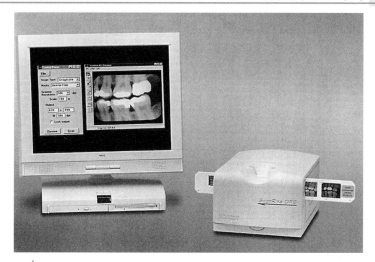

Figure 15-20. | Optical scanning digital radiography unit. *(Courtesy Scanrite Systems, Fremont, CA.)*

LEGAL ASPECTS

One of the major concerns raised about all electronic information, including digital images, has been the reliability of the information and the possibility of *image manipulation*. Disturbing as it may be, the fact that digital images could be altered by an unethical practitioner to justify unnecessary treatment must be faced.

Radiographs have been admitted in court as evidence in much the same way photographs have. With digital imaging, there is a possibility that if a jury learns that images can be altered, they may no longer look at the digital images as hard evidence. This concern has been largely overcome as the major manufacturers build "audit indicators" into their units that signal if and when an image has been altered.

SUGGESTED READINGS

Dunn SM, Kantor ML: Digital radiology, Facts and Fictions, J Am Dent Assoc 124:38-47, 1993.

Jones GA, Behrents RG, Bailey GP: Legal considerations for digitized images, Gen Dent 44: 242-244, 1996.

Mouyen F, et al: Presentation and physical evaluation of radiovisiography, Oral Surg Oral Med Oral Pathol 68:238-242, 1989.

Tsang A, Sweet D, Wood RE: Potential for fraudulent use of digital radiography, J Am Dent Assoc 130:1325-1329, 1999.

White SC, Pharoah MJ: Oral radiology: principles and interpretation, ed 5, St Louis, Mosby, 2004.

CHAPTER 16

Advanced Imaging Systems

CHAPTER OUTLINE

EDUCATIONAL OBJECTIVES

1. Have a basic understanding and appreciation of the basic concepts of computed tomography and magnetic resonance imaging.
2. Know the roles of computed tomography and magnetic resonance imaging in dentistry.

KEY TERMS

axial plane
bone window
computed tomography
  (CT) scanning
coronal plane
CT number

Hounsfield unit
image acquisition
magnetic field
magnetic resonance
  imaging (MRI)
radiofrequency

sagittal plane
signal intensity
soft tissue window
software

With the introduction and now common use of such new and advanced imaging techniques as *computed tomography (CT) scanning, magnetic resonance imaging (MRI)*, positron emission tomography (PET), and digital imaging (see Chapter 15), the field of dental radiology has greatly expanded. These new techniques can be used by dentists to image structures in ways that were previously unobtainable. The use of CT scans for diagnosing lesions and planning implant cases and the use of MRI to visualize soft tissue components of the temporomandibular joint and assess pathologic conditions are now accepted as standard procedures in dental radiology. Although CT scanners and MRI units are not found in dental offices except in the ever-increasing dental radiology specialty practices, the dental professional should have some familiarity with these newer imaging systems because patients may have to be referred for such imaging or copies of the images may be brought to the office by the patient for opinions and interpretation. Therefore an overview of these imaging systems is included in this chapter.

Although different sources of energy are used (x-radiation in CT and radiofrequency energy in MRI), a common theme in these imaging systems is the use of tomography and the absence of film as the sensing device and the use of electronic detectors that send electrical impulses to a computer, which then stores or generates an image on a monitor.

COMPUTED TOMOGRAPHY (CT SCANNING)

Computed tomography (CT) was introduced into radiology in the early 1970s. In contrast to conventional radiographic techniques in which film or film-screen combinations are used to produce images, CT images are computer-generated. However, CT still uses ionizing radiation as the energy source.

CT scanners produce digital data measuring the extent of the x-ray penetration through the patient. The *image acquisition* is done in a tomographic mode with the source of the radiation or the detectors traveling 360 degrees around the patient. Figure 16-1 shows the comparison between tomography and CT scanning.

In CT, a finely collimated x-ray beam is directed through the patient to a series of electronic detectors or sensors. These detectors send electrical impulses that are digitized and stored by the computer. This is called the *scan*, and it is usually done in the axial plane with the patient positioned in a large doughnut-shaped unit that contains the x-ray tube and the sensors (Figure 16-2). Originally all scans were done in the axial plane, thus leading to the name "computerized axial tomography" or CAT scan. The "A" has been dropped, as some initial scans are done in other than the *axial plane*, and these images can be reformatted and viewed in the *coronal plane*, *sagittal plane*, and *axial plane* (Figures 16-3 and 16-4). Figure 16-5 is a diagram illustrating of all of the orientation planes.

The computer can generate an image based on the digitized data it has received. This image can be (1) displayed on a monitor, (2) reformatted into other planes in two or three dimensions (which cannot be done in digital dental radiography), (3) adjusted for optimum viewing of hard and soft tissue, (4) stored on a disk, (5) produced as a printout (hard copy), and (6) transmitted by phone to other locations. Once the scan has been completed, the patient can be dismissed because all subsequent image reconstruction manipulation can be done by the computer.

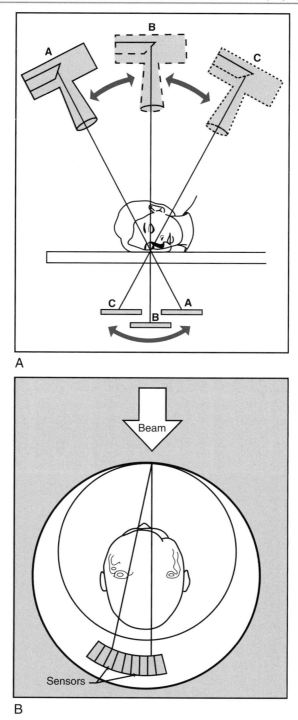

Figure 16-1. **A,** Tomography. Note the film as the image receptor. **B,** CT scan. Note the sensors as the image receptor.

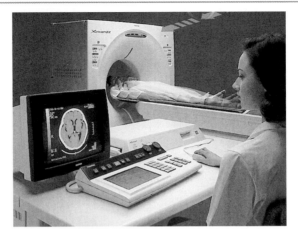

Figure 16-2. CT scanning unit. Note the patient in the scanner, the technician at the computer, and the image on the screen. *(Courtesy Toshiba America Medical Systems, Tustin, CA.)*

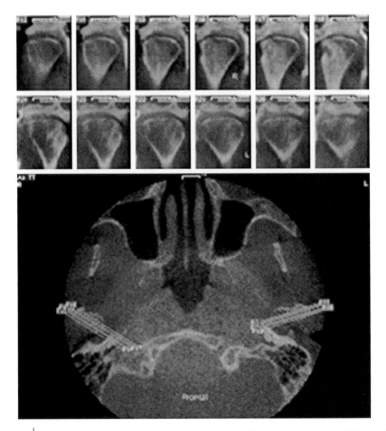

Figure 16-3. CT scan in the axial plane. Note the gray soft tissue imaging and the radiopaque bone.

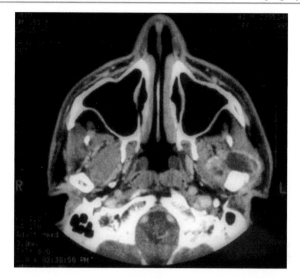

Figure 16-4. CT scan in the *axial plane*. Note the gray soft tissue imaging and the radiopaque bone.

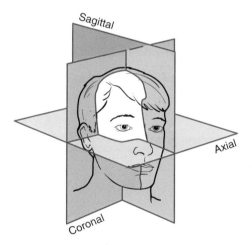

Figure 16-5. All orientation planes.

The computer collects the x-ray beam penetration data in a grid pattern called a *matrix*, much like the digital imaging described in Chapter 15. Each square in the matrix is made up of pixels, which represent the density of a small volume of tissue. Because each pixel is digitized, it can be assigned a *CT number*, which represents the density of a particular area that has been penetrated by the x-ray beam. CT numbers are also called *Hounsfield units*, in honor of one of the developers of this radiographic imaging technique. CT numbers range from +1000 to −1000, with 0 being water, bone being +1000, and air being −1000. For example, fat tissue is about 100 Hounsfield units. Because the density of tissue has been assigned a number, one can narrow the densities that can be displayed. This is called "using a window," and there can be either a *bone window* or a *soft tissue* window (Figures 16-6 and 16-7).

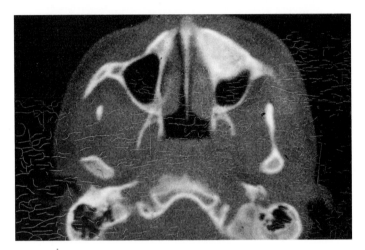

Figure 16-6. │ CT scan with a bone window. Which maxillary sinus is abnormal?

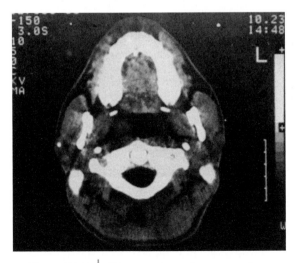

Figure 16-7. │ CT scan with a soft tissue window.

Advantages & Disadvantages

Computed Tomography

Advantages

1. Eliminates the superimposition of images of structures superficial or deep to the area in question (tomography), and this can be done in any plane. Images can be acquired in any plane, and the scan can produce images in any plane.
2. A CT scan can enable one to distinguish between tissue density that differs from 1% to 2% where at least 10% is needed for conventional films.
3. Images can be reformatted to another plane without the necessity of another scan. Some CT scanners can image the mandible and the maxilla on one scan.
4. Density and contrast can be adjusted using the CT numbers to create a bone or soft tissue window.
5. The enhanced image makes interpretation easier and more accurate.

Disadvantages

1. Increased radiation dose when compared with conventional film. Some of the newer cone beam units can reduce radiation by 90% when compared with older-design CT units. Many special software programs have been written for CT scanners that are specific for dental use in implant planning (Figure 16-8). This software directs the computer in

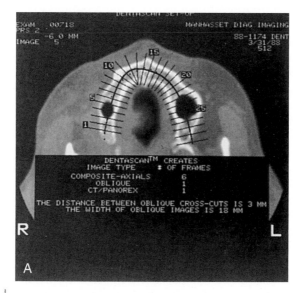

Figure 16-8. | CT scan using software designed specifically for dental implant planning.

Continued

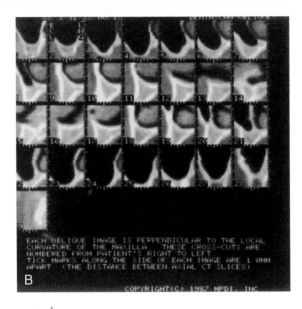

Figure 16-8—cont'd. | **A,** Axial cut with numbered orientation planes that are seen in the corresponding vertical cuts in **B.**

obtaining the desired images in three planes so that the site of the implant fixture can be determined. Not all CT units have implant software, so it is very important to inquire whether the facility has the desired software program before referring a patient to a medical facility for an implant scan. The use of CT scanning in the evaluation and planning of implant sites and evaluation of bone density has become a most common application in dentistry and is rapidly becoming the standard of care for implant planning. The American Academy of Oral and Maxillofacial Radiology in their position paper on the use of x-rays in implants has stated that "some form of cross-sectional imaging be used for implant cases," and CT is a form of cross-sectional imaging. Never before has it been possible to obtain multiple cross-sectional cuts with the speed and accuracy available now in implant evaluation.

2. The radiation dose for a CT scan of the head is about 3.4 to 5.5 rad (34 to 55 mGy), whereas a skull film done with a film-screen system has a dose of about 530 rad (5.3 mGy). However, with the film-screen technique, one has to make multiple exposures to obtain the diagnostic information contained in one scan, which also will give a better and more diagnostic image.

3. The cost to the patient for a CT scan depends on the scan but will probably be $400 to $900, in comparison with $200 for a conventional film.

4. Significant artifacts are produced by metallic objects such as metal dental restorations that are in the plane being scanned.

CONE BEAM COMPUTED TOMOGRAPHY

A new means to acquire a CT image is by cone beam computed tomography (CBCT) or cone beam volumetric tomography (CBVT). Some of these CT scanners are dedicated to maxillofacial scans (NewTom 9000; Figure 16-9, *A*). The technique involves use of a round or rectangular cone-shaped x-ray beam on a two-dimensional x-ray sensor. This new technique has the advantage of using less radiation as well as less time acquiring the image as compared with medical CT scanning. The scanned series consists of 360 images including transaxial, axial, and panoramic images. These CBCT (CBVT) units allow the patient to either be in the supine or upright position for exposure (Figure 16-9, *B*). This option allows patients to have dental scans exposed without having to lie down in a confined space.

Cone beam volumetric tomography (cone beam computed tomography) represents a new generation of FDA-approved dental scanners that generate significantly less radiation than do traditional medical CT scanning devices. These CBVT (CBCT) scanners deliver comparable diagnostic images while adhering to the ALARA principle of using the least amount of radiation to obtain a diagnostic image. CBVT (CBCT) scanners are cost-effective and more accurate than conventional medical CT scanners. CBVT (CBCT) technology has many benefits, including reduced radiation exposure while creating three-dimensional images of the anatomic structures of the mandible, maxilla, and related structures (Figure 16-10). Given the fact that CBVT (CBCT) technology has greater accuracy than a dental periapical film, a panoramic projection, or even a medical CT scan, it is suggested that CBVT (CBCT) may be used in dentistry not only for dental implant planning, but also to evaluate impacted teeth, supernumeraries, oral pathologic conditions, and many more dental applications in multiple views (Figure 16-11, *A-C*).

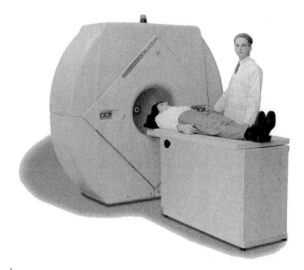

Figure 16-9. | The NewTom 9000, used specifically for imaging the head and neck.
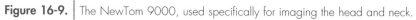

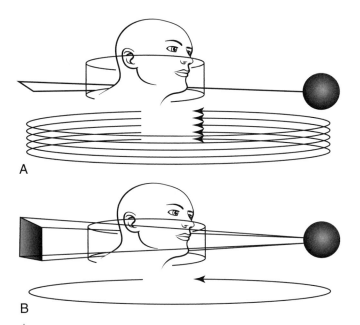

A

B

Figure 16-10. **A,** Conventional CT scan reformats series of parallel helical slices, which incorporate small errors in final scan. **B,** Cone beam volumetric tomography (BVT) captures volumes of data taken in one 360-degree rotation about a patient's head. Each volume "touches" adjacent volume to avoid distortion and error in reformatted studies.

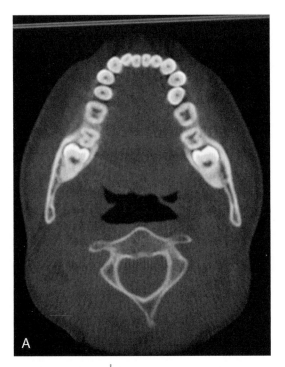

A

Figure 16-11. **A,** CBVT (CBCT) axial view.

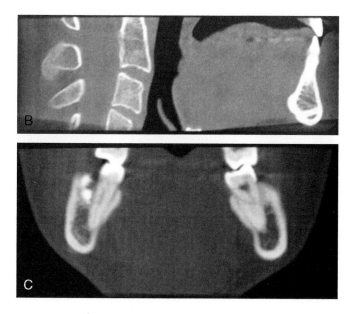

Figure 16-11—cont'd. B, CBVT (CBCT) sagittal view. C, CBVT (CBCT) coronal view.

Acquiring the Image

To take a scan, the technician places the patient in position in the CT scanner and a preliminary scout film is exposed. This scout film helps the technician determine if the patient is positioned properly and also calibrates the radiation dosage according to hard and soft tissue densities. Once the head is in the correct position, the x-ray tube rotates 360 degrees once around the patient's head to take the desired images.

Radiation Dosages

The average absorbed dose from a CBVT scanner is roughly 12.0 mSv (microsieverts), which is equivalent to or less than the radiation needed to take five dental x-rays using D-speed film. This amount of radiation is similar to one fourth of a typical panoramic machine. By comparison, medical CT scanners acquire images using effective doses 40 to 60 times these amounts; the radiation dose for medical CT scanners is based on the patient's weight, bone density, and whether one jaw or two jaws is being studied.

MAGNETIC RESONANCE IMAGING

MRI does not use ionizing radiation as the energy source but rather another type of energy wave from the electromagnetic spectrum, that is, *radiofrequency energy* (see Figure 1-1). Because these wavelengths are long and cannot cause ionization, there is no radiation dose to the patient.

The patient is placed in a large magnet that is 10,000 times more powerful than the Earth's *magnetic field*. The field is so powerful that all freestanding metal objects must be removed from the room because they can become lethal objects if affected by the magnetic field. The magnetic field temporarily changes the alignment and orientation of the protons in the patient's body. Radiofrequency waves are applied to the realigned protons, and this radiofrequency energy is absorbed. When the radiofrequency signal ends, the protons release the absorbed energy, which is received by a sensor, and the information is transmitted to a computer that generates an image. Because MRI is actually based on measurement of proton density and 70% of the human body is water, of which protons are the major component, MRI is better for visualization of soft tissues and not as good for viewing bone, which has very little water. The images produced show strong *signal intensity* (white area) for soft tissue with many water molecules and show a weak signal (black area) where there are few water molecules. This is the exact opposite of radiation-generated images, in which bone is white and soft tissue is black.

Presently the main application of MRI in dentistry has been in imaging the articular fibrous disk of the temporomandibular joint and other soft tissue lesions (Figure 16-12).

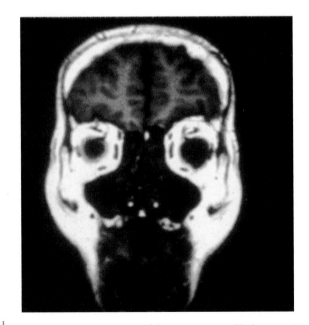

Figure 16-12. Magnetic resonance image of the temporomandibular joint. Locate and identify the condyle, articular disk, and the muscles.

NUCLEAR MEDICINE

Nuclear medicine (radionuclide scanning, bone scanning) is a diagnostic radiation procedure using radioactive compounds that have an affinity for particular tissues (target tissues). These organ-specific compounds are injected into the patient, where they concentrate in the target tissue and are detected and imaged by a sensor called a *gamma camera*. In this manner both the form and function of the target tissue can be studied. The injectable radiopharmaceutical material consists of an organic substance specific for a given tissue or structure and a nonspecific radionuclide (label). The image is recorded by a gamma camera, which detects the release of gamma rays in a given location and a given period of time. The image is displayed on a cathode ray tube or stored in a computer. Radionuclide scanning is useful for examining bone and salivary gland tissue, as well as for investigating metabolic bone disorders, infection, and bone fractures.

SUGGESTED READINGS

Brooks SL: Computed tomography, Dent Clin North Am 37:575-590, 1993.

White SC, Pharoah MJ: Oral radiology: principles and interpretation, ed 5, St Louis, Mosby, 2004.

Winter AA, et al: Cone beam volumetric tomography vs. medical CT scanners, NY State Dent J 71:28-33, 2005.

CHAPTER 17

Quality Assurance

EDUCATIONAL OBJECTIVE

1. Know the steps necessary to uphold a quality-assurance program in the dental office to ensure radiographs of the highest quality with minimum exposure to patients and dental personnel.

KEY TERMS

American Academy of
    Oral and
    Maxillofacial
    Radiology (AAOMR)

darkroom maintenance
intraoffice peer review
quality-assurance
    program

record keeping
reference film
step wedge

One of the most important protocols in a dental office is a quality-assurance (QA) program. QA is a plan of action, concern, and responsibility to ensure that the x-ray images obtained in a dental office are of the highest quality, with minimal exposure to patients and dental personnel and resulting in the maximum diagnostic yield. An effective QA policy that monitors the use of radiation in a dental office is the shared responsibility of all members of the dental team. QA programs fall into the following categories: chairside technique; monitoring of x-ray equipment; and darkroom equipment and procedures. These protocols have different time intervals, varying from daily to yearly depending on the task.

CHAIRSIDE TECHNIQUE

Maintaining high levels of chairside competence is the basis of any successful QA program. Using programs of self-evaluation, intraoffice peer review, and continuing education, superior levels of chairside technique can be attained and retained, thus keeping retakes to a minimum. One should remember that every retake that is needed doubles the radiation to the patient for that image. The ultimate goal in dental radiography is to produce the most diagnostic radiographs with the least amount of radiation exposure to the patient. The "Criteria for Radiographs" given in Chapter 10 should be followed at all times. The task of reviewing radiographs can be assigned to any member of the office staff. The ability to accept criticism and perform self-criticism is an essential trait that must be developed. There is no place for such comments as, "All of my left molar projections are always cone cut (collimator cutoff)." At that point, one should ask for help and supervision instead of repeating the error. If one does not seek self-improvement, eventually this type of undiagnostic radiograph can become inappropriately acceptable. This type of imaging is useless and does the patient a disservice if committed repeatedly.

The dental professional is likely to be the person in a dental office who takes most of the radiographs. However, the concept of peer review also applies to the dentist when applicable. The American Academy of Oral and Maxillofacial Radiology (AAOMR) has published an outline of preventive procedures for radiographic systems. The monitoring, calibrating, and inspecting of the x-ray machine would be handled by some governmental agency that might charge an inspection and registration fee. In some areas a health physicist or a certified radiation equipment safety officer (CRESO) would perform the inspection. The type of inspection and calibration included in this group would be checks on kilovoltage peak, milliamperage, output, timer accuracy, tube head stability, and x-ray beam alignment (Figure 17-1).

In most dental practices the supportive staff is most likely to be responsible for certain procedures, which the AAOMR groups into seven categories.
1. Conducting proper chairside technique
2. Properly storing and handling all films, digital sensors, cassettes, screens, grids, and processing chemicals
3. Posting current technique charts, including a time-temperature chart for processing, x-ray exposure factors, x-ray equipment measurements, and darkroom maintenance schedules
4. Keeping accurate records of films processed, mounted, and filed
5. Maintaining proper conditions of processing tanks and automatic processors
6. Maintaining optimal darkroom conditions by periodic checks for light-tightness and adequacy of safelighting, cleanliness procedures, and temperature control of solutions

NEW YORK UNIVERSITY COLLEGE OF DENTISTRY

RADIOLOGY QUALITY-ASSURANCE PROGRAM

Type of Unit: _____

Location: _____

kVp: _____

mA: _____

HVL: _____ mm of Al

FFD: _____ in

Average Exposure Time (F-speed film) _____ impulses

Output (Emission Rate) _____ mR/s

Calibration Date _____ Performed By: _____

EXPOSURES WITH EKTASPEED FILMS

Maxillary Anteriors _____ Mandibular Anteriors _____

Maxillary Premolars _____ Mandibular Premolars _____

Maxillary Molars _____ Mandibular Molars _____

Bitewings _____
Occlusals _____

Calculation of Facial Dose: Add up all exposure times
Divide by 60
Multiply by Emission Rate

DO NOT REMOVE THIS NOTICE

Figure 17-1. | Form used to monitor dental x-ray machines.

7. Maintaining the conditions of protective devices such as lead aprons, thyroid collars, barriers, and film-holding devices

Also, it is the responsibility of the dental team to enforce the office infection control policy as it concerns chairside technique and film processing.

DARKROOM

An effective QA policy for the darkroom is the shared responsibility of the dentist and the dental professional. Regardless of whether manual or automatic processing is used, a QA program in the darkroom is as important as and much easier to conduct than monitoring of the x-ray machine. First, for a darkroom QA program to be effective, the darkroom must be a darkroom and nothing else. There should be no coffee brewers or snack tables, and the room should be a dedicated space rather than a place for general storage of hats and coats or for use as a dental laboratory.

At least monthly, and depending on the workload, the dental professional should check the safelighting, light-tightness, and accuracy of the timer and thermometer. If the processing tank lid is missing or the thermometer is broken, it should be noted and ordered. Charts showing when the various QA procedures were performed and by whom should be on the wall or in a darkroom log book (Figure 17-2). The dental professional should monitor the cleanliness of the countertops, the condition of the film hangers and clips, and the level and strength of the processing solutions.

The chemical strength and level of solutions in both manual tanks and automatic processors must be monitored on a daily basis. This is the most critical part of a QA program. Processing solutions should be changed every 2 to 3 weeks depending on usage. Both manual tanks and automatic processors should be cleaned at least weekly depending on the workload of the office staff. There are better ways to determine when solutions should be changed than by just using the calendar or "eyeballing."

An easy way to obtain a rough estimate of solution strength in a dental office is to compare it with a standard or reference film (Figure 17-3). A processed periapical film of ideal density should be kept taped to the darkroom viewbox for comparison of densities of the films that are processed daily. A lessening of film density in the processed film indicates a weakened solution and signals the need for a solution change. One should not wait until the films lose their diagnostic usefulness to change the processing solutions. That approach offers little comfort to the last patient whose x-rays were taken before the solution change whose films were deemed undiagnostic and needed to be retaken.

A better and more scientifically controlled way to make a test exposure is to use a step wedge at the beginning of each work day. This test exposure is done with a step wedge or a predetermined density (Figure 17-4). The film is then processed and compared with standard film densities. In the device shown in Figure 17-5, the processed film is placed in a slot, and the measured

Quality Control
Radiographic Processing Solution

Location _____   Month/Year _____

R = Replenished
CH = Changed Solution

Week Of	Monday	Tuesday	Wednesday	Thursday	Friday
	Maintenance	Maintenance	Maintenance	Maintenance	Maintenance
	Done by:	Done by:	Done by:	Done by:	Done by:
	Maintenance	Maintenance	Maintenance	Maintenance	Maintenance
	Done by:	Done by:	Done by:	Done by:	Done by:
	Maintenance	Maintenance	Maintenance	Maintenance	Maintenance
	Done by:	Done by:	Done by:	Done by:	Done by:
	Maintenance	Maintenance	Maintenance	Maintenance	Maintenance
	Done by:	Done by:	Done by:	Done by:	Done by:

Figure 17-2. Chart used to monitor processing solutions in the darkroom.

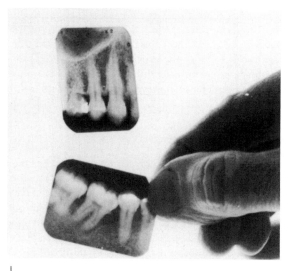

Figure 17-3. | Reference film used to check solution strength by comparing densities.

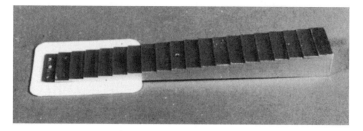

Figure 17-4. | Step wedge and film before exposure.

densities are moved until a visual match of densities is achieved. If the test densities are too light, the solutions are too weak or too cold. If the densities are too dark, the solutions are too concentrated or too warm. Either situation is unacceptable, and processing cannot begin until conditions are optimized. The strength of the fixer can be gauged by noting the time needed to clear films. Fresh, full-strength fixer clears films in 2 to 3 minutes. If clearing requires more than 4 minutes, the fixing solution is weak and should be changed. It follows that usually developer and fixer will need changing or replenishing at the same time.

Unexposed and unprocessed films as well as solutions should be stored in a cool, dry location. They never should be stored in an unventilated room near the heating system. Films should be stored at temperatures of 50°F to 70°F and between 40 and 60 relative humidity. Films should be used before their expiration date, and film boxes should be clearly marked. Older boxes should be placed on the front of the shelf in keeping with the "longest in, first out" rule.

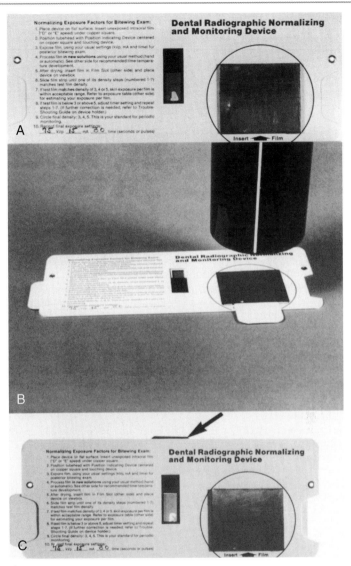

Figure 17-5. | **A,** Dental radiographic normalizing and monitoring device. **B,** Test film inserted beneath copper plate and exposure made. **C,** Processed test film (*arrow*) inserted in device and compared with numbered densities.

LEAD CONTAMINATION

Recently a potential source of lead exposure in the dental office has been identified. Although not common any longer, unexposed film was previously kept in the operatory in lead-lined boxes. Over time the lead used to line the shielded boxes may oxidize and produce a white lead powder that may contaminate the stored intraoral film. This powder is about 80% lead and may be ingested by patients and operators. Fortunately, most dental offices currently store film out of the operatory or use stable metal dispensers.

DIGITAL SENSORS

The digital sensors used with direct and indirect digital radiography must be handled with proper care and maintained in optimum condition. These efforts will ensure that they provide reliable service and adherence to infection control regulations.

The sensors used with direct digital radiography should be covered with barrier sheaths before use to prevent sensor contamination. The sensor cable is carefully uncoiled, and the operator is expected to remove all tangles and sharp bends from the cable. The operator is encouraged not to soak the sensor in sterile solution or place it in an autoclave. The sensor or cable should not be clamped with a hemostat. The dental professional should avoid stepping on or rolling over the cable with the operator chair. The sensor cable is to be gently coiled and placed in a protective case after use. The phosphor plates used with indirect digital radiography should also be covered with an infection control barrier before use. They are also not to be submerged in cold sterilizing solutions or autoclaved. All sensors are to be handled very carefully, and all effort should be made to maintain them in optimum condition to withstand years of successful daily use.

SUGGESTED READINGS

No authors listed: Recommendations for quality assurance in dental radiography, Oral Surg Oral Med Oral Pathol 55:421-426, 1983.

American Dental Association Council on Scientific Affairs: An update on radiographic practices: information and recommendations, J Am Dent Assoc 132:234-238, 2001.

Eastman Kodak Co.: Quality assurance in dental radiography, Rochester, NY, 1999, Health Science Division.

CHAPTER 18

Patient Management and Special Problems

EDUCATIONAL OBJECTIVES

1. Understand how to relate to patients in the dental environment.
2. Understand what special situations might arise in dental radiography and be able to deal with them clinically.
3. Be able to substitute alternative techniques in dental radiography when it is not possible to use the primary method.

===== KEY TERMS =====

arthrography
bedridden
buccal-object rule
disability
gag reflex
hearing impaired

localization
marking grid
physical disability
radiopaque medium
reverse bitewing
sialography

trismus
tube shift
visually impaired
wheelchair access

MANAGEMENT

Patient management is as important to all dental personnel as it is to the dentist. Patient psychology is a valuable tool in helping dental professionals perform their chairside duties. The dental team may be responsible for other patient management assignments, such as scheduling appointments, handling and screening telephone calls, and collecting fees. These duties also demand the use of patient psychology to manage patients successfully.

The dental professional encounters all types of personalities in the dental office. Some patients may be very apprehensive and tense about dental treatment, whereas others are calm and matter-of-fact. Some reveal their anxieties through behavioral and speech patterns; others may hide their anxieties.

Even with modern equipment, techniques, and attitudes, dentistry remains a stressful experience for some patients. As a profession, dentistry is still plagued by the image of the unpleasant experience. This image problem is reinforced in the public's mind by unfortunate representations on television and other media. Jokes and cartoons about dentistry raise the level of patient apprehension. It is within this societal context that dental professionals must endeavor to serve patients. With the modern technologies available and an emphasis on behavior, this goal can be met.

One of the important roles of the dental professional is to try to relax the patient—an accomplishment that makes the work easier. The dental hygienist or assistant may be the first member of the office staff to greet the patient in the reception area. Patients like to be recognized and greeted by name. However, to conform to the federal legislation (Health Insurance Portability and Accountability Act, HIPAA) patients should not be addressed by their last names to ensure privacy (see Chapter 25). It is especially important to greet new or current patients with "we shall be with you shortly" rather than "the dentist or hygienist will be with you shortly." "We" implies the team concept of treatment and stresses the importance of all of the constituents in the office, indicating that the whole dental team will take part in the active treatment.

In performing dental radiography, the dental professional also must develop a chairside manner. Patients must be made to feel comfortable and confident about the dental professional's ability to perform the radiographic examination.

In some dental offices it is routine for any of the dental professionals to perform the radiography. However, some patients may have never had dental professionals perform services and are accustomed to having the dentist do all of the procedures. These patients may be apprehensive and even object to the dental professional performing any service for them. Dental professionals should not take this attitude personally; they should regard it as a lack of patient orientation to new modes of treatment. If the patient objects strenuously, the dentist should be called in to reassure the patient. The dental professional should then perform the procedures.

As discussed in the preceding chapter, dental professionals strive for high clinical proficiency with efficient and confident work patterns. The dental professional can achieve these objectives through experience and critical evaluation by self, co-workers, and the dentist. The quality of the finished radiograph should be the same regardless of who performs the procedure. All members of the dental team should be held to the same standard of quality control.

When the dental professional is seating patients and draping them with the lead apron, some small talk may help to relax them. Patients want to know that the dental professional is interested in them and not just performing a mechanical procedure. This is not wasted time because a relaxed, confident patient is much easier to work with.

Appearance is very important. All infection control protocols must be followed. The dental professional should wear clean clothing and be well groomed. Fingernails should be kept short to avoid trauma to the patients' oral tissues. Hands should be washed; gloves, masks, protective eyewear and protective clothing worn; and the prescribed infection-control procedures followed after the patient is seated in the dental chair so that the patient can take note of these procedures. If one sneezes, coughs, picks up something from the floor, or has to leave the treatment room, regloving is mandatory before resuming work.

The dental professional should never chew gum while working with patients. If one must smoke (and as a dental professional one should not), remember that tobacco odor on the breath, hands, or clothing can be offensive to patients and co-workers. Mouthwash and hand lotions should be used to mask the tobacco residue before seeing patients. If the individual is wearing a lab coat, it should be removed during smoking. Remember, in fact, that tobacco counseling is actually now part of the dental professional's responsibility.

The dental professional should always explain to the patient what procedures are to be performed and how many films will be taken. Any questions the patient has should be answered if the dental professional feels capable of doing so. If the question involves diagnostic judgments or treatment planning that cannot be answered with confidence, it should be referred to the dentist. Patients often ask about the need for radiographs and the potential radiation risk. Because these questions are usually asked before work begins, a well-answered question will give the patient confidence and lessen apprehension about having the radiographs taken. Answers to questions of this type are found in this text, and the fears and concerns of the patient can be allayed by intelligent, meaningful answers.

The "light touch" of certain dentists and dental professionals is really nothing more than good technique and confidence developed with experience and respect for the oral tissues. No one is born with a "heavy hand"; thus there is no excuse for clumsy, uncomfortable intraoral radiographic technique.

Films and/or digital sensors must be placed in the patient's mouth, and directions must be given to the patient in a manner that indicates self-confidence. A patient likes to feel that the operator is in full control of the situation at all times. Instructions to the patient should be given in a firm but polite tone.

Dental professionals should encourage and praise patients for their cooperation. If a patient is not following instructions, such as by raising the head and altering occlusal plane orientation when necessary, the patient should be corrected. A dental professional should not accept improper patient position because of reticence about reminding patients about their movements.

Every patient is different, both in the anatomic configuration of the mouth and in physical and psychological makeup. This is the challenge of the profession: to perform one's duties and maintain standards of excellence even as the clinical situation changes. Through study, practice, and self-evaluation, these goals can be met.

PATIENTS WITH DISABILITIES AND SPECIAL NEEDS

Physical Disability

The challenges of treating the handicapped patient in the dental office vary according to the degree of *disability*. For example, the patient who has no digits or digital control cannot hold film packets in place, so a bite block or other film-holding device must be used. Because most radiographers use such devices routinely, this situation presents no problem.

The spastic patient with uncontrollable movements can present a problem. A parent, friend, or dental professional may need to hold the patient's head steady while the radiograph is taken. This person can wear lead gloves and a lead apron for radiation protection. The dental professional or the dentist, who constantly works with radiation, should never hold the patient and stand in or near the primary x-ray beam.

Developmental Disability

Patients who are mentally disabled or have other conditions, such as cerebral palsy or autism, present the greatest challenge. Remember, unless there is complete cooperation, the patient may move and render the radiograph useless. The degree of cooperation will vary among patients. Problem situations should be recognized immediately. Repeated attempts may only excite the patient, subject him or her to unnecessary radiation, and prove fruitless.

For a totally unmanageable patient or one with an extreme *physical disability*, radiographs may have to be taken with the patient under sedation or general anesthesia. These films are usually developed immediately or digital radiography is used, and the necessary dental procedures are performed while the patient is still anesthetized.

Mobility

With a patient confined to a wheelchair, it may be easier to radiograph in the wheelchair than to transfer the patient to the dental chair, as long as the patient's head can be positioned and supported. Most local building codes require *wheelchair access* to the dental operatory so that the x-ray machine and patient can be maneuvered into the proper relationship. Panoramic and extraoral projections are useful with this type of patient.

Bedridden Patients

Some homebound patients or those *bedridden* in hospitals and nursing homes may not be able to visit dental suites; their dental procedures and radiographs must be done at the bedside. Mobile dental x-ray units can be brought to the bed and radiographs taken. For the patient in the supine position, it is easier to use a film-holding device with a localizing ring. In treating a patient at home or at a site that does not have a dental x-ray unit, portable x-ray units can be adapted for dental use and assembled on site (Figure 18-1). If digital radiography is not available, then a small, portable rapid processing tank also should be brought along so that the radiographs can be processed and the patient treated during the same visit.

With the introduction of the hand-held portable dental x-ray machine, it is now possible to produce images of equal quality to previous bite block or film alignment systems. At this time the most popular of these systems is the Nomad (Figure 18-2). With this system, the film or sensor is placed in the patient's mouth while the exposure is made. The operator, while holding the device, directs it at the film in the patient's mouth and exposes the film. The use of this device raises the question of increased radiation exposure to both the patient and the operator. As a result of this technique, the patient is exposed to an increase in scatter radiation. The proponents of this technique claim that the noncompromised image placement and better image offsets the resulting increase in patient exposure. They also feel that the law of ALARA is still valid. Some states allow the use of this new device in certain clinical situations and with certain patients. Others are in the process of evaluation and are issuing temporary permits for its use. However, the operator is not 6 ft away from the source of radiation and is also not behind an acceptable barrier as described in Chapter 7.

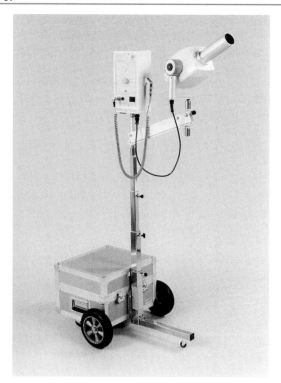

Figure 18-1. Siemens Portaray transportable x-ray examination unit. *(Courtesy M-DEC Corporation, Bellevue, WA.)*

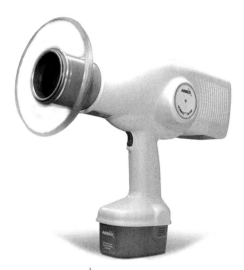

Figure 18-2. Nomad portable x-ray unit.

Hearing Impairment

The obvious challenge in treating *hearing-impaired* or deaf patients is communication, as well as realization by the operator of the disability and how it may modify usual procedures. For example, the often-used command to the patient to "hold still" as the operator leaves the room to make an exposure is not applicable for patients with a hearing impairment. Depending on the patient's method of communication, instructions may have to be given through sign language or in writing. Deaf patients can usually read lips, but the operator must be sure to remove his or her mask and always face the patient.

Vision Impairment

Visually impaired patients may have to be escorted into the operatory and directed or assisted into the dental chair. Because these patients cannot see what is going on, it is essential that the patient be kept informed of the treatment being rendered and why it is necessary. Patient education is extremely important. The dental professional must remember that the patient may have never seen a radiograph, so the explanation may require extra time and thought. In giving an explanation, pointing to an area on a radiograph is useless and only reminds the patient of the disability. Common sense and an awareness of the disability are all that is needed to treat visually impaired patients.

PEDIATRIC PATIENTS

The number and timing of radiographs for pediatric patients is discussed in Chapter 10. Dental radiography requires the complete cooperation of the patient. If the patient moves, the radiographic image is blurred and the film rendered useless. In no other area of dentistry is this absolute cooperation so necessary. If a child moves during an operative dentistry procedure, the dentist can compensate. In radiography the patient must hold still while the exposure is made. The unknown is frightening to any child, and very few children know anything about x-rays. In fact, the dental radiograph may be their first introduction to radiography. The procedure must be explained to the child in terms the child can understand. One should talk of taking a "picture" of the tooth with a "camera." Remind children that they must hold still when the picture is taken. Show children the film packet and let them put it in their mouths. Taking a picture of the child's thumb is a good way to introduce the concept of holding still and to assure the child that he or she will feel nothing when the tooth is radiographed. Of course, the x-ray machine is off when these thumb exposures are made.

Children like to see pictures, and it is sometimes helpful to show them what a radiograph of a tooth looks like. The dental professional should follow up with a promise to show them what their teeth look like on the finished radiograph. In certain instances children have even been taken into the darkroom and allowed to help process the films. Children are fascinated by the darkroom with its tanks, automatic processing machines, and chemicals. Any effort expended to relax children and make them feel at ease will reap benefits at later appointments. If there is lack of cooperation and there is no emergency that requires immediate treatment, radiographs may be postponed to a second visit, in which the children may be more cooperative as they get to feel more at home in the dental office.

Children usually tolerate periapical films, and the film can be held in place with a bite block or any film-holding device to do either the paralleling or bisecting technique. In children it is acceptable to use the bisecting technique because dimensional distortion is not critical. If the child resists periapical film placement, have the patient bite on the film and increase the vertical angulation to bisect the angle so that the procedure resembles an occlusal projection (Figure 18-3). This type of film is not as desirable as that obtained by the regular technique, but it is better than no film at all. This method will work for any area of the child's mouth, and a full-mouth series can be taken this way if necessary. Either adult-size or occlusal film can be used for this technique (Figure 18-4).

Reverse Bitewings

Some children will not tolerate placement of the bitewing film. When instructed to close on the tab, they push the lower part of the film out of the floor of the mouth with their tongue and then close their teeth on the film. If after repeated attempts proper placement meets with failure, a *reverse bitewing* technique can be substituted. In this method, the film packet is placed

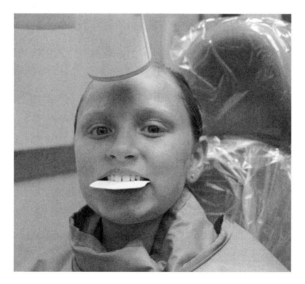

Figure 18-3. | Technique for periapical films that allows a child to bite on film. Note the increase in vertical angulation.

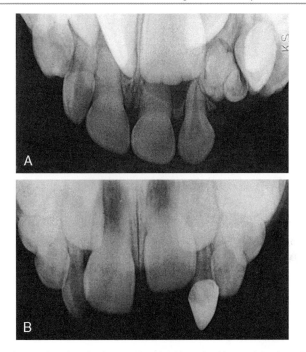

Figure 18-4. Radiographs taken by having the child bite the film packet. **A,** Adult-size periapical film packet (note odontoma blocking tooth eruption). **B,** Occlusal film.

on the cheek side of the teeth in the buccal sulcus (Figure 18-5). The child bites on the tab to hold the film packet in place, and the radiographer can position the film packet as the patient closes, without the hazard of being bitten. The x-ray beam is directed extraorally from under the opposite side of the mandible as in a lateral oblique projection (Figure 18-6). The exposure time must be increased by a factor of 4 or 5 because of the increased focal-film distance (FFD). The resulting film will not have the detail of an intraoral bitewing radiograph but will be a useful substitute (Figure 18-7).

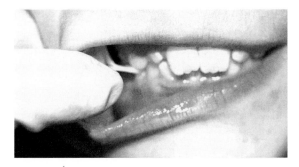

Figure 18-5. Film placement for a reverse bitewing radiograph.

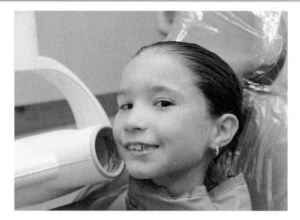

Figure 18-6. Tube position for reverse bitewing radiograph. Note that central ray is directed from underneath mandible of opposite side while being aimed at bitewing film.

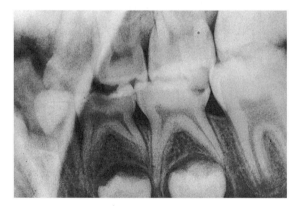

Figure 18-7. Reverse bitewing radiograph.

If intraoral film placement is not possible for the child, an extraoral film can be substituted. The view that is most diagnostic is also a slight variation of the lateral oblique technique. The cassette is positioned in the usual way, but the central ray is directed from behind the angle of the mandible on the opposite side (Figure 18-8). Again, the radiograph is not as diagnostic as an intraoral film but is better than none (Figure 18-9).

If there is no extraoral cassette in the office, a piece of occlusal film can be substituted but with the resulting increase of radiation exposure to the patient (Figure 18-10). An exposure time of nearly 1.5 second will be necessary because of the increased FFD. The radiograph produced will be of some diagnostic value (Figure 18-11). Box 18-1 provides tips to help a dental professional take radiographs of a pediatric patient.

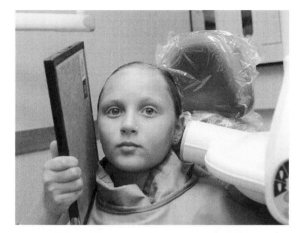

Figure 18-8. Lateral oblique technique for detecting caries and pathologic conditions in children. Note that the central ray is aimed from behind angle of mandible on opposite side.

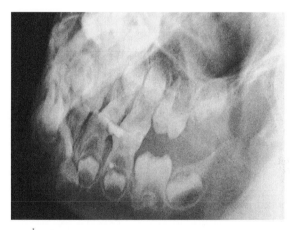

Figure 18-9. Radiograph taken through use of the lateral oblique technique.

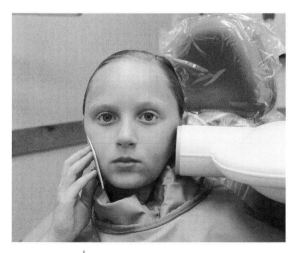

Figure 18-10. Occlusal film packet used as extraoral film.

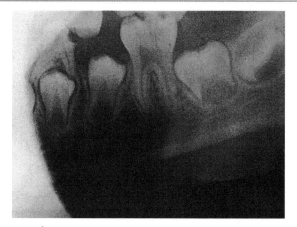

Figure 18-11. │ Radiograph made by using occlusal film packet extraorally.

Box 18-1	Helpful Hints for Radiographing the Pediatric Patient

1. Be confident. Most children react favorably to the authority of a confident and capable operator. The dental professional must secure the child's confidence, trust, and cooperation. In addition, the dental professional must be patient and must not rush through the radiographic procedures.
2. Show and tell. The typical pediatric patient is curious. The dental professional can use a "show and tell" approach to prepare the patient for radiographic procedures. Before beginning the procedure, the operator can show the child the equipment and materials that will be used and tell him or her what will happen. The child should be encouraged to touch the tube head, film holder, and lead apron.
3. Reassure the patient. Children usually fear the unknown. The operator should reassure the patient and allay any fears he or she may have about the procedures to prevent the uncooperative behavior of a frightened child.
4. Demonstrate behavior. The operator should demonstrate the desired behavior to show the child exactly what to do. For example, the radiographer can demonstrate "how to hold still" and then ask the child to do the same thing.
5. Request assistance. If a child cannot hold still or stabilize the film, the dental professional can ask the parent or accompanying adult to provide assistance. The adult can hold the film or the child during the exposure while wearing a lead glove, apron, and thyroid collar.
6. Postpone the examination. Only in emergencies and under general anesthesia should a child be forced to undergo a radiographic examination. It is much better to postpone the examination until the second or third visit rather than instill a fear of visiting the dental office.

SPECIAL PROBLEMS

Gagging

Of all the problems one may encounter in intraoral radiography, gagging is probably the most troublesome. Gagging, more properly referred to as the *gag reflex*, is a body defense mechanism. The coughing and retching produced in the gag reflex are meant to expel any foreign body from the throat and thus protect the airway from obstruction. An anesthesiologist never leaves a patient after surgery with a general anesthetic until the patient is awake and the gag reflex is restored. At this point the patient can expel any mucus or other material that might obstruct the air passage because of the action of the gag reflex. All patients have gag reflexes, with some more active than others.

The two types of stimuli for the gag reflex are psychogenic and tactile. Some patients start to feel the reflex coming on just by thinking about or anticipating the film placement. The areas that are most sensitive to tactile stimuli producing the gag reflex are the palate, base of the tongue, and posterior wall of the pharynx. Gagging occurs most often during exposure of the maxillary molar projection. The level of excitation of these reflexes varies from person to person. The patient with a low threshold for stimulation of the gag reflex presents a problem in intraoral radiography.

Very few patients, probably fewer than 0.1%, have a gag reflex so active that intraoral radiography is impossible. With this in mind, how does one deal with the remaining 99.9%? Following are a set of generally accepted suggestions and techniques that can be used to prevent gagging and overcome it when it occurs. Not all techniques are applicable, nor will they prove successful with every patient. One must be able to determine which technique best suits the individual patient. Studies have shown that the technique, authority, and self-confidence of the operator are major factors in preventing and suppressing gag reflexes during dental radiography.

Attitude

The operator should always maintain the appearance of being in control of the situation. The patient wants to believe that the operator is so competent that it would be impossible for the film to slip and lodge in the throat. Firm positioning of the film holder with decisive instructions to the patient and proper body language are all necessary.

Think positively: Never mention the possibility of gagging. The worst thing the operator can say to a patient is, "This won't make you gag" or "Do you gag?" The patient may never have thought of gagging until reminded of the possibility.

Film Order and Technique

When taking a full-mouth radiographic survey, one should start in the maxilla, taking the anterior films first and working posteriorly. The film placement in the maxillary molar area is the one most likely to excite the gag reflex. Once the reflex is excited, the patient may continue to gag even on anterior films.

When placing the film in the patient's mouth for maxillary molars and premolars, one should not slide the film along the palate. The film is placed in the desired position near the lingual surface of the teeth, and then with one decisive motion the film is brought into contact with the palate.

The exposure timing dial for the desired exposure is always set before the film is placed in the patient's mouth. The tube head is positioned on the side of the patient's face that is to be radiographed, with the position-indicating device (PID) at the approximate vertical angulation. The object is to minimize the amount of time the film packet has to remain in the patient's mouth. Preparations like these can save valuable seconds and lessen the likelihood of the patient's gagging. Generally the longer the film stays in the mouth, the greater is the likelihood of gagging.

Deep Breathing

It is often helpful to instruct the patient to take deep breaths through the nose as the film packet is placed in a gag-sensitive area, such as the palate. Why this works is debatable, but it may be that breathing through the nose prevents the rush of air across the sensitive tissues of the palate. Another explanation is that it gives the patient something to do and distracts him or her from thinking about gagging. The operator should use a firm tone of voice when instructing the patient to take these deep breaths and also may take some audible deep breaths to encourage the patient to do likewise. It is also advisable to instruct the patient to keep his or her eyes open during the procedure. This serves as a distraction as well, keeping the patient's mind off gagging.

Bite Blocks and Film-Holding Devices

Any film-holding device that requires the patient to bite and maintain pressure also may help to prevent gagging. Again, the patient is given something positive to do. Another tactile sensation, that of biting and the pressure of the bite block against the teeth, may distract the patient from thoughts of gagging. Finger-holding film techniques, which are not recommended for other reasons, tend to excite the gag reflex more than film-holding devices.

Lozenges, Gargles, and Sprays

Lozenges, gargles, and sprays may be of some help in certain situations. The key is that the patient be made to believe that the medication will have an effect. In some instances a patient was given a vitamin pill as an "antigag pill." The patient was told in advance what the pill would do, and the rate of success was very high. This placebo effect is seen also in many other areas of dental practice. Note, however, that the patient was told what would be the effect of the placebo medication.

Many viscous topical anesthetics are available for rinsing the mouth, gargling, or spraying the palate to produce a numbing sensation, intended to block the gag reflex.

An undiluted mouthwash with high alcohol concentration may have some anesthetic effects on the palate. Many cough lozenges contain some local anesthetic; having the patient suck on a lozenge before radiography may be helpful. In all these cases, it may not be so much the anesthetic vehicle used as the manner of presentation to the patient that produces the desired results.

Hypnosis

Although the practice of hypnosis is out of the province of the dental professional, its use in dentistry should be mentioned. In intractable gaggers, hypnosis by trained, competent practitioners may be necessary to permit intraoral radiography.

Convincing a patient that something (such as gagging) may not occur can be considered a form of hypnosis. An application of this principle is to tell gagging patients that the antigag nerve located in their neck is going to be pressed. There is no antigag nerve, but the patient may not know this. If the area in the neck is pressed hard, some sensation will result and the patient may become convinced that gagging will not occur. The power of suggestion often serves to foster the patient's mind control over the matter at hand.

Salt

One of the more amusing techniques described in the literature to stop gagging is to place ordinary table salt on the tip of the tongue of the gagging patient. The salt is placed in the palm of the patient's hand, and he or she is asked to touch the tip of the tongue to the salt and then raise the tongue to touch the palate. This method may be worth trying at least once in one's professional career.

For the intractable gagger, when all else fails, one must then resort to accessory techniques. Panoramic films and extraoral projections, previously discussed, because of their extraoral film placement will circumvent the gag reflex.

Localization Problems

Standard intraoral periapical and bitewing films show the teeth and bone in only two planes: superoinferior and anteroposterior. However, many clinical situations require a proper radiographic diagnosis to establish the position of structures in the buccolingual plane. Clinical examples include localization of impactions, foreign bodies, and areas of pathologic findings, as well as differentiating buccal and palatal roots in endodontic procedures (Figures 18-12 and 18-13). This information is essential to the dentist before any treatment can be instituted.

The four techniques that can be used for localization are (1) definition evaluation, (2) tube shift, (3) right-angle technique, and (4) pantomography.

Definition Evaluation

Structures that lie closer to the x-ray film have better radiographic definition than those that are farther from the film. This is true for both intraoral and extraoral films. It is sometimes possible, depending on the quality of the

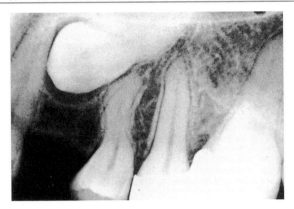

Figure 18-12. | Impacted maxillary canine. Is the tooth positioned buccally or palatally to the alveolar ridge?

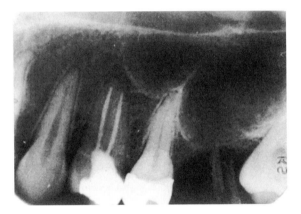

Figure 18-13. | Maxillary first premolar with endodontic filling. Which canal is buccal, and which is palatal?

radiograph, to determine the relative position of superimposed structures by determining which has better radiographic definition. Because intraoral film is positioned lingually in the patient's mouth, the superimposed structure that is more sharply defined is positioned lingually in relation to the other structures (Figure 18-14). An advantage of this technique, when compared with the others that follow, is that it requires no further x-ray exposures of the patient. It is, however, the least reliable of the techniques mentioned and is not recommended.

Tube Shift

The *tube shift* method uses what is referred to as *Clark's rule*, or the *buccal-object rule* (Figures 18-15 and 18-16). Its advantage to the practitioner is that it can be accomplished by using standard periapical technique. To determine the relative buccolingual relationship between two structures that appear

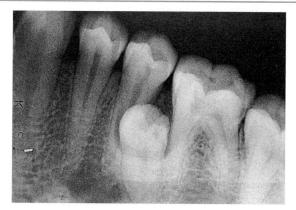

Figure 18-14. Localization by definition. Is the impacted supernumerary tooth more clearly defined than the rest of the teeth? If not, it is probably positioned buccally.

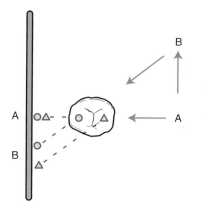

Figure 18-15. Buccal-object rule. As the tube position is shifted mesially (position *B*), the buccal object is seen to move relatively in the opposite direction, distally.

radiographically superimposed, a second radiograph is taken with a different horizontal angulation. All factors remain the same for the second exposure, except that the tube is shifted about 20 degrees either mesially or distally. The point of entry, film position, and vertical angulation remain the same as in the previous film. When the two radiographs are compared, the buccal object will appear to have moved in the opposite direction from the direction of the tube shift when compared with other structures on the radiograph (Figures 18-15 and 18-16). If the tube is shifted mesially by changing the horizontal angulation, the buccal object will appear to have moved distally. Conversely a distal shift will result in the more buccal object moving mesially. This can be demonstrated on the fingers, by holding the hand so that the second and third fingers are superimposed when sighting them from the side. Move the head either to the left or to the right (mesially or distally) and imagine the images of the

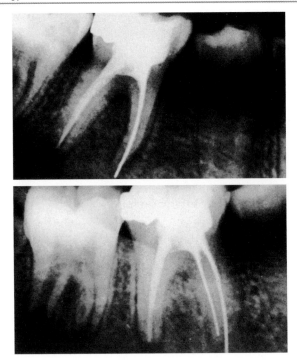

Figure 18-16. Radiographs illustrating the buccal-object rule. The tube in (B) was shifted mesially, indicating that the short endodontic point is in the mesiobuccal canal.

fingers being recorded on the film. Two distinct fingers can now be seen, and not the fingers superimposed. Now apply the buccal-object rule. The key phrase is "same lingual, opposite buccal"; the acronym is SLOB. This procedure can also be applied to objects for use in the superior inferior plane.

Right-Angle Technique
The right-angle technique uses two projections taken at right angles to each other—first a periapical film and then an occlusal film of the same area, for example. The planes radiographed are at right angles to each other. The occlusal techniques and examples are discussed in Chapter 11.

Pantomography
The redundant images produced in the anterior region by some older-model pantomographic units, such as the Panorex, can be used to localize objects in repeated areas. In viewing the film, the object in question will be seen twice (once on each half of the film). A recommended technique is to compare the relative movement of the object with adjacent structures from one side of the film to the other with the direction that the clinician reads the film (e.g., left to right). The object will seem to have moved in the same direction as the clinician's viewing movement if it is lingually positioned and in the opposite direction if it is on the buccal side (Figure 18-17).

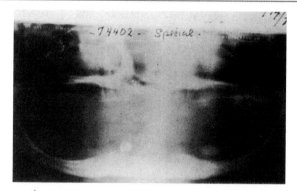

Figure 18-17. | Localization of an object by pantomographic redundant image.

Third Molar Problems

The third molars are in an area of the mouth that is difficult to radiograph. In many cases it may not be possible to position the film packet intraorally to visualize these areas adequately on radiographs. This is especially true if the teeth are impacted. In these cases it may be necessary to use the extraoral and panoramic techniques described in Chapters 12 and 13. The entire third molar area must be seen to make a complete diagnosis. This means that the entire tooth and at least 3 mm of surrounding bone in every direction must be imaged. If it cannot be seen on periapical films, other methods must be used.

Maxilla

As the film is placed more and more distally toward the patient's throat, the likelihood of exciting the gag reflex increases. It may be helpful to hold the film packet with a hemostat to maintain a minimum of contact with the palate. The film packet should be kept as parallel to the palatal vault as possible. To avoid distortion, the vertical angulation must be increased, with the resulting relationship of the central ray to the film packet looking very much like an occlusal projection.

Mandible

The most common difficulty in radiographing lower third molars is the inability to place the film packet distal enough to record the image of the whole tooth and root structure. This placement is prevented by the muscles of the floor of the mouth and tongue. To overcome this problem, the tongue can be deflected to the opposite side of the mouth by the operator's finger or a mouth mirror. The floor of the mouth is gently depressed, almost massaged, to relax the mylohyoid muscle. While this is being done, the film packet is slid along the lingual surface of the mandible as far distally as possible. In certain horizontal impactions of the mandible, it may be necessary to distort the image in the horizontal plane to visualize the entire tooth with intraoral radiography. This is done by changing the horizontal angulation of the x-ray beam so that it is not at right angles to the film packet, which is the usual procedure. Instead the beam comes from the distal side and the central ray makes an acute angle with the film.

Film Placement Problems

Narrow Arch
In some mouths it may be impossible to place anterior film packets properly without excessive bending, with resultant distortion of the radiographic image. This is a major problem when using direct digital radiography with its rigid sensor. The best way to overcome this problem is to vary the film size. The #1 narrow anterior film is recommended, although it may be necessary to use #0. There is no rule stating that one cannot use different-sized intraoral packets in the same full-mouth series. A possible problem with using a smaller film is in mounting the films specifically with a cardboard mount. The smaller or narrower films must be attached to the mount by cellophane tape or staples so that they do not slip from the window in the mount. Pediatric or narrow film may be used as the situation dictates (Figure 18-18).

If radiographs show overlapping teeth, especially in the anterior region, it does not necessarily indicate that the films were taken improperly. If the teeth are overlapped in the mouth, they appear overlapped radiographically.

Shallow Palate
The shallow palatal vault presents a problem in the paralleling technique. Fortunately this does not occur so often and severely that the bony structures make it impossible to place the film packet parallel to the long axis of the tooth

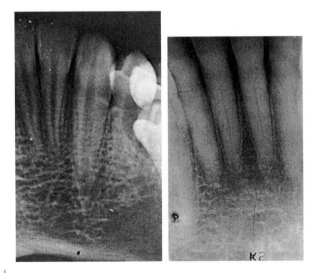

Figure 18-18. Periapical radiographs of lower anterior region using narrow anterior (#1) film seen on left and pediatric size (#0) film seen on right.

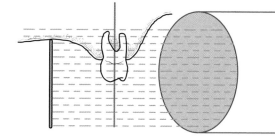
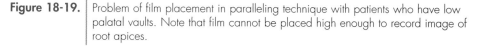

Figure 18-19. Problem of film placement in paralleling technique with patients who have low palatal vaults. Note that film cannot be placed high enough to record image of root apices.

and high enough to record the radiographic image (Figure 18-19). In these rare cases the bisecting-angle technique may be the better choice. Before changing techniques, one should always check to see that the film is in the midline where there is the greatest palatal height. The number of times that the paralleling technique cannot be used is quite small.

The bisecting-angle technique compensates for the shallow palate by increasing the vertical angulation. The film packet must be in the patient's mouth with a 3-mm border projecting beneath the incisal or occlusal edge of the teeth and the central ray bisecting the angle formed between the film packet and the long axis of the tooth (Figure 18-20). As an alternative, the operator may choose to change the film packet size.

Lingual Frenulum
It is extremely difficult to radiograph patients who have a large, tight, lingual frenulum attached close to the tip of the tongue. These patients are sometimes referred to as "tongue-tied" because they cannot protrude their tongues very far out of their mouths.

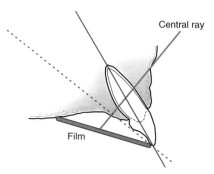

Central ray

Film

Figure 18-20. Vertical angulation overcomes the problem of a low palatal vault in the bisecting-angle technique.

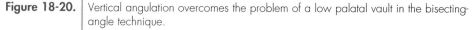

The paralleling technique is not the method of choice for these patients because the tight frenulum does not allow placement of the film packet deep in the floor of the mouth. One option is to use the bisecting technique. Because the film cannot be placed very deep in the mouth, negative vertical angulations in the range of −40 to −60 degrees can be expected. Another option is to hold the film at an angle and as the patient starts to close and the mylohyoid muscle relaxes, to slowly place the film in a more upright, parallel position.

Tori

The maxillary torus (torus palatinus), if present, usually causes no problems in periapical radiography. It is located posteriorly in the midline of the palate and does not hinder periapical film placement. The best way to radiograph a torus palatinus is by use of an occlusal projection.

The mandibular tori, or torus as the case may be, are located on the lingual aspect of the mandible in the premolar area. Their presence prevents the placement of the film packet in its usual position. This difficulty is more accentuated in the bisecting-angle technique than in the paralleling technique. The film packet cannot be depressed into the floor of the mouth and still be kept close to the lingual surface of the teeth. The only possible solution is to place the film over the torus. This increases the angle between the film packet and the long axis of the tooth; increasing the vertical angulation to bisect the angle compensates for the change. In the paralleling method with its increased object-film distances, the film is positioned behind the tori.

Canine Overlap

Overlapping the image of the mesial portion of the maxillary first premolar with the image of the distal surface of the canine is a common problem. The overlapping is caused by the large palatal cusp of the first premolar. The problem can be solved by changing the horizontal angulation so that the central ray comes more from the distal side, as in a premolar periapical projection (see Figure 18-22). Then the palatal cusp is not superimposed. Overlapping does not occur in the mandible because the first premolar has a very small lingual cusp.

Trismus

Trismus is the condition in which a patient is unable to open his or her mouth. It may be partial or complete and is usually caused by infection or trauma. To make an adequate diagnosis and identify the infected tooth or area, radiographs are necessary. If the patient's mouth cannot be opened at all, extraoral or panoramic films are necessary. If there is partial opening, it may be possible to place an intraoral film by modifying the usual technique. A hemostat is used to hold the film packet because it is much narrower than a finger or any other film-holding device. The film packet is placed in the mouth by sliding it between the partially opened anterior teeth in the horizontal plane. Once beyond the teeth, the film can be turned to its proper vertical orientation.

If possible, the patient then holds the hemostat with the film packet attached to it in position while the exposure is made.

Endodontic Problems

In patients undergoing endodontic treatment, it is necessary to take working and measurement films while the rubber dam is in place. The bisecting method can be used, with the patient supporting the film packet under the rubber dam with a finger or bite block, but it is not recommended. Using the paralleling method with the dam in place is difficult because of the lack of working space in the mouth and the patient's inability to bite on any film-holding device, because of the presence of the rubber dam clamp and protruding endodontic files from the tooth. The best course is to disengage the rubber dam frame, keeping the saliva ejector in place, and position the film packet in a hemostat or "Snap-a-Ray" parallel to the tooth and held by the patient. This is especially true for digital radiography in which the sensor is thicker and more rigid than film. Care should be taken with the sensor-holding device not to damage the fragile sensor. There are special angled film-holding devices with localizing rings made specifically for endodontic radiography (Figure 18-21).

Plastic rubber dam frames and saliva ejectors should be used to prevent superimposition of their images on the radiograph (Figure 18-23). Punching a hole in a predetermined corner of the dam makes it easier to reorient the dam in the frame once the exposure has been made.

To save time and not have the patient sit in the chair with the rubber dam in place, rapid processing, as discussed in Chapter 8, can minimize working time and can be adequately diagnostic in endodontic working films.

Digital radiography with its instantaneous image formation is a very fast and effective approach to endodontic radiography. The working image is obtained quickly and is stored for archival life.

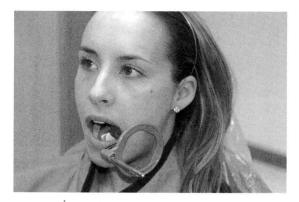

Figure 18-21. | Endodontic film-holding device with localizing ring.

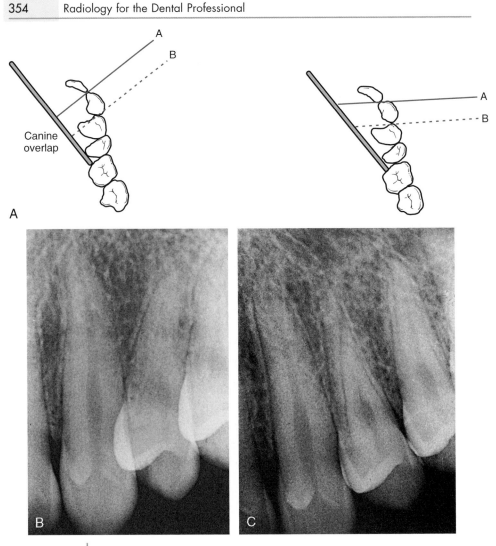

Figure 18-22. **A,** Changing horizontal angulation to prevent distal overlap of maxillary canine. **B,** Overlapped canine. **C,** Overlapping eliminated.

Grid Measurement

Some dentists use grid markings to quantify and evaluate bone levels or for endodontic measurements. Intraoral measurement grids are available that superimpose thin radiopaque or radiolucent lines in the vertical and horizontal planes in 1-mm gradations (Figures 18-24 and 18-25). The *marking grid* is affixed to the front of the film packet when the exposure is made. One manufacturer makes film packets with the grid markings incorporated into the film packet. No increase in exposure is necessary with the use of the marking grid, and the films are processed in the usual manner. The measurement or marking grid should not be confused with the grid used in extraoral projections (see Chapter 13) to absorb object scatter. Furthermore, in digital radiography

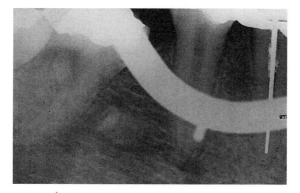

Figure 18-23. | Radiograph with superimposition of rubber dam frame.

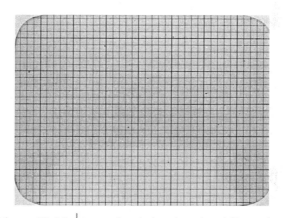

Figure 18-24. | Intraoral grid placed on dental film packet.

endodontic measurement is easily accomplished directly through use of the corresponding computer program.

Radiopaque Media

The use of *radiopaque media* has many applications in dental practice. It is used routinely in endodontics, with the radiopaque file, to determine root length. Gutta-percha or silver points can be placed in periodontal soft tissue pockets to determine pocket depth and direction. Fistulous tracts can be traced to their origin using thin, flexible wire or gutta-percha points (Figure 18-26).

The technique of *sialography* involves injecting radiopaque media into salivary ducts and glands and then visualizing these soft tissues radiographically. This method is used in diagnosing ductal and glandular obstructions, salivary stones, infections, and tumors of the major salivary glands. The contrast medium used is usually an iodine-containing formula in either an aqueous or oil suspension (Figure 18-27). Contrast media are also used in radiographing the temporomandibular joint to visualize the articular disk, a procedure called arthrography (Figure 18-28). Because the disk is fibrocartilage, it is not seen

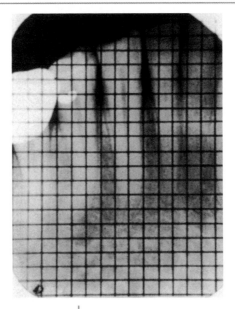

Figure 18-25. │ Radiograph with grid markings.

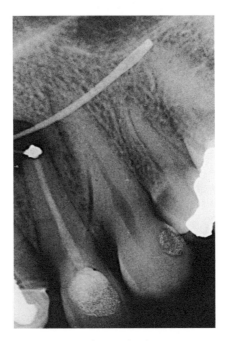

Figure 18-26. │ Fistulous tract traced back from palatal opening to its origin by insertion of gutta-percha point.

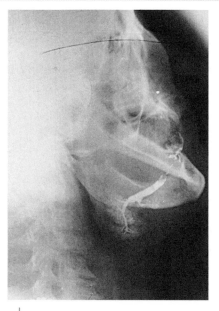

Figure 18-27. Sialograph outlining submandibular duct and gland.

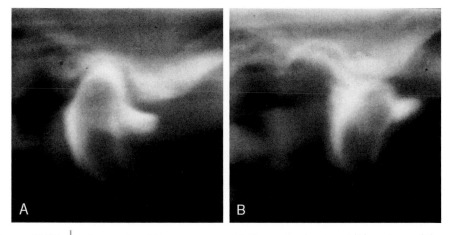

Figure 18-28. Arthrography of the temporomandibular joint in the closed **(A)** and open **(B)** positions. Note the radiolucent space between radiopaque areas that represents the articular disk.

on radiographs, but if a radiopaque medium is injected into the upper and lower joint spaces, then the void between them represents the articular disk (see Chapter 14).

SUGGESTED READINGS
Sewrine I: Gagging in dental radiography, Oral Surg Oral Med Oral Pathol 58:725-728, 1984.

CHAPTER 19

Film Mounting and Radiographic Anatomy

EDUCATIONAL OBJECTIVES

1. Understand what determines the radiographic appearance of teeth and the alveolar processes of the maxilla and mandible.
2. Recognize radiographic landmarks of the mandible and maxilla as seen on periapical and bitewing films.
3. Recognize normal radiographic anatomy seen on panoramic and occlusal films.

KEY TERMS

alveolar bone
alveolar crest
anterior nasal spine
anterior palatine foramen
arch
bone marrow
buccinator shadow
cancellous bone
cementum
concavity

concha
coronoid process
cortical bone
dentin
enamel
external oblique ridge
floor of the maxillary sinus
floor of the nasal cavity
foramen
fossa

genial tubercle
hamular notch
hamular process
hamulus
incisive foramen
internal alveolar canal
internal oblique ridge
labial mounting
lamina dura
lateral fossa

lingual foramen

lingual mounting

mandibular canal

maxillary sinus

maxillary tuberosity

median palatine suture

medullary spaces

mental foramen

mental ridge

mounts

mylohyoid ridge

nasal cavity

nasal septum

nutrient canals

periodontal ligament

pulp canal

pulp chamber

ridge

septa

sinus

submandibular fossa

trabeculae

tuberosity

viewbox

x-ray

zygoma

zygomatic process

The mounting of processed dental radiographs is another important function of the dental professional. It is much easier to view and diagnose radiographs when the films are placed in mounts in their proper anatomic orientation than it is to look at them on a film hanger or sort them from an envelope. Properly mounted films make charting and examination a more orderly procedure. The mounted films are kept with or in the patient's chart, and at each subsequent visit the radiographs are placed on the viewbox for the dentist's referral. Care should be taken not to handle the mounted radiographs or the chart with contaminated gloves.

The finished radiographs are identified and oriented as to the position in the mouth by the raised portion of the dot, tooth, and bony structures visible on each film. A thorough understanding of radiographic anatomy makes mounting an interesting and challenging procedure, not one that is done automatically. Mistakes are made and the work becomes tedious when the dental professional has no basic understanding of radiographic anatomy.

DESCRIPTIVE TERMINOLOGY

Because this chapter deals with the processed radiograph in mounting and interpretation, certain terms are needed to describe the shades of black, white, and gray that appear. The appearance of any area (e.g., tooth, bone) on a radiograph is determined by the density of that area, the quality of the x-ray photons, and hence the penetration of the x-ray beam that reaches the film. With these terms, one can more accurately describe the radiographic findings. The black areas, where there is greater penetration of x-rays that reach the radiographs, are called radiolucent (RL), and the white areas, where there is little or no penetration, are called radiopaque (RO). All structures are either radiolucent or radiopaque, but each category includes gradations. For instance, metallic fillings are more radiopaque than enamel, but both are still radiopaque. Caries appear radiolucent because the decay causes a lessening of density when compared with enamel and dentin.

One should never refer to a radiograph as an x-ray. One may say "x-ray film" or better still, "radiograph," but the term *x-ray* should be used only when referring to the beam of energy that is aimed at the film packet in the patient's mouth. The film then is processed to produce a radiograph.

MOUNTS

Various types of dental film mounts are available. *Mounts* are made for both pedodontic and adult surveys and come with a full range of numbers of windows (Figure 19-1). In addition to full-survey mounts, single-film, double-film, and bitewing survey mounts are also available (Figure 19-2). In digital imaging the arrangement of the images is determined by the digital template

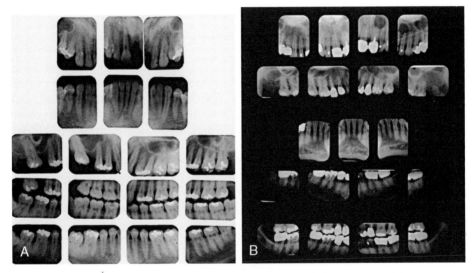

Figure 19-1. Full-mouth series mounted in clear celluloid (**A**) and opaque (**B**) mounts.

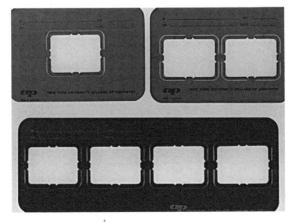

Figure 19-2. Bitewing and single-film mounts.

selected. Film mounts usually are made of cardboard or a celluloid-like material. The overall size and shape of the mount are made to fit the various types of view boxes found in dental offices. The area around the film windows may be clear or opaque. The opaque mounts are preferred because the light is concentrated behind the radiographs and viewing is easier and more diagnostic. If the number of radiographs taken does not fill the mounts, the unused windows should be covered to prevent the light from distracting the viewer. The black opaque wrapper from the periapical film packet is ideal for this because it is the correct color and size and is easily placed in the mount.

The patient's name, chart number (if applicable), date, and number of films taken (optional) must be recorded on each mount.

MOUNTING

Placement of the radiographs in their correct position in the mounts may seem baffling at first. However, if one develops a system based on understanding, this problem can be mastered in a short time. The operator must always work on a clean, dry, light-colored tabletop so that he or she can see the radiographs easily when they are laid out. The radiographs are viewed on an illuminator or *viewbox* placed on or in front of the surface where the mounting is being done.

Every radiograph has an embossed or raised dot to help indicate the film orientation. The film packet is placed in the patient's mouth so that the side with the dot is always nearest the occlusal or incisal surfaces of the teeth. Manufacturers position the film in the packet so that the raised portion of the dot faces the x-ray machine when the exposure is made (Figure 19-3).

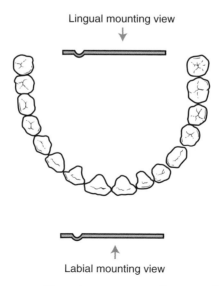

Lingual mounting view

Labial mounting view

Figure 19-3. | Raised dot on x-ray film and its orientation in film mounts for labial or lingual viewing.

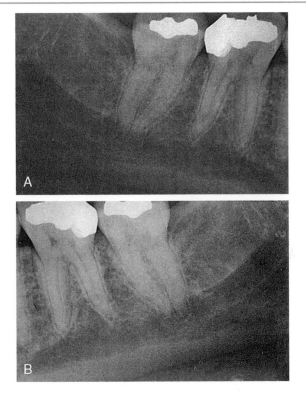

Figure 19-4. | Periapical radiograph of right mandibular molar area. **A,** Labial mounting. **B,** Lingual mounting.

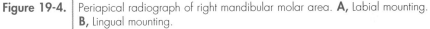

If the operator mounts the radiographs so that the raised portion of the dot is toward him or her, the operator is looking at the film as if he or she were facing the patient; the patient's left side is on his or her right. This is called *labial mounting* (Figure 19-4, *A*). If the film is mounted so that the depressed side of the dot is toward the operator, he or she are looking at the films as if viewing them from a position on the patient's tongue looking out; the patient's left side is on the operator's left. This is called *lingual mounting* (Figure 19-4, *B*). Both mounting systems are used in dentistry today, but the trend has been to adopt labial mounting as the universal system. The American Dental Association recommends labial mounting for use by all dental offices. When receiving mounted radiographs from another dental office, one should always feel for the orientation dot to confirm the position of the film in the mount.

PROCEDURE

The proper size and number of film mounts is selected. The patient's name or identification number and the date the films were taken are entered on the mount. The patient's films are laid out on the clean, dry tabletop, and the empty mount is placed on the viewbox. Maxillary teeth are placed in the mount with their roots facing up and the mandibular teeth with their roots facing down. The films are placed so that the dots are all one way, either facing toward or away from the operator. The films are then divided into three groups: bitewings, anterior periapical, and posterior periapical. The bitewing films are easily identified because the crowns of both the upper and lower teeth are seen. The anterior and posterior periapical films are differentiated by the vertical orientation on the film for anterior teeth and the horizontal orientation for posterior teeth. It is suggested that the anterior periapical films are mounted first.

Dental professionals can differentiate the maxillary anterior films from the mandibular anterior films on the basis of root and crown shape and anatomic landmarks, which are discussed later. To determine whether a film is from the patient's right or left side, the film is held up to the mount, and one imagines that the mount is the patient's face. Then it is decided which is the mesial and which is the distal side of the radiograph, and the film is placed accordingly. When the anterior films have been placed in their proper position in the mount, the same routine is repeated for the posterior films.

The bitewing films are mounted last. Because they show only the crowns of the teeth, there are no root shapes and surrounding bony landmarks to aid in anatomic identification. Once the periapical films are mounted, fillings and missing teeth can be used to help identify and orient the bitewing films. However, the bitewing films can be mounted easily by orienting the curve of Spee for correct placement. Another method is to mount the bitewings first, then the posterior periapical radiographs, using the restorations on the bitewings to identify the posterior periapical projections. With this method, the anterior periapicals are mounted last.

Some generalizations can be made about crown and root shapes seen on radiographs. The following hints will aid the novice in mounting films:

1. Crowns of upper anterior central and lateral incisors are wider and have longer roots than those of lower central and lateral incisors. Because they are wider, the maxillary anteriors do not fit on one film as do the mandibular incisors.

2. Maxillary premolars usually have two roots; mandibular premolars have one root.

3. Mandibular first and second molars usually have two divergent curved roots with bone clearly visible between them. This is particularly true of the first molar. Maxillary molars have three roots: two buccal and one palatal. The large palatal root obscures the interradicular bone.

4. Most roots curve distally.

5. The occlusal plane as it goes distally curves up in what is called the curve of Spee. When looking at the bitewing, one should imagine that the patient has a smile as the curve rises and an unhappy look if the curve incorrectly curves downward (Figure 19-5).

Remember, all radiology patients are happy patients!

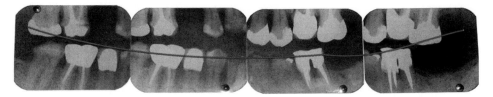

Figure 19-5. | The "smile" appearance created by the curve of Spee.

These aids, along with the anatomic landmarks that are described next, enable the dental professional to properly orient radiographs in the x-ray film mount.

NORMAL RADIOGRAPHIC ANATOMY

To fully use and properly interpret radiographs, the dental staff must be thoroughly familiar with normal radiographic anatomy. This includes all of the structures seen on periapical, bitewing, occlusal, panoramic, and extraoral projections. The first consideration in diagnosing a suspected lesion should be to differentiate it from a normal structure. Often this may be difficult because of wide variations of normal gross anatomy in regard to size, shape, and location that may be further modified by age and use. Radiographically these variations may be further exaggerated by the projection and angulation used. Not all landmarks are always demonstrated on every full-mouth survey or individual film. When one is confronted by a suspicious lesion, the first things to consider are the anatomic landmarks normally seen in that particular area. Normal anatomy should be ruled out first when making a differential pathologic diagnosis.

In interpreting radiographic landmarks, dental professionals should keep in mind the gross configuration of the structure. A thick, bony structure such as a ridge or muscle attachment appears more radiopaque because of increased object density. Any foramen, cavity, or *concavity* of bone produces an area represented on the film as radiolucent because of decreased density. Radiographs, as two-dimensional representations of three-dimensional objects, produce superimpositions of many normal structures that can be misleading, and the dental professionals should remember this when interpreting films.

Because radiographs are two-dimensional representations of a three-dimensional object, they do not portray depth; teeth may be superimposed on anatomic structures in the mandible, maxilla, or skull that may be millimeters in front of or in back of them. The best example is the roots of the maxillary molars and the maxillary sinus. Maxillary molar roots are rarely actually in the sinus, although they may appear that way on almost all molar radiographs (see Figure 19-10).

RADIOGRAPHIC TOOTH ANATOMY

The component structures of the tooth and its supporting structures are well defined on the dental radiograph because of their differences in density (Figure 19-6).

Enamel is the densest and thus the most radiopaque of the natural tooth structures. It is seen as a radiopaque band that covers the crown of the tooth and ends in a fine edge at the cementoenamel junction.

Dentin is the next layer of tooth structure. It is not as highly calcified as enamel and thus not as radiopaque. It composes the major part of the tooth structure and is seen in both the crown and the root portions. On a radiograph with poor contrast, it is difficult to see the border between enamel and dentin (the dentinoenamel junction).

Cementum is the thin, calcified covering on the surface of the root of the tooth. It is difficult to distinguish cementum from dentin because it is thin and its density is not very different from that of dentin. Cementum is best seen in the pathologic condition known as hypercementosis, which is an overgrowth of cementum.

The *pulp chamber* and pulp canal are seen as a continuous radiolucent space in the center of the crown and root of the tooth. The fingerlike projections in the coronal portion are called pulp horns. They are seen most often in young patients because the pulp chambers of teeth become smaller with age and in some cases may be totally obliterated by secondary dentin.

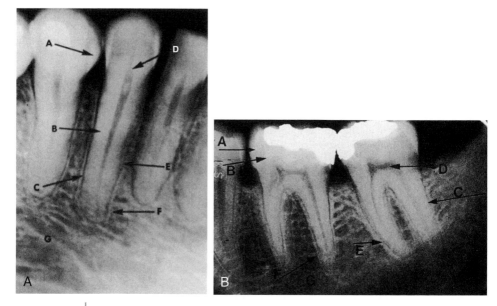

Figure 19-6. | Normal radiographic tooth anatomy, anterior (A) and posterior (B) tooth: A, Enamel. B, Dentin. C, Periodontal membrane. D, Pulp chamber. E, Cementum. F, Lamina dura. G, Alveolar bone.

The *periodontal ligament (membrane)* is seen as a radiolucent line approximately 0.5 mm wide between the cementum of the root of the tooth and the lamina dura. There is always a periodontal ligament attaching the tooth to bone, but the periodontal membrane may not always be seen clearly on every root surface because of differences in horizontal angulation when the radiograph was taken.

The *lamina dura* is a radiopaque line of cortical bone that surrounds the periodontal ligament. It represents the bony wall of the tooth socket. As with the periodontal ligament, it may not be seen on every surface because of angulation.

The *alveolar bone* is the bone that supports the tooth. It is composed of cancellous and cortical-compact bone. The *cancellous bone* is seen as a series of small radiolucent compartments called *medullary spaces*. These spaces are separated by a radiopaque honeycomb pattern called *trabeculae*. The occlusal part of the alveolar bone is referred to as the *alveolar crest*, which is composed of cortical bone. The mandible is a much denser bone than the maxilla; hence the medullary spaces are smaller, and there is greater trabeculation in the mandible.

The *cortical bone* is seen as a dense radiopaque structure that comprises the buccal and palatal plates of the maxilla, the buccal and lingual plates, the inferior border of the mandible, the lamina dura, and the alveolar crest.

(Text continues on page 381)

RECOGNIZING AND UNDERSTANDING RADIOGRAPHIC ANATOMY OF MAXILLA AND MANDIBLE

MAXILLA

Maxillary Incisor Area (Figure 19-7)

The nasopalatine (incisive) foramen is seen as an oval radiolucency between the roots of the maxillary central incisors. In some radiographs the incisive canal can be seen leading to the foramen. The *foramen* is actually in the anterior portion of the palate, but superimposition makes it appear to be located between the roots of the central incisors. The position of the nasopalatine foramen on the radiograph may vary from just above the crest of the alveolar ridge to the level of the apices of the teeth because of anatomic variations and vertical angulation. In some cases the shadow of the foramen may be superimposed on the apex of a central incisor and must be differentiated from periapical disease. This is done by taking another radiograph at a different horizontal angulation or

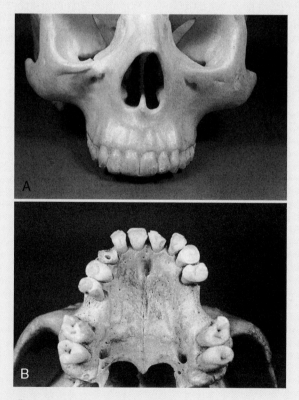

Figure 19-7. Maxillary central incisor area. **A** and **B,** Skull. **C,** Radiographs: *A,* Nasopalatine foramen. *B,* Median palatine suture.

PROCEDURE 19-1

PROCEDURE 19-1

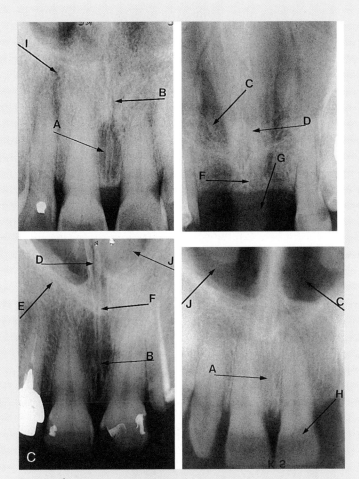

Figure 19-7—cont'd. *C,* Nasal fossa. *D,* Median nasal septum. *E,* Floor of nasal cavity. *F,* Anterior nasal spine. *G,* Columella of nose. *H,* Lip line. *I,* Lateral fossa. *J,* Inferior concha.

testing pulp vitality. Another option is to trace the lamina dura and periodontal ligament space. These structures will be completely intact if it is a foramen and interrupted if a periapical pathologic condition is present.

The *median palatine suture* is seen as a thin radiolucent line running vertically between the roots of the maxillary central incisors. It must be differentiated from a fracture line, nutrient canal, and fistulous tract.

The nasal *fossa* is the paired radiolucent structure superior to the apices of the incisor teeth. The fossa is also seen on the canine projection, where it may overlap or appear to adjoin the maxillary sinus. The radiopaque band that separates the left and right nasal fossa is called the median *nasal septum*. The septum ends inferiorly in the V-shaped radiopaque *anterior nasal spine*.

The radiopaque anterior nasal spine is near or superimposed on the *incisive foramen*. The radiopacity that sometimes projects into the nasal fossa from its lateral wall is the inferior *concha* (turbinate). The concha is not calcified, so it does not appear as radiopaque as the walls of the *nasal cavity*. When the concha is very large, however, the thickness of the soft tissue may make it look slightly opaque.

The soft tissue and cartilaginous shadow of the tip of the nose and the soft tissue outline of the lip may be superimposed from the crest of the ridge to the crowns of the teeth. These soft tissue shadows are seen most clearly on edentulous films in which even the nares (openings) of the nose and the columella (separating column) are seen.

The *lateral fossa* is a depression in the labial plate in the lateral incisor region. It appears as radiolucent between the lateral incisor and canine because it represents an area of thin bone.

Maxillary Canine Area (Figure 19-8)

In the maxillary canine region, two large radiolucent areas are seen. The more mesial area is the lateral aspect of the nasal fossa, and the more distal is the anterior extent of the maxillary sinus. In edentulous films the radiopaque Y, formed by the anterior and inferior border of the maxillary sinus as the arms and the *floor of the nasal cavity* as the stem, is useful in mounting orientation.

The radiopaque soft tissue shadow of the nose may also show on canine area radiographs. In some projections a radiolucent area is seen distal to the canine and represents the nasolabial fold.

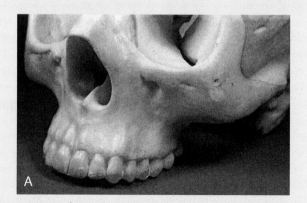

Figure 19-8. | Maxillary canine area. **A,** Skull. **B,** Radiographs:

Continued

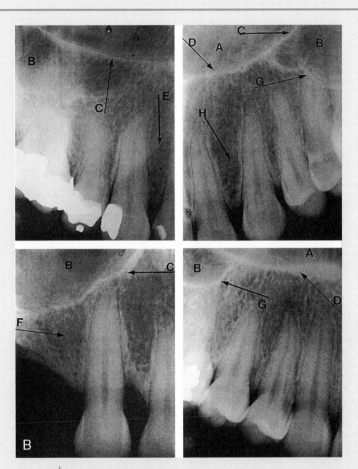

Figure 19-8—cont'd. *A,* Nasal fossa. *B,* Maxillary sinus. *C,* Septum of bone separating maxillary sinus and nasal septum. *D,* Floor of nasal cavity. *E,* Shadow of the nose. *F,* Nasolabial fold. *G,* Floor of maxillary sinus. *H,* Lateral fossa.

Maxillary Premolar Area (Figure 19-9)

In the maxillary premolar area the radiolucent maxillary sinus may be seen either superimposed on, between, or above the apices of the teeth. It is not always visible because of vertical angulation of the x-ray beam and because the size and position of the maxillary sinus may vary from patient to patient. The *floor of the maxillary sinus* appears as a radiopaque line running horizontally along its lower border.

The floor of the nasal fossa may be seen as a radiopaque line running horizontally at the superior portion of the maxillary sinus. Nutrient canals may be seen in the alveolar bone along with grooves for vessels in the walls of the maxillary sinus. Bony septum also may be seen in the maxillary sinus.

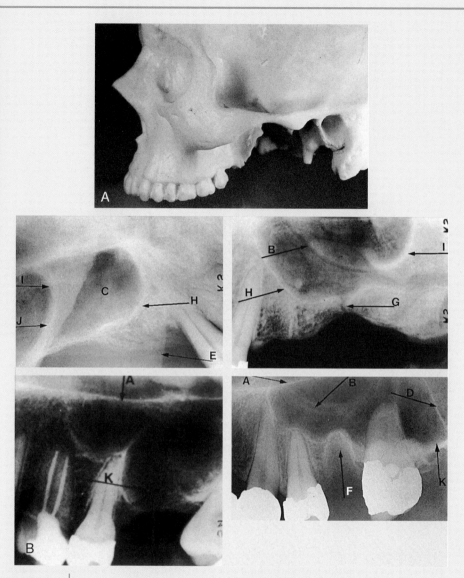

Figure 19-9. | Maxillary premolar area. **A,** Skull. **B,** Radiographs: *A,* Floor of nasal fossa. *B,* Nutrient canals in sinus wall. *C,* Maxillary sinus. *D,* Sinus septum. *E,* Buccinator shadow. *F,* Extraction socket. *G,* Oral-antral communication. *H,* Floor of maxillary sinus. *I,* Zygomatic process of maxilla. *J,* Zygomatic arch. *K,* Pneumatization.

The edentulous premolar radiograph is identified by the presence of the maxillary sinus. It differs from the molar radiograph in the absence of the maxillary sinus in the mesial part of the film and the start of the radiopaque zygomatic arch band at the distal portion of the film.

In some edentulous films the shadow of the buccinator muscle is seen. The *buccinator shadow* makes part of the normally radiolucent area below the ridge appear radiopaque because of the increased density of the muscle.

Maxillary Molar Area (Figure 19-10)

The *maxillary sinus* is a radiolucent area that always appears on periapical projections of the maxillary molar region. The sinus may be unilocular or compartmentalized by bony *septa*. Radiopaque spurs or *ridges* may project into the sinus; radiolucent tracts or grooves, representing blood vessel positions, may be seen in the walls of the sinus. The size of the maxillary sinus varies greatly because of age, morphology, radiographic projection, and vertical angulation used. A patient's sinuses may be asymmetric and may tend to enlarge or grow into areas of the alveolar ridge where teeth have been extracted. This process is called

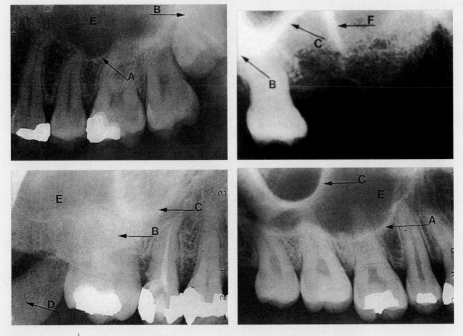

Figure 19-10. Maxillary molar area. *A,* Floor of sinus. *B,* Zygomatic arch. *C,* Zygomatic process of maxilla. *D,* Coronoid process of mandible. *E,* Maxillary sinus. *F,* Septum in sinus.

PROCEDURE 19-1

pneumatization. Just distal to the third molar ridge area is the *maxillary tuberosity.* This area of cancellous bone also may contain the posterior extension of the maxillary sinus. The large, fibrous buildup of soft tissue above the tuberosity may cause a slightly radiopaque shadow on the radiograph and is called the *tuberosity pad.*

The *zygomatic process* of the maxilla is seen as a U-shaped radiopacity superimposed on the roots of the first and second molars and the maxillary sinus. The malar bone (*zygoma*), which is a continuation of the zygomatic process, appears as a broad, uniform radiopaque band that extends posteriorly. Together with the zygomatic process of the temporal bone they make up the zygomatic *arch.*

The *hamular process* (*hamulus*) is the radiopaque projection that extends downward distal to the posterior surface of the maxillary tuberosity. It is the inferior end of the medial pterygoid plate of the sphenoid bone. The radiolucent area between the tuberosity and the hamular process is referred to as the *hamular notch* (Figure 19-11).

In the distal inferior portion of maxillary molar radiographs, a large radiopaque structure may be seen. This is the *coronoid process* of the mandible. When an edentulous series is mounted, this landmark is helpful in determining which is the most distal of the maxillary radiographs.

The maxillary torus (torus palatinus) is a lobulated bony growth in the midline of the palate. On a periapical radiograph, it appears as a dense, well-demarcated, radiopaque area (Figure 19-12).

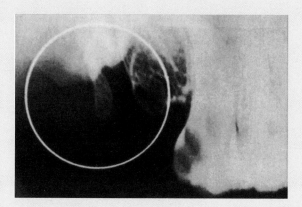

Figure 19-11. | Posterior part of maxillary molar region. In the circle are maxillary tuberosity, hamular notch, and hamular process.

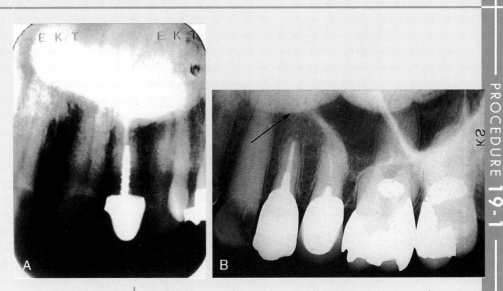

Figure 19-12. | Maxillary torus. **A,** Anterior periapical. **B,** Posterior periapical.

MANDIBLE

Mandibular Incisor Area (Figure 19-13)

In the mandibular central incisor area, just below the apices of the central incisors in the midline, there is often a somewhat circular radiopacity. This is the *genial tubercle*, which represents a bony growth on the lingual surface of the mandible to which the genioglossus and the geniohyoid muscles are attached. In the middle of the genial tubercle, a small circular radiolucency may be seen. This is the *lingual foramen*, which is the exit point from the mandible for the

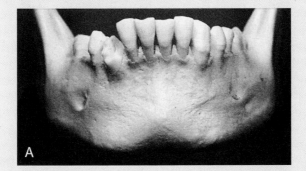

Figure 19-13. | Mandibular incisor area. **A** and **B,** Skull. **C,** Radiographs:

Continued

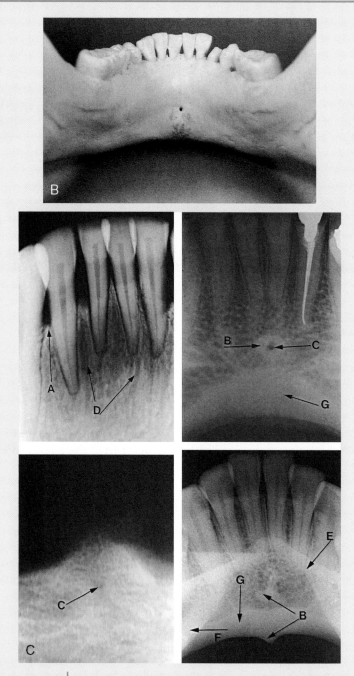

Figure 19-13—cont'd. A, Alveolar ridge. B, Genial tubercles. C, Lingual foramen. D, Nutrient canals. E, Mental ridge. F, Mylohyoid ridge. G, Inferior border of mandible.

lingual branches of the incisive vessels. *Nutrient canals*, although found in all areas of the mandible and maxilla, are seen most easily in this area and must be differentiated from fistulous tracts or fracture lines. They appear as radiolucent lines that run vertically in the alveolar bone and terminate in small, circular, radiolucent nutrient foramina. The nutrient canals are pathways for blood vessels and nerves.

The *mental ridge* is a broad V-shaped radiopaque band that represents a ridge of bone on the labial aspect of the mandible. It arises bilaterally below the apical area of the canine and incisors and runs medially and upward toward the mandibular symphysis. The ridge, if superimposed on the apices of the teeth, may hinder diagnosis. The ridge should be differentiated from the *internal oblique ridge*.

The shadow of the lip is seen on anterior radiographs. That portion of the film not covered by the lip appears darker than the rest of the film because there is no soft tissue attenuation in the area. The lip line, unless identified as such, can hinder radiographic interpretation.

The inferior border of the mandible is seen as a broad radiopaque band that represents the thick cortical bone of this area.

Mandibular Canine Area (Figure 19-14)

The anterior extension of the internal oblique ridge and submandibular fossa can be seen in the canine area.

The edentulous mandibular canine may be difficult to orient in the mount. One should look for the genial tubercle on the mesial part of the film and possibly the mental foramen in the distal part. The edentulous alveolar ridge crest slopes downward as it goes distally.

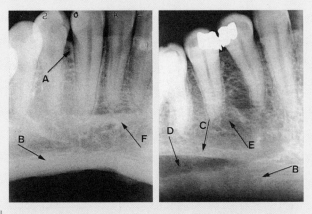

Figure 19-14. | Mandibular canine area. *A*, Alveolar ridge. *B*, Inferior border of mandible. *C*, Internal oblique ridge. *D*, Submandibular fossa.

Continued

PROCEDURE 19-1

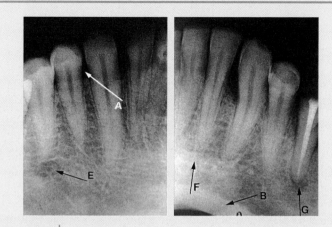

Figure 19-14—cont'd. | *E*, Mental foramen. *F*, Mental ridge. *G*, Periapical pathologic condition.

Mandibular Premolar Area (Figure 19-15)

The mental foramen is seen as a round or oval radiolucency near the apices of the premolars. The *mental foramen* may be found between, below, or even superimposed on the apices of the premolars. The mental foramen may not be seen on all premolar periapicals because of horizontal angulation of either the central ray or the position of the foramen itself. It is through this foramen that the mental nerves and blood vessels emerge. In some cases the radiolucent mandibular canal may be seen leading directly to the foramen. The mental foramen, in many cases because of its superimposition on the apices of the premolar, must be differentiated from a periapical pathologic condition. Tracing the lamina dura and periodontal ligament

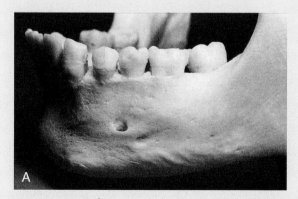

Figure 19-15. | Mandibular premolar area. **A,** Skull.

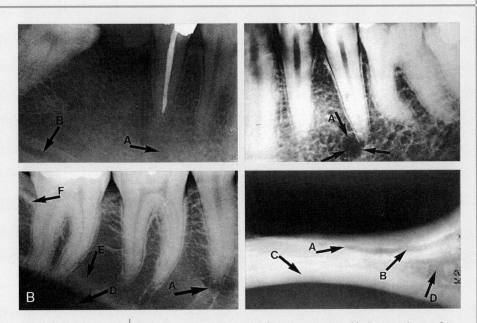

Figure 19-15—cont'd. | **B,** Radiographs: *A,* Mental foramen. *B,* Mandibular canal. *C,* Inferior border of the mandible. *D,* Submandibular fossa. *E,* Internal oblique ridge. *F,* External oblique ridge.

space will again be helpful in distinguishing normal anatomy from a pathologic condition.

The termination of the external oblique ridge can be seen in this area, along with the internal oblique ridge, submandibular fossa, and inferior border of the mandible.

The mandibular tori (torus mandibularis), although not strictly considered normal landmarks, are included in this section because of their frequency. They are seen singularly or multiply, usually bilaterally on the lingual aspects of the mandible in or near the premolar region. They appear as clearly outlined radiopacities (Figure 19-16).

The edentulous premolar film is identified and oriented for mounting by the presence of the mental foramen and the ending of the external oblique ridge. The crest of the edentulous alveolar ridge tends to rise as it goes mesially.

Mandibular Molar Area (Figure 19-17)

The *mandibular canal* (*internal alveolar canal*) is seen as a radiolucent band below the apices of the posterior teeth. It originates at the mandibular foramen and runs downward and forward to end at the mental foramen. It is bordered by thin radiopaque lines.

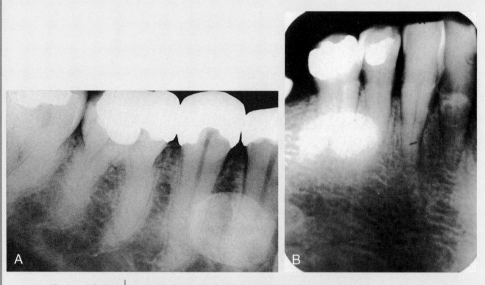

Figure 19-16. | Mandibular tori. **A,** Premolar projection. **B,** Canine projection.

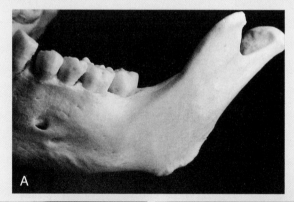

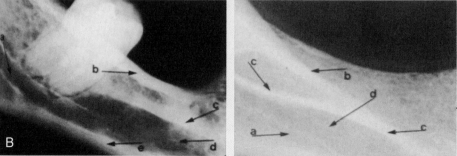

Figure 19-17. | Mandibular molar area. **A,** Skull. **B,** Radiographs: *a,* Mandibular canal.

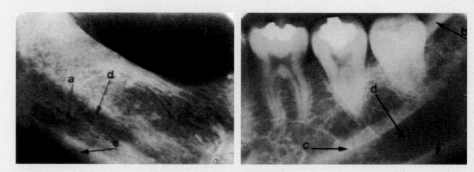

Figure 19-17—cont'd. *b,* External oblique ridge. *c,* Internal oblique ridge. *d,* Submandibular fossa. *e,* Inferior border of mandible.

The oblique ridges refer to the internal and *external oblique ridges.* The external ridge, a continuation of the anterior border of the ramus, is seen as a radiopaque line that passes diagonally down and forward across the molar region. The internal oblique or *mylohyoid ridge* is a radiopaque line that runs from the medial and anterior aspect of the ramus downward and forward to end at the lower border of the symphysis. When these two ridges are seen together, the internal oblique ridge is the lower of the two radiopaque lines.

Helpful Hint: The external oblique ridge is higher and shorter, whereas the internal oblique ridge is lower and longer.

The submandibular fossa is seen as a radiolucent area below the internal oblique (mylohyoid) ridge. It represents an area of reduced thickness of bone caused by a depression on the medial surface of the mandible. This radiolucency may be accentuated by a prominent mylohyoid ridge and a thick, opaque, inferior border of the mandible.

Nutrient canals are seen commonly in the molar region, especially when it is edentulous.

RESTORATIONS

As with tooth and bone structure, the density of the restoration determines its appearance on radiographs. Metallic restorations such as gold inlays, crowns, foils, posts, pins, or silver amalgam are the most radiopaque areas seen on radiographs (Figures 19-18 and 19-19). One can identify them only on the basis of size and shape, not on the degree of radiopacity. The synthetic restorations used in anterior teeth (e.g., glass ionomers, laminates, composites,

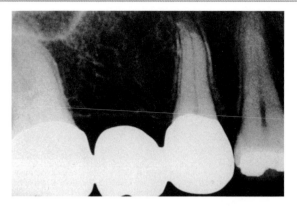

Figure 19-18. Fixed bridge and amalgam restoration. Note that acrylic facing of pontic does not appear on radiograph. Also note difference in radiopacities between amalgam and the cement base in the premolar.

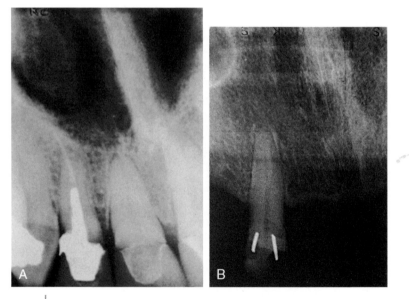

Figure 19-19. **A,** Gold post and core under porcelain jacket. **B,** Metallic pins under synthetic restoration.

and acrylics) appear radiolucent and may be mistaken radiographically for caries (Figure 19-20). Some manufacturers of some synthetic restorations now incorporate radiopaque particles in their preparations to distinguish the restorations from caries (Figure 19-21). Temporary or sedative fillings and cavity liners, such as zinc oxide, calcium hydroxide, and zinc oxyphosphate cement, appear radiopaque because they contain some metallic elements (see Figures 19-20 and 19-21). Porcelain jackets appear slightly radiopaque

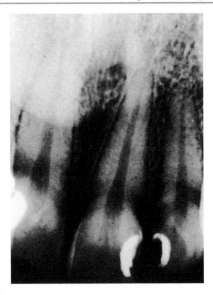

Figure 19-20. Radiolucent anterior synthetic restorations with cement bases.

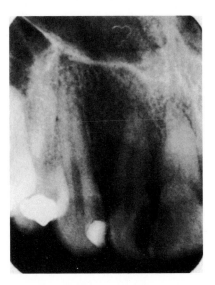

Figure 19-21. Radiopaque anterior synthetic restoration mesial to the canine. Mesial to the lateral incisor is a radiolucent synthetic restoration.

because the silicate from which they are made is a metal, with the radiopaque cement being more apparent (Figure 19-22, *A*). Porcelain-fused-to-metal crowns appear with distinct outlines of the metal, with the porcelain seen poorly or not at all (see Figure 19-22). Endodontic fillings appear as radiopacities in the pulp and root canal chambers. Of the two types of endodontic

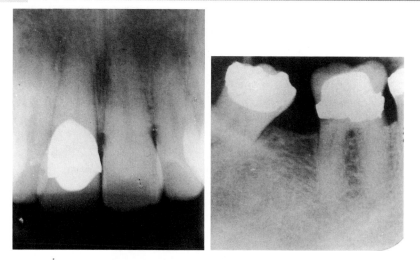

Figure 19-22. Porcelain-fused-to-metal (PFM) crowns on anterior and posterior teeth. Note the different densities of the metal and porcelain.

fillings most commonly used, the silver cones appear more radiopaque than the gutta-percha points. Compare the endodontic filling in Figure 19-19, *A*, with the filling in Figure 19-23. Other materials that can be seen are fracture wires (Figure 19-24) and orthodontic bands and wires (Figure 19-25).

RADIOGRAPHIC ANATOMY FOR PANORAMIC FILMS

The normal radiographic anatomy for panoramic films is shown in Figure 19-26. Some of the anatomic landmarks listed were described in the preceding section on periapical radiographs. Those landmarks commonly seen on panoramic films that are diagnostically important are also discussed here.

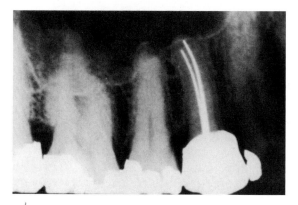

Figure 19-23. Silver cones used as endodontic filling material in the first premolar.

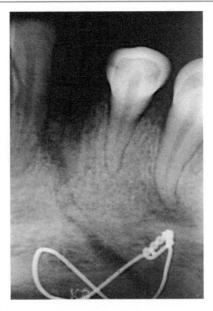

Figure 19-24. Healing mandibular fracture with intraosseous wires in place.

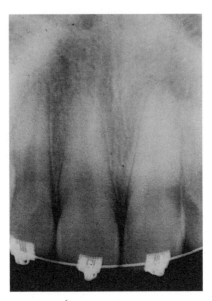

Figure 19-25. Orthodontic brackets and wires.

Mandibular Foramen

The mandibular foramen appears as an oval radiolucency at the origin of the mandibular canal at the midpoint of the ramus of the mandible.

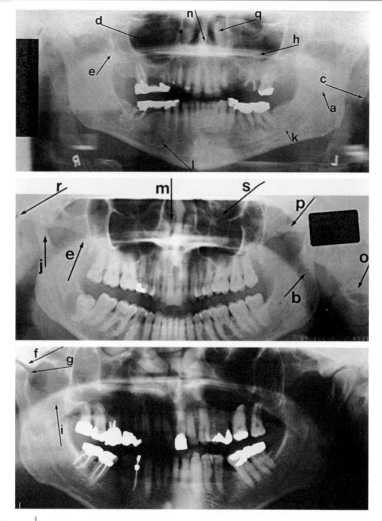

Figure 19-26. Panoramic film. *a,* Mandibular foramen. *b,* Pharyngeal airspace. *c,* Styloid process. *d,* Maxillary sinus. *e,* Coronoid process. *f,* Articular eminence. *g,* Glenoid fossa. *h,* Hard palate. *i,* Mental foramen. *j,* Mandibular condyle. *k,* Mandibular canal. *l,* Mental foramen. *m,* Nasal fossa. *n,* Nasal septum. *o,* Cervical vertebra. *p,* Zygoma. *q,* Inferior turbinate. *r,* External auditory meatus. *s,* Orbit.

Pharyngeal Airspace

The pharyngeal airspace appears as a bilateral, symmetric, radiolucent band between the radiopaque palatal line and the apices of the maxillary posterior teeth. It runs posteriorly and downward across the ramus and into the soft tissues of the neck. The appearance of the airspace on radiographs varies depending on the position of the tongue and thus the air above it and the state of contraction of the pharyngeal muscles. The diagnostic key for the airspace is the bilateral and symmetric appearance that can be followed running distally off the bone into the soft tissue.

Styloid Process

The styloid process is a radiopaque projection that may be seen bilaterally projecting downward just posterior to the ramus of the mandible. The styloid ligaments attached to the process may calcify and give the appearance of an abnormally long styloid process. The calcification of the ligament may not be continuous or may start at the attachment of the ligament to the styloid process, giving the appearance of a fracture of the styloid process (Figure 19-27).

Mandibular Condyle

The condyle, condylar neck, sigmoid notch, and coronoid process of the mandible are seen on panoramic films. Unless the unit has a variable focal plane, this is not the best way to view the condyle because it does not lie within the usual focal trough. At best the panoramic film can be considered a "scout film" to enable looking for gross changes in the maxilla or mandible.

OCCLUSAL RADIOGRAPHS

When interpreting occlusal films, dental professionals must remember that the projection is in the superoinferior plane ("axial") and shows the third dimension not seen in periapical, bitewing, and panoramic films (Figures 19-28 and 19-29). The type of occlusal projection used, right-angle or topographic (65 degrees), also should be considered because the position of the landmarks varies depending on the angulation used.

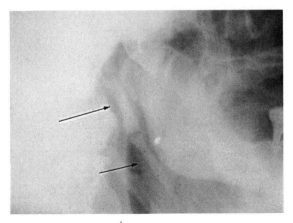

Figure 19-27. | Calcified styloid ligament.

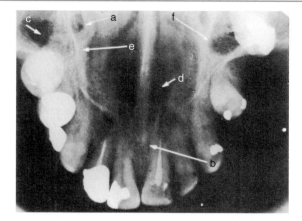

Figure 19-28. Maxillary occlusal film. *a,* Nasolacrimal duct. *b,* Anterior palatine foramen. *c,* Maxillary sinus. *d,* Nasal fossa. *e,* Lateral wall of nasal fossa. *f,* Lateral wall of maxillary sinus.

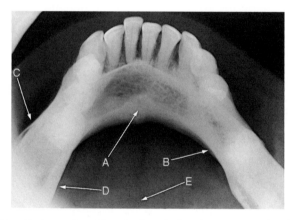

Figure 19-29. Mandibular occlusal film. *A,* Genial tubercles. *B,* Interior border. *C,* Buccal cortical plate. *D,* Lingual cortical plate. *E,* Shadow of tongue.

EXTRAORAL PROJECTIONS

The most commonly seen and important landmarks for the extraoral techniques described in Chapter 13 are illustrated in Figures 19-30 to 19-34.

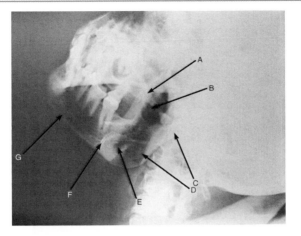

Figure 19-30. Lateral oblique projection of mandible. *A*, Coronoid process. *B*, Sigmoid notch. *C*, Condyle. *D*, Pharyngeal airspace. *E*, Mandibular foramen. *F*, Mandibular canal. *G*, Mental foramen.

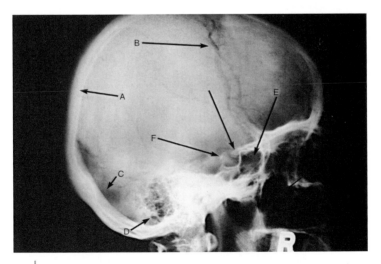

Figure 19-31. Lateral skull projection. *A*, Inner and outer table. *B*, Vascular markings. *C*, Lateral venous sinus. *D*, Mastoid air cells. *E*, Sphenoid sinus. *F*, Anterior and posterior clinoid processes and sella turcica.

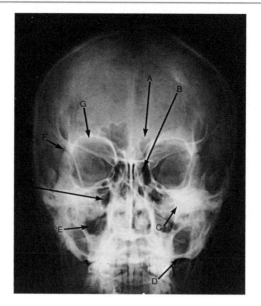

Figure 19-32.   Posteroanterior view. *A,* Frontal sinus. *B,* Ethmoid sinus. *C,* Petrous ridge. *D,* Base of skull. *E,* Maxillary sinus. *F,* Frontozygomatic suture. *G,* Orbit.

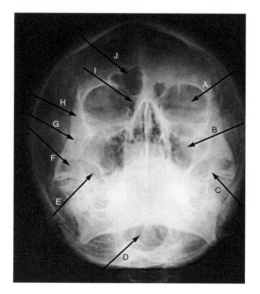

Figure 19-33.   Posteroanterior view of sinuses (Waters' view). *A,* Orbit. *B,* Maxillary sinus. *C,* Coronoid process. *D,* Foramen magnum and vertebra. *E,* Lateral wall of maxillary sinus. *F,* Zygomatic arch. *G,* Malar bone. *H,* Frontozygomatic suture. *I,* Ethmoid sinus. *J,* Frontal sinus.

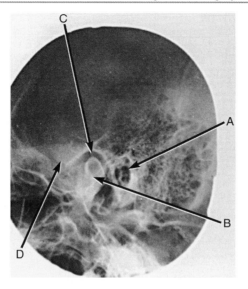

Figure 19-34. | Normal temporomandibular joint. *A,* External auditory meatus. *B,* Condyle. *C,* Articular fossae. *D,* Articular eminence.

SUGGESTED READINGS

White SC, Pharoah MJ: Oral radiology: principles and interpretation, ed 5, St Louis, Mosby, 2004.

CHAPTER 20

Principles of Radiographic Interpretation

EDUCATIONAL OBJECTIVES

1. Understand the steps to be taken in interpreting radiographs and their importance in establishing a diagnosis.
2. To understand how the patient's signs and symptoms relate to radiographic diagnosis.

KEY TERMS

benign lesion
bilateral lesion

differential diagnosis
interpretation

unilateral lesion
vitality testing

DIFFERENTIAL DIAGNOSIS

The inclusion of five chapters on interpretation in this text is not meant to imply that it is the dental professional's role to make the final radiographic diagnosis, but rather to stress that interpretation is only one step in making a diagnosis. This step should be shared by all of the dental clinicians. At present the final diagnostic role legally rests with the dentist, but certainly help and input from other members of the dental team should be encouraged.

The dictionary defines *interpretation* as "an explanation" and *diagnosis* as "the art or act of identifying a disease from its signs and symptoms." The interpretation of radiographs gives signs or symptoms on which to build a diagnosis. Other signs or symptoms that may be part of a diagnosis are gathered by using the patient's chief complaint, dental and medical history, clinical examination, *vitality testing*, advanced imaging, biopsy, and laboratory tests. The steps that are to be taken in forming a diagnosis are: (1) identification of an area or structure that is questionable; (2) interpretation of what has been identified; and (3) diagnosis based on the interpretation. Because the role of dental professionals is in steps 1 and 2, they need to develop interpretive skills to identify all normal anatomic structures, both tooth and bone, and artifacts that may be visible on interior radiographs and pantomographs. The dental professional also must be able to differentiate deviations in radiographic form and density from normal structures.

To produce adequate diagnostic films, the dental professional must know what relevant information is being sought from the radiograph. This base of knowledge makes taking the radiographs a more challenging, interesting, and rewarding process. If dental professionals know how periapical pathologic conditions appear radiographically, they also will understand the necessity of seeing the entire periapical area of the tooth in question to make a proper diagnosis. For example, if dental professionals know how difficult and in some cases how impossible it is to interpret caries on radiographs with horizontal overlapping of the teeth, they will be motivated to prevent or correct this error in technique to produce adequate diagnostic films.

The purpose of Chapters 19 through 24 is to give dental professionals some basic understanding of radiographic interpretation to stimulate interest and show the importance of producing an adequate diagnostic radiograph.

DIAGNOSTIC QUESTIONS

There are certain radiographic findings or questions that diagnosticians should ask themselves and be able to answer to help make a proper differential diagnosis. The list that follows is recommended clinical and radiographic information with which diagnosticians should be familiar.

- What is the patient's chief complaint? Often this will give important information that will help focus the diagnosis.
- What were the clinical findings that prompted the ordering of the radiographs? Is a bone or soft tissue pathology suspected?
- What does the vitality test reveal? About 70% of all pathologic conditions seen in the jaws are the result of nonvital teeth and their sequela.
- What radiographic projections are available, and what additional films should be ordered?

One should start with the basic intraoral films, then progress if necessary to an occlusal projection, extraoral radiograph, panoramic view (Figure 20-1), and finally a CT scan or in some cases a magnetic resonance image.
- Is the lesion radiolucent, radiopaque, or mixed (Figures 20-2 to 20-4)?
Most lesions are radiolucent.
- Have periapical and bitewing radiographs been taken recently?

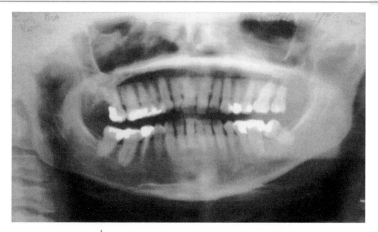

Figure 20-1. | Panoramic radiograph with third molar impaction.

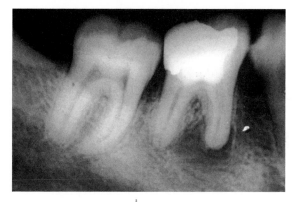

Figure 20-2. | Radiolucent lesion.

Previous films may give a history of treatment (e.g., signs of pulp capping bring periapical pathologic process to the forefront of the diagnostic possibilities) (Figure 20-5).

• Could the suspected "lesion" be an anatomic landmark (Figure 20-6)?
Landmarks are located in specific areas throughout the oral cavity and are well within normal limits.

• Where is the lesion located? Is it in the mandible, the maxilla, or elsewhere?
Certain lesions are seen more in one jaw than the other or in one location (e.g., a nasopalatine cyst) (Figure 20-7).

• Is the lesion a unilateral or bilateral lesion (Figure 20-8)?
Most bilateral findings are normal anatomic landmarks.

• What is the size and shape of the lesion (expressed in millimeters)?
• Are the borders of the lesion well defined (Figure 20-9)?

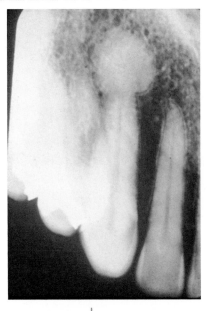

Figure 20-3. | Radiopaque lesion.

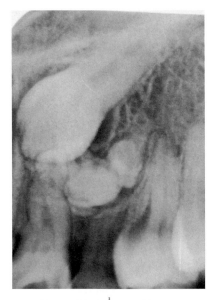

Figure 20-4. | Mixed lesion.

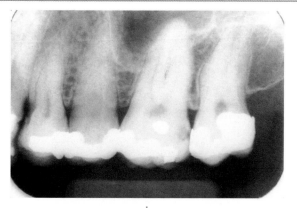

Figure 20-5. | Pulp capping.

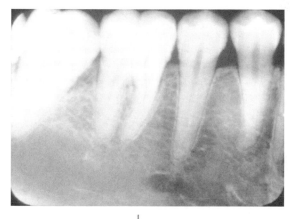

Figure 20-6. | Normal anatomy.

Well-defined lesions are the signs of a benign lesion, whereas poorly defined borders suggest a malignant growth.

- Is the lesion unilocular or multilocular (Figure 20-10)?
- How has it affected the teeth in the area? Has there been root resorption or just root displacement (Figure 20-11)?
- Can the lesion been seen in the three planes? If not, then further imaging is needed.
- Can all the borders of the lesion be visualized (Figure 20-12)? If not, then further imaging is necessary.
- If previous films of the lesion are available, what is the rate of growth of the lesion?

Certain lesions (e.g., malignancies) have rapid growth, whereas cysts and benign lesions grow slowly.

- Have all impacted teeth and edentulous areas been visualized?

Just because the area is edentulous does not mean that radiographs are unnecessary. An occult pathologic process may be present.

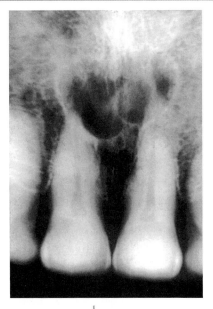

Figure 20-7. │ Nasopalatine cyst.

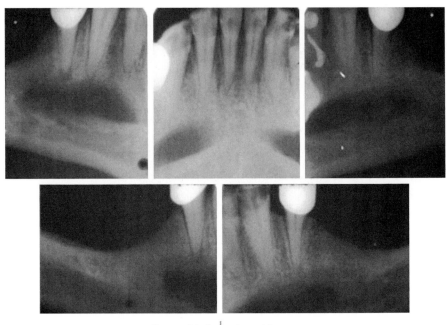

Figure 20-8. │ Bilateral lesion.

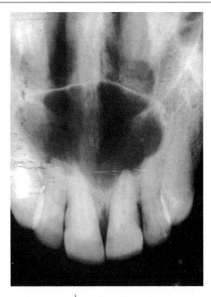

Figure 20-9. Lesion with distinct borders.

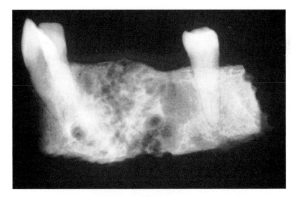

Figure 20-10. Multilocular lesion.

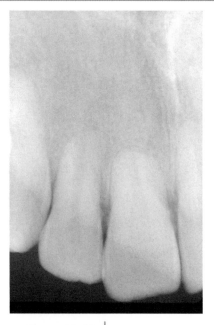

Figure 20-11. | Root resorption.

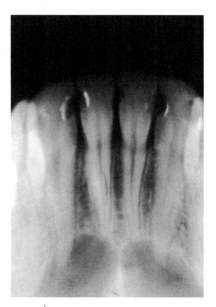

Figure 20-12. | All the borders of the lesion are not seen.

SUGGESTED READINGS
White SC, Pharoah MJ: Oral radiology: principles and interpretation, ed 5, St Louis, Mosby, 2004.

CHAPTER 21

Caries and Periodontal Disease

CHAPTER OUTLINE

EDUCATIONAL OBJECTIVES

1. Understand the effect of caries and periodontal disease on the radiographic appearance of teeth and alveolar bone.
2. Recognize caries on radiographs, correlate clinical findings with radiographic findings, differentiate caries from anatomic features and restorative materials, as well as judge the extent of caries.
3. Be aware of the limitations of radiographs in caries detection.
4. Identify the signs of periodontal disease on radiographs.
5. Be able to diagnose the extent of bone loss and identify predisposing factors.

KEY TERMS

abrasion
advanced caries
attrition
buccal caries

calculus
caries
cementoenamel junction
cervical burnout

composite
crown-root ratio
cupping
filling overhang

furcation	lingual caries	triangulation
horizontal bone loss	occlusal caries	vertical bone loss
incipient caries	open contact	
infrabony pocket	periodontal abscess	
interproximal caries	periodontal disease	

CARIES

Before beginning this discussion of caries interpretation, it must be stressed that all areas interpreted as caries must be confirmed by clinical examination. Many conditions can resemble caries, and such simple errors as reversed mounted films or viewing the wrong patient's radiographs can be prevented by following the essential routine.

Detection of caries is probably the most common reason for taking dental radiographs. Caries is seen on radiographs as a radiolucency in the crowns and roots of teeth. The caries process is one of demineralization of the hard tooth structure with subsequent destruction. This decrease in density allows greater penetration of the x-rays in the carious area and resultant radiolucency on the film. The degree of radiolucency on a given film is determined by the extent of the caries in the buccolingual plane in relation to the density of the overlying tooth structure. Radiographic interpretation of caries can be misleading in regard to relative depth and position in the tooth, as well as differentiation from other radiolucencies. For this reason, technique factors, such as proper vertical and horizontal angulation, and all of the other factors discussed in Chapter 10 are very important. Caries always is advanced further clinically than the radiographs indicate because the bacterial penetration of the dentinal tubules and early demineralization do not produce significant changes in density to affect the penetration pattern. The depth of the caries in relation to the pulp also can be misleading. Because the radiograph portrays a three-dimensional object in two planes, what may seem to be an obvious pulpal exposure radiographically may be the result of superimposition of images or improper horizontal angulation.

Incipient Caries

Caries that has only penetrated halfway through the enamel is called *incipient* caries (Figure 21-1). This type of caries may be difficult to detect radiographically because the size and density of the tooth structure have not undergone any great change. In fact, some clinicians, because of the possibility of remineralization, may elect not to restore these areas and just observe them for further changes.

Most advanced caries involving dentin in either the crown or the root of the tooth will appear on properly taken radiographs. However, small, deep occlusal, buccal, or lingual carious lesions may not be seen because the decrease in

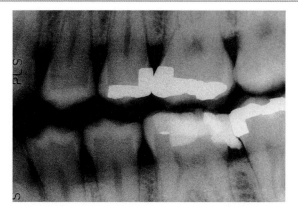

Figure 21-1. Bitewing radiograph showing incipient caries on the distal of the maxillary first premolar and the mesial of the maxillary second premolar. Note temporary filling and excess on the distal of the mandibular first molar.

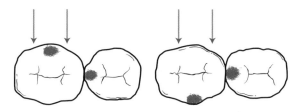

Figure 21-2. Buccal and lingual caries and relative effects on object thickness and the penetration of the x-rays when compared with interproximal caries.

density caused by the caries is small compared with the total buccolingual density of the tooth (Figure 21-2).

Interproximal Caries

It is in the diagnosis of interproximal decay that radiographs are most important. Interproximal caries is best seen on bitewing radiographs (Figure 21-3). If the paralleling technique is used, caries also appears clearly and undistorted on periapical films (Figure 21-4). In the bisecting-angle technique, the vertical angulation may distort or even mask interproximal caries. This is especially true of recurrent decay under old restorations. Bitewing radiographs are also useful in detecting poor contact, fit, and contour of metallic fillings, as well as filling overhangs and broken fillings (see Figures 21-3 and 21-5). To repeat, all these findings may be obscured because of incorrect horizontal angulation, which results in an overlapped image that does not show the interproximal surfaces clearly and therefore is of no diagnostic value (Figure 21-6).

The first radiographic sign of interproximal caries is a notching of the enamel, usually just below the contact point. As the caries progresses inward,

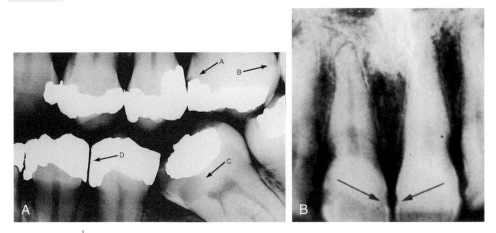

Figure 21-3. **A,** Interproximal caries on bitewing radiograph. *A,* Recurrent; *B,* incipient; *C,* advanced; *D,* open contact. **B,** Caries seen on periapical film of maxillary incisors.

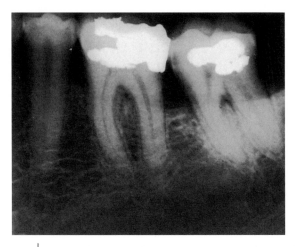

Figure 21-4. Periapical radiograph showing caries, mesial second molar.

it assumes a triangular shape, with the apex of the triangle toward the dentoenamel junction. As it invades the dentin, the caries spreads along the dentoenamel junction and proceeds toward the pulp in a roughly triangular pattern (Figure 21-7).

The radiographic appearance of interproximal caries is affected by the size and shape of the contact of the tooth involved. A tooth with a broad contact point does not show the caries as well as one with a narrow contact point because of the greater density of the tooth structure surrounding the caries (Figure 21-8).

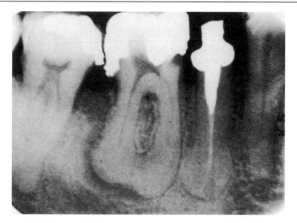

Figure 21-5. Caries seen on periapical radiograph. Note faulty contour on restorations and periapical radiolucency.

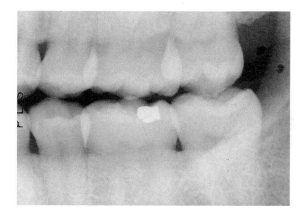

Figure 21-6. Bitewing radiographs showing horizontal overlapping.

Occlusal Caries

A careful clinical examination with a mouth mirror and an explorer will detect occlusal caries earlier than will radiographic interpretation. The absence of radiographic findings is a result of the superimposition of the dense buccal and lingual cusps on the relatively small carious area in the occlusal pits and fissures. Occlusal caries is not seen radiographically until it has reached the dentoenamel junctions, at which point it appears as a horizontal radiolucent line. As the decay progresses into the dentin, it appears as a diffuse radiolucent area with poorly defined borders. This appearance differentiates it from advanced buccal or lingual decay, which has more defined borders. This radiographic differentiation is always confirmed clinically (Figure 21-9).

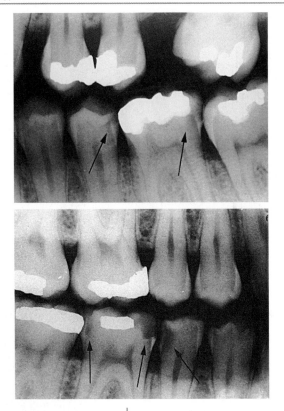

Figure 21-7. | Interproximal caries.

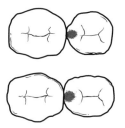

Figure 21-8. | The effect of contact point on caries interpretation.

Very often, radiographs of teeth with deep or broad occlusal pits and fissures show radiolucencies that resemble caries. These normal variants can be differentiated by examination with a mirror and an explorer.

Buccal and Lingual Caries

Early lesions on buccal and lingual surfaces may be very difficult, if not impossible, to detect radiographically because of the superimposition of the

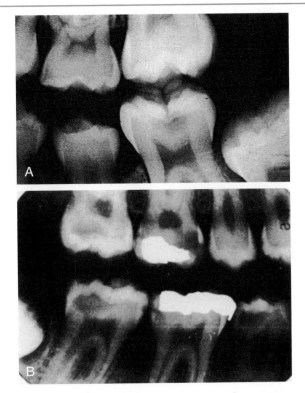

Figure 21-9. | **A,** Occlusal caries in mandibular first molar. **B,** Advanced occlusal caries in maxillary second molar and pulpal exposure in mandibular second molar. List the other carious lesions shown on this film.

densities of normal tooth structures. As the caries progresses, the radiolucency is characterized by its well-defined borders. Although it is theoretically possible to differentiate radiographically between buccal and lingual decay on the basis of sharpness of the image, it is not clinically important. The differentiation is identified more easily with a mirror and an explorer. It is impossible to judge the relationship of buccal or lingual caries to the pulp on radiographs because the depth of the caries lies in a geometric plane that is not recorded radiographically (Figure 21-10).

Conditions Resembling Caries

Many radiolucencies seen on dental radiographs may be mistaken for caries. The final diagnosis of caries is always made by corroborating the clinical examination with the radiographic findings.

Cervical Burnout
Cervical burnout appears as a radiolucent band at the neck of the tooth. It is contrasted because the part of the tooth apical to it is covered by bone and

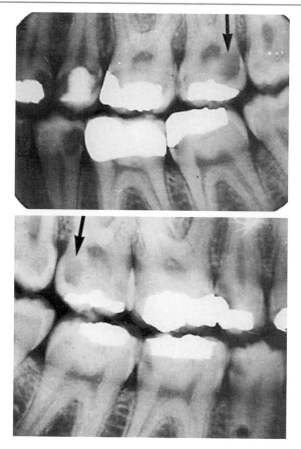

Figure 21-10. | Buccal caries as indicated by arrows. List the other carious lesions on these films.

hence is more radiopaque, whereas the area of the tooth occlusal to it is covered by enamel and is also radiopaque. In addition to these differences in densities caused by enamel and bone, the concave root contours below the cementoenamel junction appear as radiolucencies. Cervical burnout is most often observed when there has been no loss of the alveolar bone that provides the radiographic contrast. It is seen most often in the mandibular incisors and molars (Figure 21-11).

Abrasions and Attrition

Radiographically, cervical *abrasion* may resemble caries because it causes a wearing away of root structure and results in a decrease in density in the affected area. The radiolucency produced by the abrasion is usually a well-defined horizontal defect seen at the cementoenamel junction. Evidence of secondary dentin formation and pulp recession in response to the irritant also may be seen radiographically.

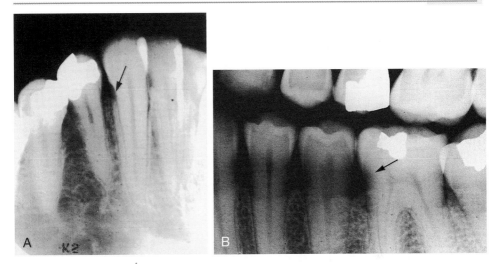

Figure 21-11. | Cervical burnout (*arrows*). **A,** Anterior teeth. **B,** Posterior teeth.

Attrition, which is defined as occlusal wear on teeth, is easily visualized clinically and radiographically by the absence or thinning of the occlusal enamel and dentin. This loss of tooth material is seen as a radiolucent area (Figure 21-12).

Indirect Pulp Capping

A radiolucent shadow under a metallic restoration may not always indicate recurrent decay but may indicate a previous indirect pulp capping. To avoid a carious pulp exposure in this technique, the last remaining portion of decayed tooth is not excavated. A sedative base and permanent restoration

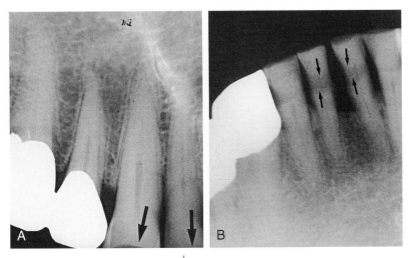

Figure 21-12. | **A,** Attrition. **B,** Abrasion.

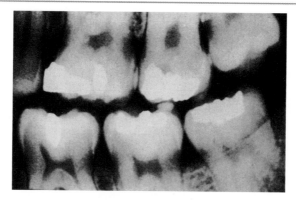

Figure 21-13. Indirect pulp capping. Note radiolucent area under restoration in maxillary second molar.

are placed with the hope that secondary dentin will be laid down to protect the pulp, and, because of the seal and anaerobic conditions, caries will not progress any further. Radiographically, the indirect pulp-capping procedure shows the radiolucent band of the unexcavated decay near the pulp chamber with a sedative base and permanent restoration (Figure 21-13).

Restorative Materials

Restorative materials such as silicates, acrylics, and some composites may resemble caries radiographically (Figure 21-14). Recently some brands of composite filling material have had radiopaque materials added to their formulation.

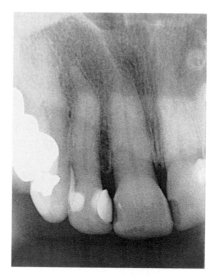

Figure 21-14. Radiolucent restorations in central incisors. The mesial and distal surfaces of the lateral incisor have synthetic restorations with radiopaque material added.

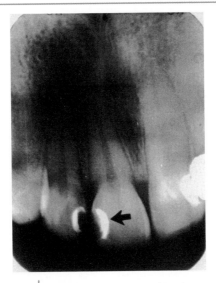

Figure 21-15. Synthetic restorations with radiopaque bases.

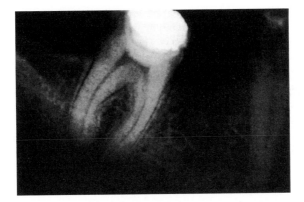

Figure 21-16. Radiopaque base and pulpotomy under metallic restoration.

One can differentiate between caries and the radiolucent filling on the basis of the regular geometric outline of a cavity preparation and the presence of a radiopaque cement base (Figure 21-15). However, all base and pulp-capping formulations that have a metallic component (e.g., zinc oxyphosphate, zinc oxide, calcium hydroxide) appear radiopaque (Figure 21-16).

PERIODONTAL DISEASE

The proper diagnosis and evaluation of periodontal diseases can be made only with a combination of radiographic and clinical examinations. Periodontal disease has both soft tissue and bony components. There are radiographic limitations in both aspects of the disease process. Soft tissue (gingival) changes such as inflammation, hypertrophy, and recession do not appear on radiographs because all soft tissue is radiolucent. Bone loss in some areas may not be seen because of superimpositions of buccal and lingual alveolar bone. Dental professionals should remember that the radiograph portrays a three-dimensional disease process in two planes. Radiographic images of bone changes almost always show less bone loss than there is.

Despite these limitations, a proper periodontal diagnosis cannot be made without a full-mouth survey of radiographs. Radiographs serve to (1) identify the risk factors, (2) detect early to moderate bone changes where treatment can preserve the dentition, (3) approximate the amount of bone loss and its location, (4) help in evaluating the prognosis of affected teeth and the restorative needs of these teeth, and (5) serve as baseline data and as a means of evaluating posttreatment results.

Normal Periodontal Structures

To recognize disease one must know normal anatomy. Periodontal anatomic structures identifiable on radiographs include such supporting structures as lamina dura, alveolar bone, periodontal ligament space, and cementum (see Figure 19-6).

The normal crest of interproximal bone runs parallel to a line drawn between the cementoenamel junctions on adjoining teeth at a level 1 to 1.5 mm apical to the cementoenamel junction (Figure 21-17). The shape of the alveolar crest is primarily determined by the contact area of adjacent teeth and the shape of the cementoenamel junction. The alveolar crest is flatter in the posterior areas and more convex and pointed in the anterior region. The interdental bone septum can be narrow in cases of close root proximity. In some patients the roots of adjacent teeth are so close that there may be little to no cancellous bone present.

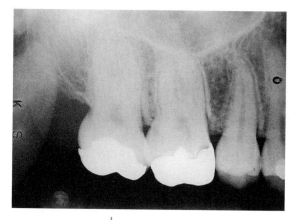

Figure 21-17. | Ideal level of interseptal bone.

The lamina dura is seen radiographically as a thin radiopaque line surrounding the entire tooth and is continuous with the alveolar crest. The lamina dura represents the alveolar bone that lines the tooth socket. It may not be visible in all radiographs.

The periodontal ligament fibers traverse from the cementum to the alveolar bone. Because these fibers are soft tissue, they are not seen on radiographs, but the space the fibers occupy is seen and referred to as the *periodontal ligament space*. Evaluating the width of the periodontal ligament space is an important part of a periodontal examination. The normal ligament space is about 0.5 mm. In situations of occlusal trauma, an increase in the size of the periodontal ligament space is often seen.

Techniques

The paralleling technique with an appropriate focal-film distance is the best method for evaluating periodontal disease. A full periapical survey taken in this manner and augmented by posterior, anterior, or vertical bitewings is the technique of choice. Vertical bitewings are especially useful for detecting bone loss of 5 mm or more radiographically.

The use of the bisecting technique with its inherent dimensional distortion provides a distorted representation of the level of bone present (see Figure 10-11).

Panoramic films are of some value in the diagnosis of periodontal disease, especially in the most advanced cases. Panoramic films should only be used if intraoral films cannot be taken.

Risk Factors in Periodontal Disease

The detection of local risk factors is one of the most important roles of radiography in periodontal disease. The management or prevention of early periodontal disease is much easier and has a higher success rate than efforts made once the disease has progressed. The detection and elimination of local irritants are essential steps in prevention or actual periodontal therapy. Reducing local risk factors increases the host response to disease.

Calculus
Both subgingival and supragingival calculi are the most common of all local irritants. Early deposits, small and not fully calcified, are not seen radiographically. Even when calcified, supragingival calculus, which is seen most often on the lingual surface of lower anterior teeth and the buccal surface of upper molars, is not seen clearly in its early stage because of superimposition of tooth structure (Figure 21-18). Subgingival calculus on the proximal surfaces is detected more easily than supragingival calculus, although both are not easily observed in the early calcified stages. The calculus appears as an irregularly pointed radiopaque projection from the proximal root surfaces (Figure 21-19). Horizontal bitewing radiographs are most helpful in

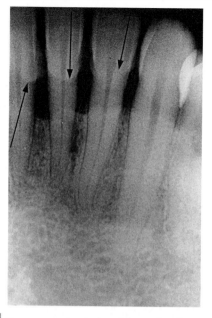

Figure 21-18. Supragingival calculus on lingual surfaces of lower incisors.

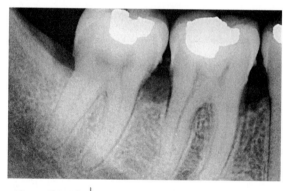

Figure 21-19. Subgingival calculus. Note bone loss.

discerning interproximal calculus in the posterior areas or vertical bitewings in the anterior or posterior areas.

Restorations
Radiographic examination reveals restorations with open contacts, poor contours, overhanging and deficient margins, and caries, all of which are significant risk factors in periodontal disease (Figures 21-20 to 21-22).

Anatomic Configurations
Only through radiographic examination can information about the size, shape, and position of the roots and the bone level of periodontally involved

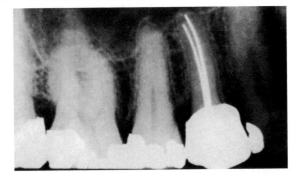

Figure 21-20. | Overcontoured crown on premolar and bone response.

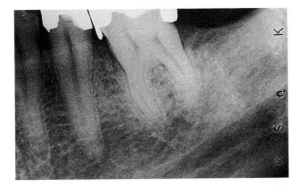

Figure 21-21. | Restoration with open contact and overhang. Note bony response.

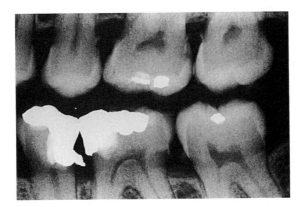

Figure 21-22. | Restoration with overhang. Note heavy calculus formation in other areas.

teeth be obtained. These factors are important in evaluating the present condition and planning periodontal and restorative therapy.

The crown-root ratio refers to the length of root surface embedded in bone compared with the length of the rest of the tooth. The greater the length of the

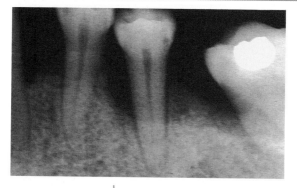

Figure 21-23. | Unfavorable crown-root ratio.

tooth embedded in bone, the better the prognosis (Figure 21-23). This becomes a critical factor when designing both fixed and removable prostheses.

Teeth that have an anatomically short root have a poorer prognosis periodontally than teeth with long roots. Teeth with bulbous roots have more area for attachment than those with fine, tapered roots. In multirooted teeth, the space between the roots is important; teeth with widely spaced roots have a better periodontal prognosis. Adjoining teeth whose roots are close together have a poorer prognosis than those with adequate areas of interseptal bone.

Stages of Periodontal Disease

Gingivitis

Because gingivitis is a soft tissue change, there are no radiographic findings other than the presence of predisposing factors. Existing deep pockets, if there is no bone loss, will not be seen. Postoperative radiographs of extended surgery only show the new bone level and do not indicate healthy tissue and lack of pocket depth. Among the risk factors for gingivitis are medications that may cause gingival hyperplasia and inflammation.

Early

The early stage of periodontal change is characterized radiographically by changes in the crest of the interproximal bone septum and triangulation of the periodontal membrane. Triangulation is the widening of the periodontal membrane space at the crest of the interproximal septum that gives the appearance of a radiolucent triangle to what is normally a radiolucent band. As mentioned, the normal crest of the interseptal bone runs parallel to a line drawn between cementoenamel junctions on adjoining teeth at a level 1 to 1.5 mm below the cementoenamel junction. The crest of the septa normally has a distinct radiopaque border. Fading of the density of the crest with cup-shaped defects appears in the early stages of periodontal disease (Figure 21-24).

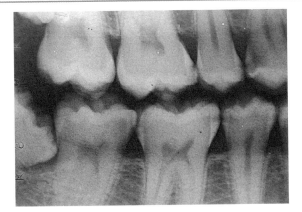

Figure 21-24. Early periodontal bone loss. Note fading of density of the alveolar crest, slight cupping, and triangulation.

Moderate

In the moderate stages, bone loss shows up in both horizontal and vertical planes. Radiolucencies appear in the furcations of multirooted teeth, indicating bone loss in these critical areas (Figure 21-25). *Horizontal bone* loss is resorption that occurs in a plane parallel to a line drawn between the cementoenamel junctions on adjoining teeth (Figure 21-26). In *vertical bone* loss the resorption on one tooth root sharing the septum is greater than on the other tooth, the so-called infrabony pocket (Figure 21-27). In this stage the horizontal bone loss on the buccal or lingual surfaces may go undetected because of superimposition. Careful examination of the radiograph may reveal a difference in density, indicating different levels of bone on the buccal and lingual surfaces (Figure 21-28).

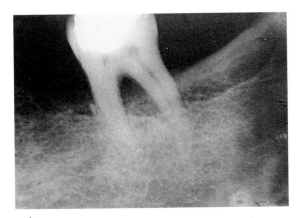

Figure 21-25. Moderate to advanced bone loss showing bifurcation involvement.

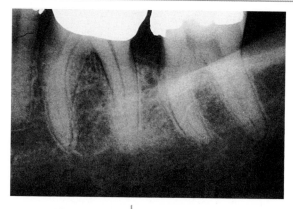

Figure 21-26. | Horizontal bone loss.

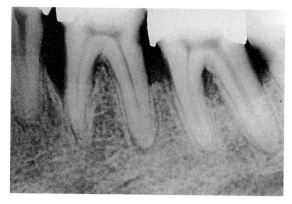

Figure 21-27. | Vertical and horizontal bone loss. Note the early bifurcation involvement on the second molar.

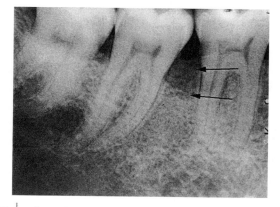

Figure 21-28. | Different levels of buccal and lingual bone as indicated by arrows.

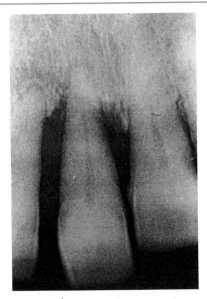

Figure 21-29. | Advanced periodontal bone loss.

Advanced

The advanced stage of periodontal disease is easily identified radiographically by the advanced vertical and horizontal bone loss, furcation involvement, thickened periodontal membranes, and indications of changes in tooth position (Figures 21-29 and 21-30).

Periodontal Abscess

The radiographic signs of a periodontal abscess vary greatly. Such a diagnosis is dictated by an acute clinical manifestation. *Periodontal abscess* is caused by

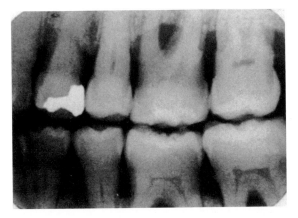

Figure 21-30. | Trifurcation bone loss, upper first molar; bifurcation bone loss, lower first and second molars.

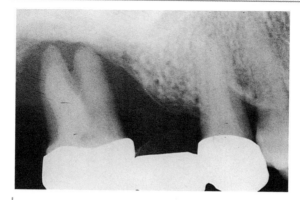

Figure 21-31. | Periodontal abscess. Patient had acute buccal swelling and facial edema.

the blockage of an existing pocket; therefore the radiograph of the acute episode may not differ greatly from previous films of the existing condition that produced the pocket. In other instances there may be signs of rapid and extensive bone destruction (Figure 21-31).

SUGGESTED READINGS

White SC, Pharoah MJ: Oral radiology: principles and interpretation, ed 5, St Louis, Mosby, 2004.

CHAPTER 22

Pulpal and Periapical Lesions

EDUCATIONAL OBJECTIVES

1. Understand the process and sequelae of pulpal necrosis and its radiographic findings.
2. Be able to radiographically diagnose periapical pathologic conditions and differentiate between it and normal anatomy, as well as other apical findings.

KEY TERMS

calcification
dentoalveolar abscess
external resorption
internal resorption
periapical cemental
  dysplasia (periapical

cemental osseous
  dysplasia)
periapical condensing
  osteitis
periapical cyst
periapical granuloma
periapical lesions

pulp calcification
pulp denticle
residual cyst
residual granuloma
root resorption
secondary dentin

PULPAL LESIONS

The most commonly seen pathologic condition after caries and periodontal disease is pulpal necrosis and subsequent periapical bone lesions. In fact, most pulpal and periapical lesions are the sequelae of caries, trauma, intrabony lesions, and advanced periodontal disease.

Anatomy

As shown in Chapter 19, the pulp chambers and pulp canals of teeth are seen radiographically as radiolucent areas because they contain noncalcified material and are hence less dense than the tooth structure that surrounds them (Figure 22-1). High pulp horns and large pulp chambers can occur in all age groups, not just in young patients in whom these findings are characteristic. The normal size and shape of the pulp chamber and canals change with age, in certain developmental anomalies, and in response to local irritants. The radiographic densities of pulp chambers and canals differ because of size, position in the tooth, and radiographic angulation, but not because of vitality. Gradual reduction in the size and shape of the pulp chamber and canal is marked by the deposition of secondary dentin at the walls of the chamber and canals and the appearance on radiographs of a radiopacity to replace the radiolucent area (Figure 22-2). Radiographically, secondary and regular dentin appear the same and can only be differentiated by the changes in the shape of the chamber and canals that accompany aging. The formation of

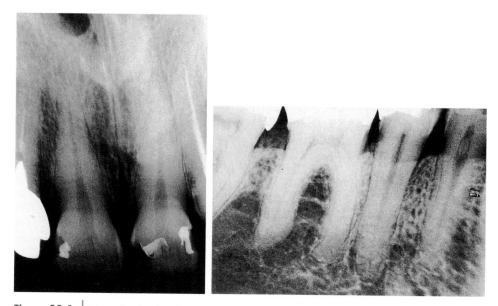

Figure 22-1. Normal pulp chambers in anterior and posterior teeth. Note different shapes and densities and presence of pulp denticle in first premolar.

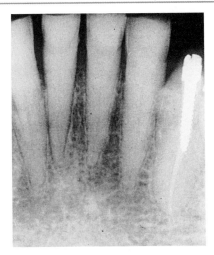

Figure 22-2. | Pulp chambers receded with age. Secondary dentin formation.

secondary dentin with the resulting obliteration or narrowing of the pulp chamber and canals can be caused by different types of irritants. The most common causes are deep caries, pulp capping, deep-seated restorations, attrition, abrasion, and a healed tooth fracture (Figure 22-3). This decrease in pulp and root chamber size also can be seen in the developmental disturbances dentinogenesis imperfecta and dentinal dysplasia (Figure 22-4).

Pulp denticles (stones) or calcifications appear as well-defined radiopacities within the pulp chamber (Figure 22-5). A radiolucent line may be seen separating the stone from the pulpal wall and give the appearance of a "free-floating" denticle, but it really is attached to the floor or wall of the chamber. The stones, which are composed of either dentin or calcified salts, have the density and appearance of dentin. Other than blocking endodontic access, pulp calcifications have no clinical significance and do not cause pulp strangulation as was once thought.

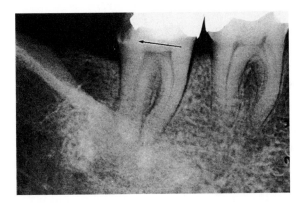

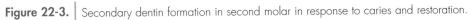

Figure 22-3. | Secondary dentin formation in second molar in response to caries and restoration.

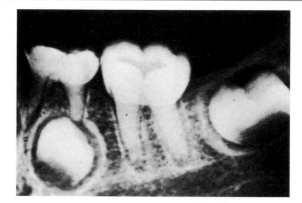

Figure 22-4. | Dentinogenesis imperfecta. Note early calcification of pulp chamber and canals.

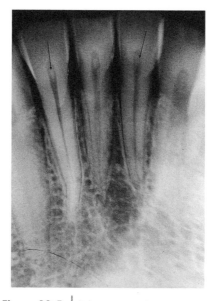

Figure 22-5. | Pulp stones in lower incisors.

Pulpitis

There are no radiographic signs of pulpitis in the pulp chamber. Normal, inflamed, or necrotic pulp all appear the same because their densities are the same. The only possible radiographic findings in pulpitis are the causative factors such as caries, pulp exposure, tooth fracture, previous pulp capping, or deep restorations (Figure 22-6). The pulps of teeth may vary in radiographic density. This is not because of differences in vitality, but because of the differences in object density of the overlying tooth structure.

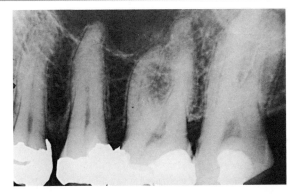

Figure 22-6. | Pulpitis with no apical changes. Second premolar was acutely sensitive to thermal stimulation and found to be partially nonvital.

PERIAPICAL LESIONS

Periapical Pathologic Conditions

Periapical lesions are seen in the apical tissues surrounding the tooth after the pulp has become necrotic. The periodontal membrane, lamina dura, and alveolar bone are the affected tissues. This necrosis, or degeneration of the pulp, may be a result of carious invasion of the pulp, tooth fracture, and physical or chemical trauma (Figure 22-7). The exudate from the pulp first spills into

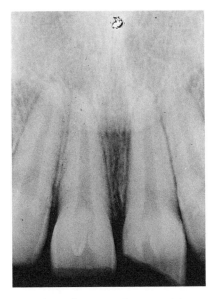

Figure 22-7. | Fractured crowns of maxillary central incisors. Note proximity of fracture lines to pulp chambers.

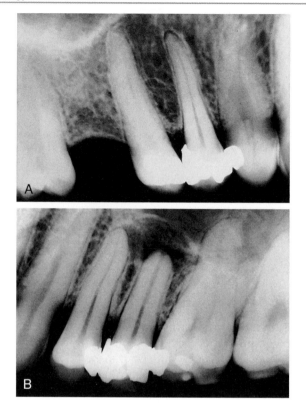

Figure 22-8. | **A,** Thickened periodontal membrane and early apical bone change on maxillary first bicuspid. **B,** Early apical bone resorption.

the periodontal ligament, causing a thickening that can be seen radiographically. The pressure then causes resorption of the lamina dura and alveolar bone (Figure 22-8). Depending on certain factors, a cyst, granuloma, or dentoalveolar abscess may develop at this point. If the exudate reacts with some residual epithelial rests, then a periapical cyst will form. The strength and type of bacteria and the tissue resistance determine whether a granuloma or abscess will develop. It is almost impossible to differentiate radiographically between a periapical granuloma and a periapical cyst (Figures 22-9 and 22-10). The dentoalveolar abscess may cause root resorption and a more diffuse radiolucency (Figure 22-11). If present, a fistulous tract leading from the abscess to the oral cavity is very difficult to see on radiographs because of its tortuous course through the bone, and it would only be evident if the fistulous tract and the central ray were in the same cross-sectional plane.

Periapical Condensing Osteitis

Periapical condensing osteitis is recognized by the formation of dense bone around the apex of a tooth in response to low-grade pulpal necrosis. This

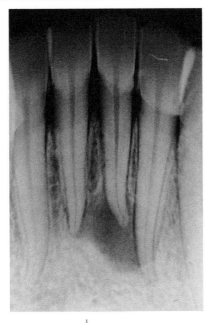

Figure 22-9. | Periapical granuloma.

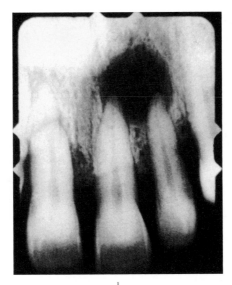

Figure 22-10. | Periapical cyst.

radiopaque asymptomatic condition is seen most often at the mandibular pre-molar and molar apices (Figure 22-12). In almost all cases the teeth are shown to be nonvital through pulp testing. Although the condition may be asymp-tomatic, it should be considered a radiopaque type of periapical pathologic condition and treated accordingly with either root canal therapy or extraction.

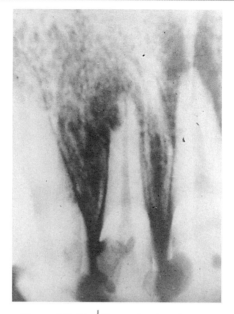

Figure 22-11. | Dentoalveolar abscess.

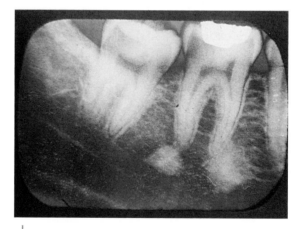

Figure 22-12. | Periapical condensing osteitis on mesial and distal roots of first molar.

Residual Periapical Lesions

Residual periapical lesions are radiolucencies that appear in edentulous areas of either the maxilla or the mandible. They represent pathologic areas that arose from teeth extracted in the area. If a granuloma or cyst that surrounds the apex of a nonvital tooth is not curetted out at the time of extraction, it may remain, grow, and destroy bone or move and possibly devitalize teeth. Such a lesion is considered either a residual cyst or granuloma

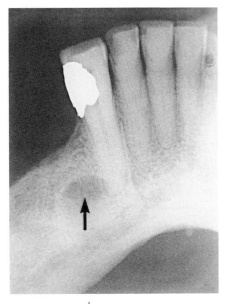

Figure 22-13. Residual cyst of mandible.

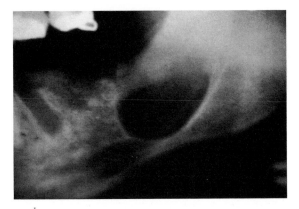

Figure 22-14. Residual cyst of left mandible seen on portion of panoramic film.

(Figures 22-13 and 22-14). Residual periapical lesions are quite common and are always considered in a diagnosis of an infrabony lesion.

Root Resorption

Root resorption can be caused by chronic periapical or periodontal infection, trauma, pressure from tumors or cysts, or rapid excessive orthodontic pressure, or it can be idiopathic (Figures 22-15 to 22-18). In a differential diagnosis, it is important to distinguish between smooth (cysts, tumors) and rough root resorption (infection, trauma).

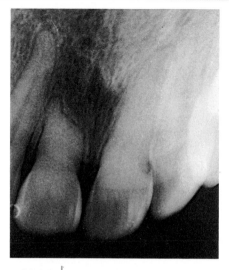

Figure 22-15. | Root resorption resulting from trauma.

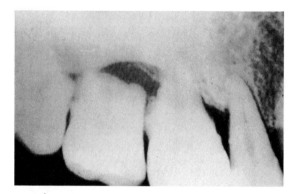

Figure 22-16. | Root resorption resulting from chronic periodontal infection.

Internal Resorption

The cause of the destructive process known as *internal resorption* (Figure 22-19) is unknown. The pulpal tissue resorbs the dentin surrounding the pulp chamber or canal and eventually perforates to the periodontal ligament. The radiographic findings of internal resorption are irregularities and widening of the usually smooth, tapered outline of the root chamber. In advanced cases the irregular outline of the resorption can be seen perforating the root structures and reaching the periodontal ligament.

External Resorption

The cause of *external resorption* (Figure 22-20) is also unknown. In this case, the cells of the periodontal ligament resorb the cementum and dentin of the root or pulp chambers to reach the pulp. Radiographically, teeth with external

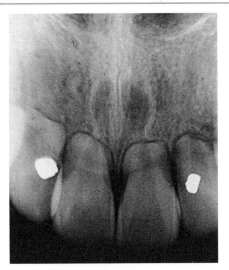

Figure 22-17. Root resorption resulting from excessive and rapid orthodontic movement.

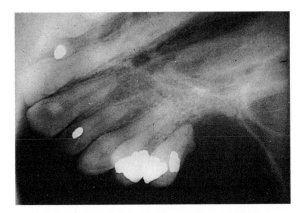

Figure 22-18. Root resorption resulting from a malignant tumor.

resorption have a round or oval radiolucency lateral to or superimposed over the pulp canal. If it is superimposed, the outline of the normal canal can be seen through the superimposition. If the radiolucency is lateral to the pulp canal, it can be seen leading from the periodontal ligament. It does not affect the pulp canal in its early stages; however, it perforates into the pulp canal and devitalizes the pulp tissue in its later stages.

Periapical Cemental Dysplasia/Periapical Cemental Osseous Dysplasia

Periapical cemental dysplasia (PCD)/periapical cemental osseous dysplasia (PCOD) (Figure 22-21) is a three-stage lesion that is asymptomatic and

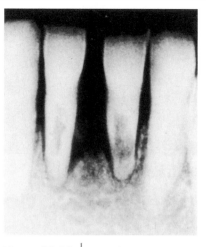

Figure 22-19. | Internal root resorption.

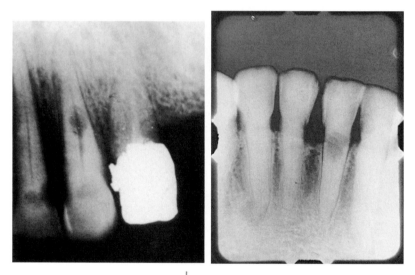

Figure 22-20. | External root resorption.

self-limiting and for which no treatment is indicated. It occurs at the apical region of vital teeth and originates in the periodontal membrane of the tooth. In its first stage it is radiolucent and resembles periapical disease. The second stage is mixed because the radiolucent lesion starts to calcify. In its third stage it is totally radiopaque. Clinically the teeth always test vital, and in all cases no treatment is indicated. PCD/(PCOD) must be differentiated from periapical pathologic conditions and condensing osteitis by vitality testing.

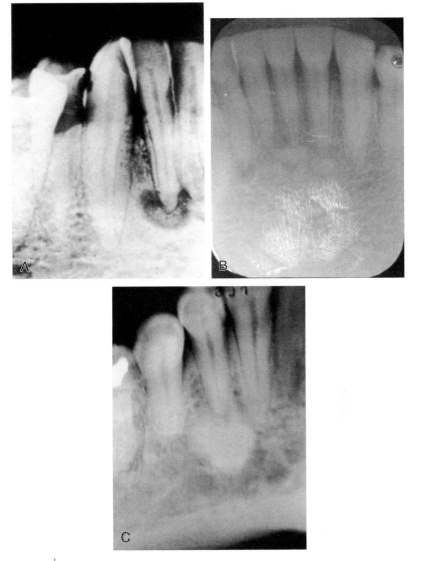

Figure 22-21. | **A,** First-stage periapical cemental osseous dysplasia resembles periapical disease. **B,** Second-stage (mixed) radiolucent lesion starts to calcify. **C,** Third-stage radiopaque area surrounds tooth apex. All teeth test vital in all stages.

SUGGESTED READINGS

White SC, Pharoah MJ: Oral radiology: principles and interpretation, ed 5, St Louis, Mosby, 2004.

CHAPTER 23

Developmental Disturbances of Teeth and Bone

EDUCATIONAL OBJECTIVES

1. Understand the formation and radiographic appearance of developmental lesions of teeth and bone.
2. Recognize developmental lesions of teeth and bone and know which radiographic projections are necessary to formulate a diagnosis.

KEY TERMS

amelogenesis imperfecta
anodontia
cleft
concrescence
cyst
deciduous
dens invaginatus
dental papilla
dentigerous

dilaceration
distodens
enamel pearls
eruption
fusion
gemination
hypercementosis
hypodontia
impaction

malposed
mesiodens
oligodontia
overretention
primordial cyst
root sack
taurodontia
transposed

The recognition of developmental conditions of tooth and bone is an important part of the dental professional's diagnostic responsibility. Most of the lesions can be detected radiographically, and their early recognition can prevent further problems. The most common conditions are discussed in this chapter. There are many developmental conditions that are linked to systemic problems, and an atlas or textbook of such lesions will complement the material presented here.

TOOTH DEVELOPMENT

The developing tooth can be seen at all stages on radiographs. The tooth germ (Figure 23-1) before calcification appears as a round or oval radiolucency in the body of the maxilla or mandible. As crown formation progresses, the radiolucent follicle is seen surrounding the crown of the tooth (Figure 23-2). After the tooth erupts, the *dental papilla* appears at the forming apices (Figure 23-3).

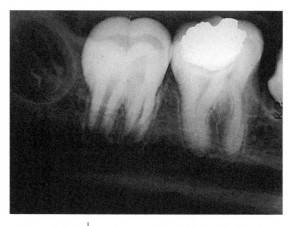

Figure 23-1. | Tooth germ of mandibular third molar.

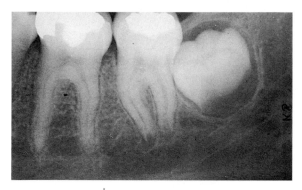

Figure 23-2. | Follicle of mandibular third molar.

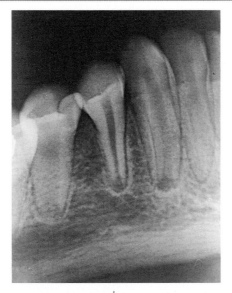

Figure 23-3. | Dental papilla.

Radiographic examination by either the standard full-mouth series or panoramic films is essential in determining the progress and pattern of tooth *eruption* (Figures 23-4 and 23-5). In this manner, conditions such as premature loss of primary teeth, anodontia, hypodontia, overretained teeth, ankylosis, tumors, and supernumerary teeth, which can affect the eruption pattern, can be identified (Figures 23-6 and 23-7).

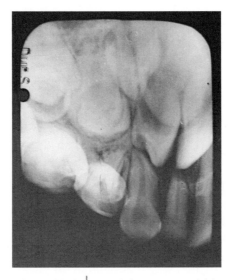

Figure 23-4. | Mixed dentition in a child.

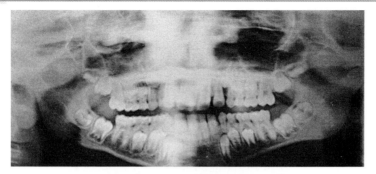

Figure 23-5. | Mixed dentition on panoramic film.

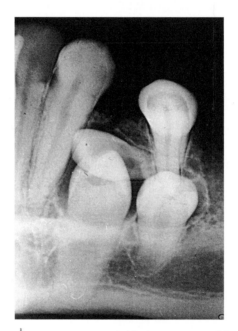

Figure 23-6. | Supernumerary tooth blocking eruption of first premolar.

ERUPTION OF TEETH

Periapical radiographs of patients up to age 12 reveal some evidence of a mixed dentition. The permanent teeth or tooth buds are seen apical to the *deciduous* teeth they will replace (Figures 23-8 and 23-9). The first, second, and third permanent molars, which have no deciduous predecessors, also can be seen in various stages of formation (Figure 23-10). The force of the erupting permanent tooth causes resorption of the deciduous roots, with resulting loosening and loss of the tooth (Figure 23-11). If root formation

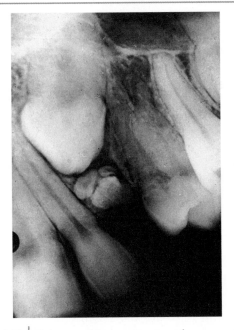

Figure 23-7. | Odontoma blocking eruption of permanent canine.

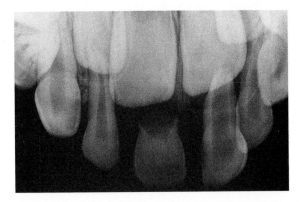

Figure 23-8. | Maxillary central incisor area in a child. Permanent teeth are seen in bone. Note root resorption of deciduous central incisor resulting from an eruptive force.

is not complete, a radiolucent area may appear around the root tip. This radiolucency is the dental *root sack* and should not be confused with periapical pathologic conditions (Figure 23-12). There is a range of ±9 months in the normal development and eruption time of the dentition. Systemic diseases such as hypopituitarism and hypothyroidism cause delayed development; other diseases, such as cleidocranial dysostosis, can cause *overretention* of the primary teeth and postponed permanent tooth eruption (Figure 23-13).

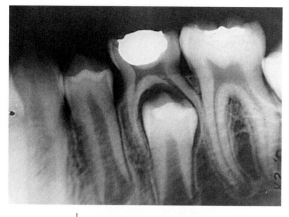

Figure 23-9. | Mixed dentition in mandibular molar area.

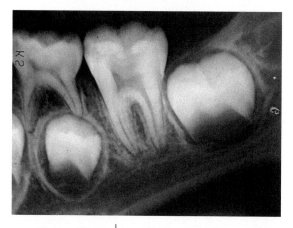

Figure 23-10. | Mandibular mixed dentition.

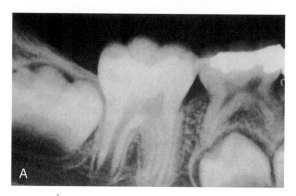

Figure 23-11. | Root resorption of deciduous second molar. **A,** Early.

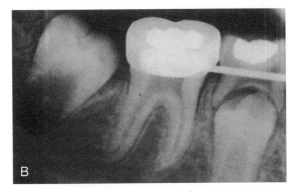

Figure 23-11—cont'd. | **B,** Late.

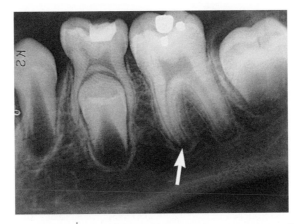

Figure 23-12. | Root sack on developing first permanent molar.

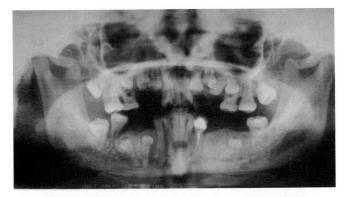

Figure 23-13. | Overretention of primary teeth as seen in an 18-year-old with cleidocranial dysostosis.

IMPACTED TEETH

The radiograph is the prime diagnostic tool in locating and defining the relative position of the impacted tooth because most impacted teeth are not visible on intraoral examination. The maxillary and mandibular third molars are the most common *impactions*. These teeth must be localized not only in their mesiodistal position by periapical, panoramic, or lateral oblique films, but also in the buccolingual relationship by right-angle (90-degree/cross-sectional) occlusal films and/or computed tomographic scanning.

Radiographically, the bony impaction may be seen completely or partially covered by bone (Figure 23-14). A soft tissue impaction is not covered by bone. In some cases the outline of the covering soft tissue appears on the radiograph (Figure 23-15).

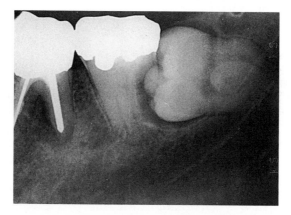

Figure 23-14. Bony impaction of mandibular third molar. Note relationship of tooth to mandibular canal and root resorption of second molar.

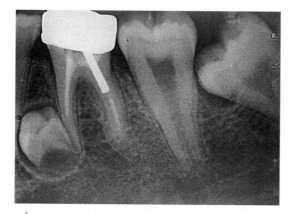

Figure 23-15. Soft tissue impaction. Note supernumerary tooth in premolar area.

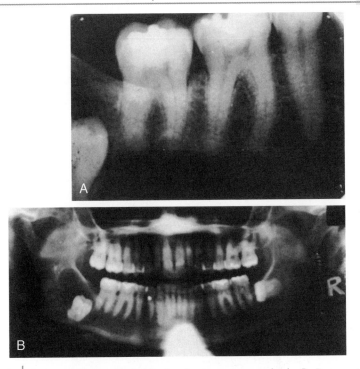

Figure 23-16. **A,** Impacted mandibular third molar not seen completely. **B,** Panoramic radiograph shows extent of dentigerous cyst.

Periapical radiographs of impacted teeth must show the entire tooth and at least 2 to 3 mm of surrounding bone. If periapical projections cannot accomplish this, panoramic or another extraoral projection should be used. If the entire tooth is not seen, a lesion such as the *dentigerous* cyst seen in Figure 23-16 might be missed, with resulting disastrous consequences for the patient.

SUPERNUMERARY TEETH (HYPERDONTIA)

Supernumerary or extra teeth, and their relative position to other teeth, are easily detectable on the proper radiographs. As with impacted teeth, the buccolingual relationship can be established by the use of right-angle occlusal films. The most common supernumerary teeth are mandibular premolars, maxillary incisors, and fourth molars (see Figures 23-15 and 23-17). If the supernumerary tooth occurs between the maxillary central incisors, it is called a *mesiodens* (Figure 23-18). If it is positioned distal to the third molar, it is referred to as a *distodens* (paramolar or fourth molar).

Supernumerary teeth may erupt into the mouth or remain impacted. They may delay or prevent the eruption of the normal dentition. Supernumerary

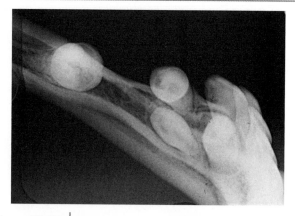

Figure 23-17. | Supernumerary premolar seen on occlusal view.

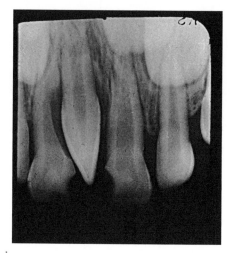

Figure 23-18. | Mesiodens. Supernumerary tooth between the central incisors.

roots also can occur on teeth and may or may not be detected radiographically (Figure 23-19).

CONGENITALLY MISSING TEETH

Hypodontia is the failure of teeth to develop. It can occur in either the primary or adult dentition. It can be a single missing tooth, many missing teeth (*oligodontia*), or complete absence of teeth (*anodontia*). Missing teeth can be detected clinically. The diagnosis of hypodontia can be made definitively only by radiographic examination of the underlying bone (Figure 23-20).

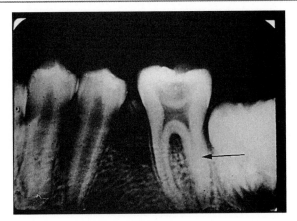

Figure 23-19. | Supernumerary roots. After extraction, two distal roots were found on the first molar. Note how wide the distal root is.

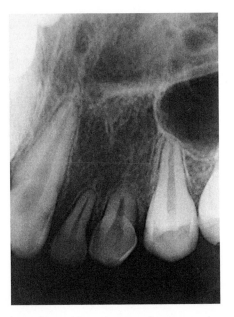

Figure 23-20. | Partial anodontia. Note absence of permanent lateral incisor and canine.

MALPOSITION OF TEETH

Teeth that do not occupy their normal position in the mouth are said to be *malposed*. Tumors, cysts, supernumerary teeth, or lack of space may keep a tooth from achieving its proper position. If a tooth occupies the normal position of another tooth, it is said to be *transposed* (Figure 23-21).

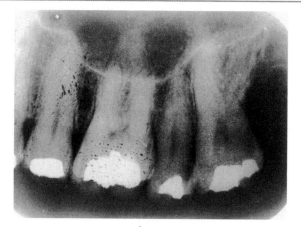

Figure 23-21. | Tooth transposition.

HYPERCEMENTOSIS

Hypercementosis is a condition characterized by the buildup of cementum on the root of the tooth. Normally it is difficult to distinguish cementum from dentin because of its thin layers and similar densities. The buildup of cementum makes the root appear club-shaped instead of its usual conical appearance (Figure 23-22). This condition can be seen in patients who have Paget's disease of bone.

ENAMEL PEARLS

Enamel pearls (enameloma) are small, spherical-shaped pieces of enamel attached to the roots of teeth. Enamel pearls usually are seen at the trifurcation

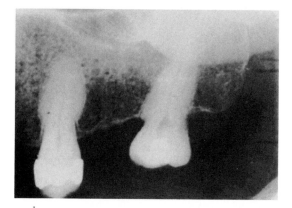

Figure 23-22. | Hypercementosis. Note club-shaped root on second premolar.

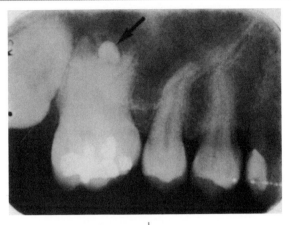

Figure 23-23. Enamel pearl.

of maxillary molars or the bifurcation of mandibular molars. They are asymptomatic and are usually discovered through routine radiographic examination (Figure 23-23).

FUSION

Fusion is a condition that occurs when two teeth join early in their development. The result is usually a single large crown with two root canals (Figure 23-24).

GEMINATION

Gemination occurs when a single tooth germ splits during its development. It usually appears as two crowns with a common root canal (Figure 23-25).

CONCRESCENCE

Concrescence is the joining of two or more teeth by cementum. Although seen radiographically, it may be very difficult to differentiate concrescence from teeth in close contact or those superimposed on one another.

DENS INVAGINATUS

Dens invaginatus, or dens in dente, is not a "tooth within a tooth," as it is commonly referred to, but an invagination of the enamel organ within the

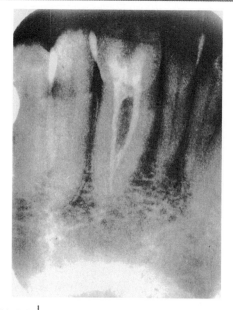

Figure 23-24. | Fusion. Note single crown with two root canals.

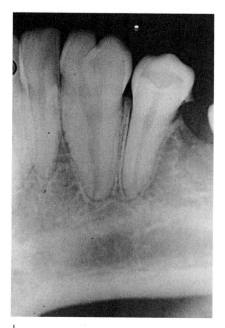

Figure 23-25. | Gemination. Note two crowns with common root canal.

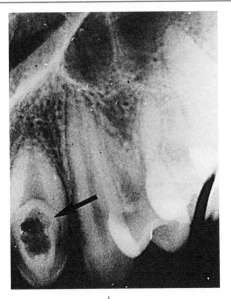

Figure 23-26. | Dens invaginatus.

body of the tooth. The point of invagination of the enamel is usually the cingulum of the tooth (Figure 23-26).

DILACERATION (S-SHAPED ROOT)

Dilaceration is a permanent distortion of the shape and relationship of either the crown or the root of the tooth. This abnormality would only present a problem if the tooth required root canal therapy or extraction. It is thought to be caused by trauma during development of the tooth (Figure 23-27). It is important to distinguish between dilaceration and a distorted or bent image

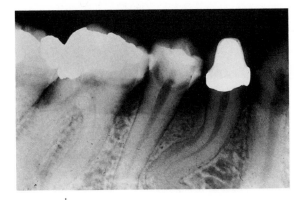

Figure 23-27. | Dilaceration. Note the curved root on first premolar.

caused by overbending of the film packet during film placement. In dilaceration only one part of the image is distorted, whereas the rest of the structures are normal.

TAURODONTIA

In *taurodontia* the body of the tooth is elongated with the extension of the pulp chamber into the elongation; the roots are short, but the size of the crown is normal (Figure 23-28). It acquires its name because of a likeness to a bull.

AMELOGENESIS IMPERFECTA

Amelogenesis imperfecta is a hereditary disturbance that affects both the primary and secondary dentition. The dentin and root formation are normal. The enamel on the teeth is thin and of poor quality and may fracture away completely. Radiographically, the absence of enamel or thin enamel is apparent (Figure 23-29).

DENTINOGENESIS IMPERFECTA

Dentinogenesis imperfecta is also a hereditary disturbance that affects both the primary and secondary dentition. It is characterized by poor enamel that may wear thin or chip, early calcification of the pulp chambers and canals, and short roots especially noticeable in the permanent teeth (Figure 23-30).

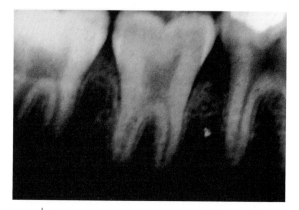

Figure 23-28. | Taurodontia. Note the longitudinal distortion and short roots.

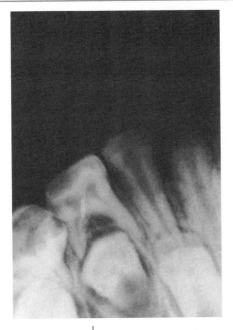

Figure 23-29. Amelogenesis imperfecta.

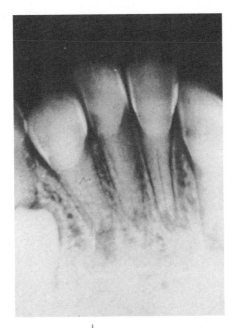

Figure 23-30. Dentinogenesis imperfecta.

FISSURAL CYSTS

Fissural cysts are always found in predictable anatomic locations because they develop along embryonic suture lines. The nasopalatine cyst where the teeth are vital appears as a radiolucency in the midline near the apices of the maxillary central incisors and must be differentiated from periapical pathologic processes. The globulomaxillary cyst is always seen as a pear-shaped radiolucency between the maxillary lateral incisor and canine. The median palatine cyst is seen as an oval radiolucency in the midline of the palate. The nasopalatine and globulomaxillary cysts appear on periapical films of their respective areas; the median palatine cyst is seen best on occlusal films (Figures 23-31 to 23-33).

CLEFT PALATE

The failure of embryonic processes to fuse in development causes *clefts*. These clefts can occur in the hard palate, soft palate, or both. Clefts can disturb the dental lamina, resulting in anodontia, malposition, or supernumerary teeth. Radiographically, the cleft appears as a radiolucent area in which one would expect to find bone (Figure 23-34).

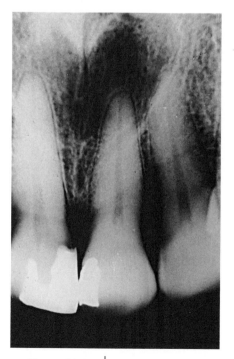

Figure 23-31. | Nasopalatine cyst.

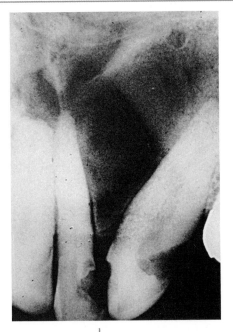

Figure 23-32. │ Globulomaxillary cyst.

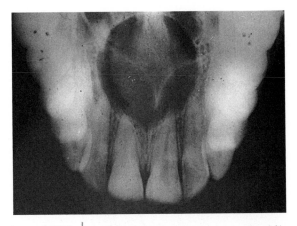

Figure 23-33. │ Median palatine cyst seen on occlusal film.

DENTIGEROUS CYST

A dentigerous cyst forms when the developing tooth bud undergoes cystic degeneration. The cyst may surround or be lateral to the developing tooth. It is most commonly seen in association with third molars. A cyst that forms from the dental lamina before the tooth bud forms is called a *primordial cyst* (Figures 23-35 and 23-36).

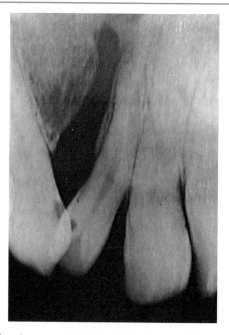

Figure 23-34. | Cleft palate. Note radiolucent defect between lateral incisor and canine.

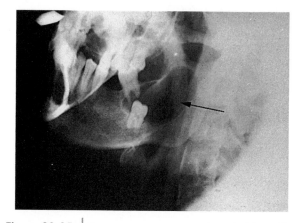

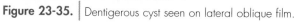

Figure 23-35. | Dentigerous cyst seen on lateral oblique film.

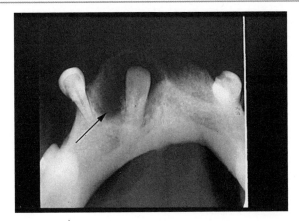

Figure 23-36. | Dentigerous cyst seen on mandibular occlusal film.

SUGGESTED READINGS

White SC, Pharoah MJ: Oral radiology: principles and interpretation, ed 5, St Louis, Mosby, 2004.

CHAPTER 24

Bone and Other Lesions

EDUCATIONAL OBJECTIVES

1. Recognize bone lesions and differentiate their appearance from normal.
2. Understand which radiographic projections are needed to formulate a complete radiographic diagnosis of bone lesions.

KEY TERMS

benign
extraction socket
fracture
hyperostotic lines

malignancy
metabolic condition
mixed lesions
radiolucent lesion

radiopaque lesion
sialoliths
trabecular pattern

DESCRIPTION OF LESIONS

This portion of the text applies the principles of diagnosis that were discussed previously. After discovering a lesion radiographically, the diagnostician must know certain facts about its radiographic appearance. In gathering this information, more radiographs may be required to assemble all the information necessary to make the final diagnosis. The following is a repetition of certain diagnostic criteria and categories that illustrate the diagnostic procedures.

Radiolucent versus Radiopaque

In describing or, in some cases, categorizing bone lesions, they are referred to as radiopaque, radiolucent, or mixed. A *radiopaque lesion* indicates an increase in the density of the bone or new calcified material being formed (e.g., osteoma), whereas a radiolucent lesion indicates a decrease in density or destruction of bone (e.g., cyst). The *mixed lesions* have both processes occurring (e.g., periapical cemental dysplasia).

Location

In making a diagnosis of a pathologic bone condition, location is very important because some lesions have a predilection for certain areas of the mouth (e.g., ameloblastoma in the mandibular third molar region).

Extent of the Lesion

The diagnostician must see the entire lesion and be able to define its borders and extent in three planes before any type of treatment is instituted. Large pathologic areas often require the use of panoramic, extraoral, computed tomographic, or magnetic resonance projections to obtain this information.

Benign versus Malignant

The possibility of *malignancy* always must be considered when diagnosing an unknown lesion. In general, malignancies tend to have poorly defined radiographic borders and destroy normal anatomic structures (Figure 24-1). *Benign* tumors and cysts expand slowly with clearly defined borders referred to as *hyperostotic lines*. Their slow growth tends to displace rather than destroy structures. As seen on occlusal films, benign lesions expand the buccal and lingual cortex of bone, whereas malignant lesions perforate and invade neighboring tissue (Figure 24-2). This effect on the buccal and lingual cortices can be seen best on right-angle occlusal projections of the maxilla and mandible as well as on computed tomographic scans.

CYSTS AND TUMORS

All cysts located in bone are seen as radiolucent areas. Tumors can appear radiolucent, radiopaque, or mixed. When the cyst and the tumor appear radiolucent, the lesion has destroyed normal bone and replaced it with less dense cystic or tumor tissue (Figure 24-3). If the lesion is radiopaque, this signifies that the new tumor tissue being formed has a greater density or size than the tissue it is replacing (Figure 24-4). The mixed lesion may have a variety of densities. Tumors of bone and cartilage appear radiopaque, whereas all other tumors appear radiolucent. The odontoma has a variety of

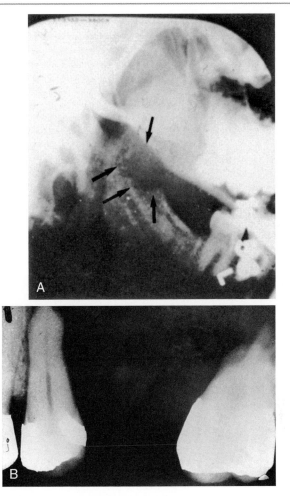

Figure 24-1. | **A,** Lateral oblique radiograph showing destruction of coronoid process by malignant tumor. **B,** Periapical radiograph of maxillary premolar area showing complete bone destruction as evidenced by the radiolucent malignant lesion.

densities corresponding to the densities of tooth structure (i.e., enamel, dentin, cementum, and pulp) (Figure 24-5).

METABOLIC BONE LESIONS

Many *metabolic conditions* manifest themselves with changes of the trabecular pattern and lamina dura of bone in the mandible and maxilla. Examples of this type of disease process are Paget's disease (cotton wool bony appearance), hyperparathyroidism, and certain types of anemia. The dental professional's role is not to diagnose these diseases, but rather to recognize the change from

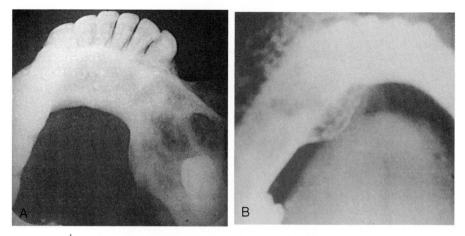

Figure 24-2. **A,** Occlusal radiograph showing expansion of buccal and lingual plates of mandible caused by benign tumor. **B,** Occlusal radiograph showing perforation and spread through the buccal and lingual cortices by a malignant tumor.

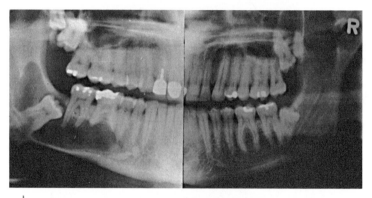

Figure 24-3. Radiograph of tumor (ameloblastoma) enveloping teeth on the right side of mandible.

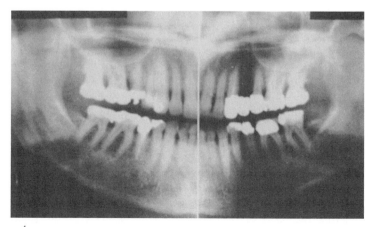

Figure 24-4. Panoramic radiograph showing well-defined radiopaque tumor in left maxillary sinus. Compare right and left maxillary sinuses.

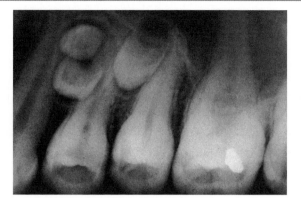

Figure 24-5. | Radiograph of an odontoma. Note the densities that correspond to tooth structures.

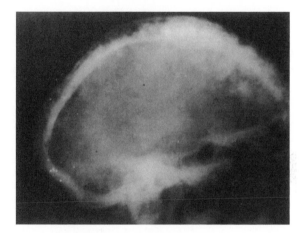

Figure 24-6. | Paget's disease. Lateral skull projection showing the characteristic "cotton wool" appearance of Paget's disease of bone.

normal as seen on the radiographs (Figures 24-6 to 24-8) and then refer the client for treatment.

TRAUMATIC INJURIES

Fractures of teeth, especially anterior teeth, are very common. Clinically and radiographically, a fracture of the crown of a tooth is easier to detect than a root fracture. The fracture appears on the radiograph as a radiolucent line, or the missing part of the tooth is apparent (see Figure 24-7). A root fracture also is seen as a radiolucent line, but is much more difficult to visualize because of superimposition of alveolar bone trabeculation (Figures 24-9 and 24-10). Tooth and root fractures can lead to pulp damage and ensuing

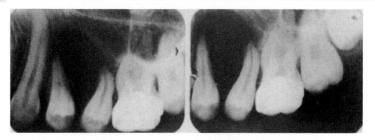

Figure 24-7. | Radiolucent lesion of hyperparathyroidism seen between roots of premolars.

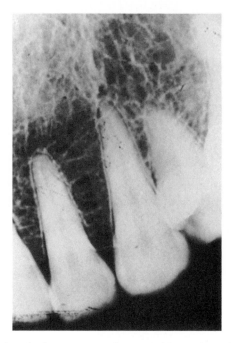

Figure 24-8. | Trabecular bone pattern of anemia. Note enlarged medullary spaces.

periapical pathologic conditions. Fractures of the maxilla and mandible may be seen in part on periapical film (see Figure 18-23), but larger views, such as panoramic or extraoral films, are needed for complete visualization (Figures 24-11 and 24-12). The fracture appears as a radiolucent line, and radiographs may show displacement of the fracture segments.

FOREIGN BODIES AND ROOT TIPS

Any sort of foreign body can be embedded in the jawbones. Only those that are radiopaque can be seen radiographically. Metallic foreign bodies are the

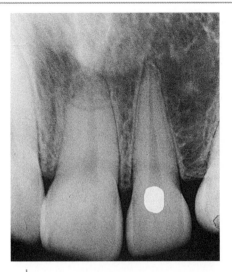

Figure 24-9. | Root fracture near apex of maxillary central incisor.

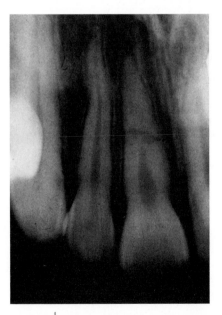

Figure 24-10. | Root fracture, maxillary central incisor.

easiest to see and the most common. These radiopacities may be amalgam, burrs, broken instruments, needles, metallic fragments from an external source (Figure 24-13), wires used to reduce fractures, or metallic implants (Figures 24-14 and 24-15).

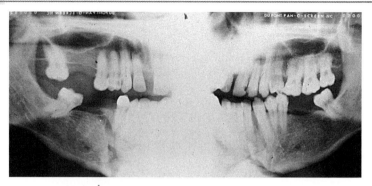

Figure 24-11. | Panoramic radiograph showing fractured mandible.

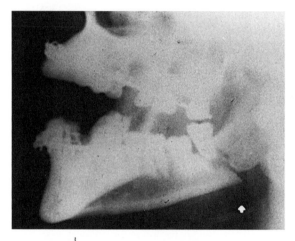

Figure 24-12. | Fracture of mandible on a lateral oblique film.

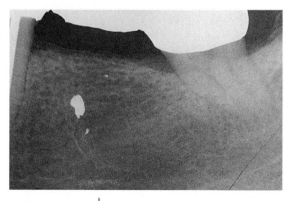

Figure 24-13. | Metallic foreign body in mandible.

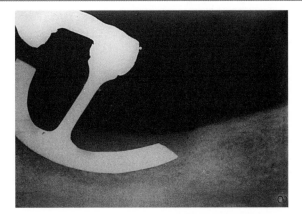

Figure 24-14. Metallic implant of the mandible serving as distal abutment. Note thinning of bone indicating start of rejection process.

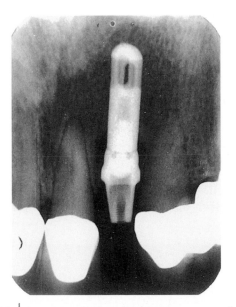

Figure 24-15. Osseointegrated implant seen on periapical radiograph.

Retained root tips have the density of tooth structure (Figure 24-16), so sometimes it is difficult to distinguish between the retained root tip and dense areas of bone. One way to differentiate is by the appearance of a pulp canal or the conical shape of a root tip. These root tips should be localized radiographically in three dimensions before treatment is attempted.

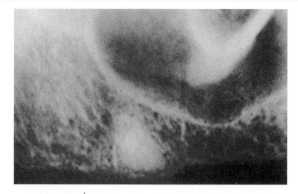

Figure 24-16. | Retained root tip in maxillary molar region.

EXTRACTION SOCKETS

Extraction sockets may be radiographically evident in the bone up to 6 months after surgery. They initially appear as radiolucent areas, and then the area eventually fills in with bone in the normal *trabecular pattern* (Figure 24-17).

SALIVARY STONES

Although not a bone lesion, salivary stones are included here because salivary gland disease is often treated by the dentist and can be seen on dental radiographs. Although the salivary glands and ducts are soft tissue, radiographs are still important in the diagnostic workup. Salivary stones (*sialoliths*) are a common cause of obstruction, secondary swelling, and infection. Because the sialolith is calcified, it can be seen on radiographs. Stones in the submandibular duct can be seen best on a mandibular occlusal film (Figure 24-18).

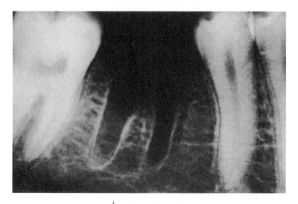

Figure 24-17. | Extraction socket in mandible.

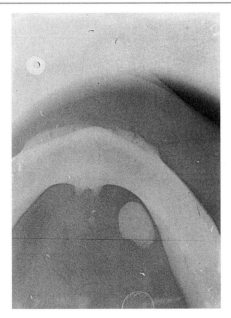

Figure 24-18. | Occlusal radiograph of edentulous mandible showing radiopaque salivary stone in submandibular duct in floor of mouth.

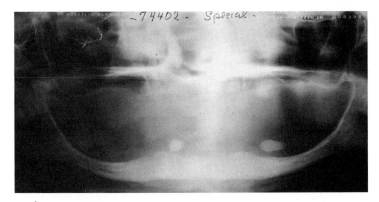

Figure 24-19. | Salivary stone seen on panoramic film. The stone is seen twice as this "Panorex" unit produces a redundant image.

Stones also can be seen on panoramic radiographs and periapical films (Figure 24-19). For the parotid gland, in which stones are not so common, a lateral oblique, posteroanterior, computed tomographic scan, or soft tissue film placed in the mucobuccal fold can be employed.

SUGGESTED READINGS

White SC, Pharoah MJ: Oral radiology: principles and interpretation, ed 5, St Louis, Mosby, 2004.

Legal Considerations

EDUCATIONAL OBJECTIVES

1. Describe and be able to differentiate between state and federal regulations as they pertain to dental radiology and licensure.
2. Understand the concept of informed consent.
3. Understand the concepts of risk management as they apply to patient relations, ownership and retention of radiographs, and the medical and radiation history.
4. Understand the legal status of insurance forms and the dental records.

KEY TERMS

confidentiality
direct supervision
disclosure
federal regulations
general supervision
Health Insurance
   Portability and

Accountability Act
   (HIPAA)
informed consent
liability
licensure
negligent
radiation inspection

records
respondeat superior
risk management
standard of care
statute of limitations

It may be a sign of the times, but no discussion of a subject in the health sciences can be considered complete today without mentioning the legal aspects that affect the profession. Radiology is no exception; it is probably the most regulated discipline within dentistry, with its registration and certification of x-ray machines, laws, and special testing for operators of the equipment. Therefore one must understand the laws and regulations, both local and federal, that govern the use of radiation in this profession.

The legal considerations with which the dental professional should be familiar regarding the use of ionizing radiation in dentistry fall into three major categories: (1) federal and state regulations regarding x-ray equipment and its use; (2) licensure and periodic inspection for users of x-ray equipment; and (3) risk management.

FEDERAL AND STATE REGULATIONS

All dental x-ray machines either manufactured or sold in the United States after 1974 must meet the federal regulations (federal government's performance standards), which include safety specifications for minimum filtration and accuracy and reproducibility of the milliamperage time and kilovoltage settings. These standards are discussed in Chapters 1 and 3.

Actually, all x-ray equipment, regardless of the date of manufacture, is subject to state, county, or city radiation health codes. These codes may include regulations concerning barriers, film speed, position of the operator, and, more recently, film processing. It is not unusual for the registration of x-ray machines to be required and a fee charged for such a permit.

Many states or other jurisdictions require biannual or triennial radiation inspections of the x-ray machines in the dental office, for which a fee is charged. Violations of the radiation code can lead to fines or suspension of a dentist's radiation permit. The positive aspect of these inspections is that they serve as a quality assurance (QA) procedure. The inspectors, as they measure for violations, perform recommended QA procedures that dentists could not do themselves because of the need for sophisticated radiation-monitoring equipment.

LICENSURE

Regarding licensure, each state has its own policy for the user of dental radiation. The dental hygienist, who in all states is a licensed professional, may or may not have to take an additional examination to be certified to perform dental radiography. The dental assistant may be required to take a radiology examination other than the national certifying examination to be authorized to perform dental radiography. Some states have exceptions in their radiation rules that allow an uncertified dental assistant to take radiographs under the direct supervision of a dentist. Direct supervision means that the dentist is physically present in the office when the radiographs are taken. Hygienists may take radiographs under the general supervision of a dentist, which means the hygienist is performing these tasks in a licensed dentist's office or clinic and can be reached if necessary. In most states, dental assistants cannot take extraoral films other than a panoramic film.

Each state deals with dental radiography differently. It is not the purpose of this text to compile lists of these requirements because they change rapidly. The dental professional should be knowledgeable about the rules and regulations of the state or jurisdiction in which he or she is working and should not assume that all state regulations are the same.

RISK MANAGEMENT

By far the most important legal aspect of dental radiology is risk management. Everyone knows about the increase in the number of malpractice suits against professionals. Dentistry has not been excluded from this trend, and malpractice actions have increased in number and the amount of awards over recent years. Risk management concerns the policies and procedures designed to reduce the likelihood of suits for malpractice against dentists. All members of the dental staff must be aware of and participate in the risk management efforts of the office if they are to be effective.

First, it must be pointed out that liability, both professionally and legally, rests with the dentist and not the dental hygienist or dental assistant. This is called the doctrine of *respondeat superior*, or the "captain of the ship" principle; more simply put, the captain of the ship is responsible for the actions of the sailors. The dental professional may be named in a lawsuit, but the liability is ultimately with the employing dentist.

A dental hygienist falls under the doctrine of respondeat superior if she or he is an employee. If the hygienist is the one found to be negligent, the dentist's insurance company may decide to subrogate (sue the hygienist's company for a share of the award) the payment of the claim against the hygienist or the hygienist's insurance company. Therefore the hygienist is well advised to carry professional liability insurance. If the hygienist is an independent contractor, then he or she may be sued alone.

Patient Relations

Avoiding misunderstandings is a critical component of risk management. Dental office staff must communicate in advance to patients about how the office policy deals with financial arrangements, payments, recall procedures, and the filing of insurance claims.

Dental professionals should never say anything negative about equipment, procedures, staff, or anything else in the office. If the equipment is not working correctly, one should not complain in front of or to the patient. Remarks such as "this timer is always off" or "these films weren't processed properly" are unnecessary. These comments are considered "admissions against interest," also known as the theory of *res gestae*. Statements made by anyone spontaneously at the time of an alleged negligent act are admissible as evidence.

Informed Consent

The dental professional may participate in the process of obtaining informed consent, which entails explaining to the patient the nature and purpose of the procedure. This is called *full disclosure*. In the case of taking radiographs, full disclosure entails explaining to the patient, in lay terms, the risks and benefits to be derived. Recent legal decisions have noted that it is equally important to inform the patient of the risks of not having a specific procedure. In this case the patient must be told about the diseases that might go undetected without radiography and the possible consequences. If the patient is a minor, the parent or guardian must consent.

If a patient refuses a recommended radiographic examination, this should be entered into his or her record to justify why treatment will not be rendered. There are few if any dental procedures that should be done without current and diagnostic radiographs because their use is now the accepted standard of care. Patient refusal is not a valid reason for treating without radiographs.

Health Questionnaire

The dental professional always should review the patient's health history and questionnaire and update as necessary. He or she should call to the dentist's attention any information that might contraindicate or change the number and type of radiographs that are to be taken.

RECORDS

It has been said that the three most important parts of a defense in a malpractice suit are "records, records, records." Dental radiographs are considered part of the patient's dental record and so are considered legal documents. The number and quality of the radiographs may be an important issue in any litigation. If the quality is poor and nondiagnostic and the procedures in question are based on the radiographs, this substantially weakens the defense. If the radiographs are lost or misfiled or do not have archival life, then again the case for the defense is seriously compromised.

The most common error is the failure to make an entry in the patient's record when radiographs are taken; the date, number, and type of radiograph should always be recorded. There are no exceptions to this rule. Postoperative, working endodontic, or retakes must be recorded, or the records will be deemed incomplete. Individual radiographs, pantomograms, and full-mouth series should be labeled and dated. If it is a single film in a coin envelope, care should be taken that the envelope is labeled and placed securely in the chart folder. One can easily recognize the role of the dental professional in this phase of risk management. The issue of the legal status of digital radiographs and possible alterations of the images is discussed in Chapter 15.

Confidentiality

The patient's records are confidential. The contents or findings in these records should never be discussed or shown to anyone outside the office. Confidentiality also pertains to any radiographs or photographs that are part of the record. Since April 2000 it has also been necessary that all records comply with the *Health Insurance Portability and Accountability Act* (*HIPAA*) (Box 25-1).

Box 25-1 | **Health Insurance Portability and Accountability Act of 1996**

The Health Insurance Portability and Accountability Act (HIPAA) of 1996 was signed into law by President Bill Clinton on August 21, 1996. Conclusive regulations were issued on August 17, 2000, to be instated by October 16, 2002. HIPAA requires that the transactions of all patient healthcare information be formatted in a standardized electronic style. In addition to protecting the privacy and security of patient information, HIPAA includes legislation on the formation of medical savings accounts, the authorization of a fraud and abuse control program, the easy transport of health insurance coverage, and the simplification of administrative terms and conditions.

HIPAA encompasses three primary areas, and its privacy requirements can be broken down into three types: privacy standards, patients' rights, and administrative requirements.

1. *Privacy Standards.* A central concern of HIPAA is the careful use and disclosure of protected health information (PHI), which generally is electronically controlled health information that can be distinguished individually. PHI also refers to verbal communication, although the HIPAA Privacy Rule is not intended to hinder necessary verbal communication. The U.S. Department of Health and Human Services (USDHHS) does not require restructuring, such as soundproofing, architectural changes, and so forth, but some caution is necessary when exchanging health information by conversation.

   An Acknowledgment of Receipt Notice of Privacy Practices, which allows patient information to be used or divulged for treatment, payment, or health care operations (TPOs), should be procured from each patient. A detailed and time-sensitive authorization can also be issued, which allows the dentist to release information in special circumstances other than TPOs. A written consent is also an option. Dentists can disclose PHI without acknowledgment, consent, or authorization in very special situations, such as perceived child abuse, public health supervision, fraud investigation, or law enforcement with valid permission (i.e., a warrant). When divulging PHI, a dentist must try to disclose only the minimum necessary information to help safeguard the patient's information as much as possible.

Continued

| Box 25-1 | Health Insurance Portability and Accountability Act of 1996—cont'd |

It is important that dental professionals adhere to HIPAA standards because healthcare providers (as well as healthcare clearinghouses and healthcare plans) who convey electronically formatted health information via an outside billing service or merchant are considered covered entities. Covered entities may be dealt serious civil and criminal penalties for violation of HIPAA legislation. Failure to comply with HIPAA privacy requirements may result in civil penalties of up to $100 per offense with an annual maximum of $25,000 for repeated failure to comply with the same requirement. Criminal penalties resulting from the illegal mishandling of private health information can range from $50,000 and/or 1 year in prison to $250,000 and/or 10 years in prison.

2. *Patients' Rights.* HIPAA allows patients, authorized representatives, and parents of minors, as well as minors, to become more aware of the health information privacy to which they are entitled. These rights include, but are not limited to, the right to view and copy their health information, the right to dispute alleged breaches of policies and regulations, and the right to request alternative forms of communicating with their dentist. If any health information is released for any reason other than TPO, the patient is entitled to an account of the transaction. Therefore, it is important for dentists to keep accurate records of such information and to provide them when necessary.

The HIPAA Privacy Rule determines that the parents of a minor have access to their child's health information. This privilege may be overruled, such as in cases in which there is suspected child abuse or the parent consents to a term of confidentiality between the dentist and the minor. The parents' rights to access their child's PHI also may be restricted in situations in which a legal entity, such as a court, intervenes and when a law does not require a parent's consent. For a full list of patient rights provided by HIPAA, be sure to acquire a copy of the law and understand it well.

3. *Administrative Requirements.* Complying with HIPAA legislation may seem like a chore, but it does not have to be so. It is recommended that dental professionals become appropriately familiar with the law, organize the requirements into simpler tasks, begin compliance early, and document their office's progress in compliance. An important first step is to evaluate the current information and practices of the office.

Dentists will need to write a privacy policy for their office, a document for their patients detailing the office's practices concerning PHI. The American Dental Association's HIPAA Privacy Kit includes forms that the dentist can use to customize a privacy policy. It is useful to try to understand the role of healthcare information for patients and the ways in which they deal with the information while they are visiting the dental office. The dentist should train the staff, making sure they are familiar with the terms of HIPAA and the office's privacy policy and related forms. HIPAA requires that the dentist designate a privacy officer, a person in the office who will be responsible for applying the new policies, fielding complaints, and making choices involving the minimum necessary requirements. Another person with the role of contact person will process complaints.

A *Notice of Privacy Practices*—a document detailing the patient's rights and the dental office's obligations concerning PHI—also must be drawn up. Furthermore any role of a third party with access to PHI must be clearly documented. This third party is known as a business associate (BA) and is defined as any entity who, on behalf of the dentist, takes part in any activity that involves exposure of PHI. The *HIPAA Privacy Kit* provides a copy of the USDHHS "Business Associate Contract Terms," which provides a concrete format for detailing BA interactions.

The main HIPAA privacy compliance date, including all staff training, was April 14, 2003, although many covered entities who submitted a request and a compliance plan by October 15, 2002, were granted 1-year extensions. The dentist can contact the local branch of the ADA for details. It is recommended that dentists prepare their offices ahead of time for all deadlines, which include preparing privacy polices and forms, business associate contracts, and employee training sessions.

For a comprehensive discussion of all of these terms and requirements, a complete list of HIPAA policies and procedures, and a full collection of HIPAA privacy forms, contact the ADA for a HIPAA Privacy Kit. The relevant ADA Web site is www.ada.org/goto/hipaa. Other Web sites that may contain useful information about HIPAA are:

- USDHHS Office of Civil Rights (www.hhs.gov/ocr/hipaa)
- Work Group on Electronic Data Interchange (www.wedi.org/SNIP)
- Phoenix Health (www.hipaadvisory.com)
- USDHHS Office of the Assistant Secretary for Planning and Evaluation (http://aspe.os.dhhs.gov/admnsimp/)

Data from: HIPAA Privacy Kit and http://www.ada.org/prof/prac/issues/topics/hipaa/index.html. (From *Mosby's Dental Dictionary*, St Louis, Mosby, 2004.)

OWNERSHIP

The dentist is the guardian and keeper of dental records, and such records are the property of the dentist. Patients may request a copy of their radiographs, and this request should be written and signed by the patient. A fee may be charged for this duplication. Laws differ from state to state on whether a dental office must give the radiographs to the patient if the fee for this service has not been paid. In some states the radiographs or copies must be given to the patient even if the fee has not been paid. The dentist may pursue collection but only after giving the radiographs to the patient. This is not true in all states and only underscores that one must be familiar with the laws regulating practice in the state in which one works.

The dentist should be informed of this request and an entry made in the record of when and to whom the duplicate radiographs were sent. Never under any circumstances should the original radiographs be given or sent to a patient. There is no defense if there are no radiographs. One should not make the assumption that "this is an old and loyal patient who would never dream of taking legal action." That is a poor risk management assumption. However, on occasion the court may request or subpoena the original radiographs, and with this order one must comply.

Retention

Dental radiographs should be kept for 7 years after the patient ceases to be a patient in the office, depending on state laws. Ideally they should be kept forever. Actions that can be brought against a dentist depend on the statute of limitations. The usual time limitation for an adult is 3 years after the discovery of the injury or when the injury should have been discovered. For children, it is 3 years after they reach their maturity, which in some states is 21 years. Suits therefore can be brought many years past the mandated 7 years of retention of radiographs.

INSURANCE CLAIMS

It is the legitimate right of the insurance company to request copies of pretreatment radiographs to evaluate a treatment plan. The original radiographs should never be sent to the insurance company because they may be lost in the mail or by the insurance company. In either case the dentist is left without an important part of the patient's record, and in case of litigation, the fact that the originals were lost is no defense.

As mentioned in Chapter 6, radiographs should never be taken to prove to the insurance company that the services have been performed. The result of this action would be an administrative radiograph, which is considered unsuitable.

SUGGESTED READINGS
Weissman BJ, Serman NJ: The law and who can expose dental radiographs, Oral Surg Oral Med Oral Pathol Oral Radiol Endod 90:663-665, 2000.

Common Error Summaries

COMMON PROCESSING ERRORS (See also Chapter 8)

Common Processing Error	Appearance	Cause	Remedy
Fogged film	Overall gray appearance due to diminished contrast.	Darkroom errors: light leaks, improper safelight, improper film storage, and outdated film.	Check for light leaks. Check safelight with "coin test." Store film in cool area and away from sources of scatter radiation. Check expiration date on film box and use old film first.
Underdeveloped film (thin image)	Light (thin) in appearance.	Insufficient developing time. Cold developing solution. Weak developing solution.	Change solution every 2-3 weeks (or more frequently if necessary). Use time-temperature method of developing. Utilize "reference film," step wedge, or dental radiographic normalizing and monitoring device to check solution strength.
Overdeveloped film (dense image)	Dark (dense) in appearance.	Prolonged developing time. Hot developing solution.	Use time-temperature method of developing. Perform daily QA checks on solution strength.
Developer cutoff	A straight radiopaque border on what was the upper edge of the top film on the processing rack or was not exposed to developing solution in the automatic processor.	This represents an undeveloped area of the film. When the solutions are allowed to deplete in the processing tanks, the films on the top positions of the racks may not be covered by solution when the racks are placed in the tanks.	Keep processing tanks full. If the level of solution has dropped, do not add water. Add replenisher solution to maintain the desired levels. This error can also occur in automatic processing.

Clear films	No image is seen. Emulsion is removed completely.	This error should be differentiated from collimator cutoff, which will give a curved radiopaque border if circular collimation is used and a straight border if rectangular collimation is used. In collimator cutoff, the film portion is unexposed. In developer cutoff the film portion is undeveloped. Films remain in the water bath from 24 to 48 hours. Films are in the fixer for prolonged periods of time. Film is unexposed. Films are placed in the fixer before the developer.	Films should be removed from the water bath before the end of the day. Films should not be left in the fixer overnight or for prolonged periods. Keep unexposed and exposed films separated. Remember to plug the machine in and turn it on before exposures are performed. Do not process unexposed films. If processing manually, place the films in the developer solution before the fixer. Make sure the fixer solution is after the developer in the automatic processors.
Stained films	Splotches on the film. (Dark spots = developer; lightspots = fixer.)	Wet or dirty working surface.	Keep all surfaces in the darkroom clean and dry.

Continued

COMMON PROCESSING ERRORS—Cont'd

Common Processing Error	Appearance	Cause	Remedy
Discolored films	Yellowish brown films.	Inadequate fixation.	Fix film optimally for at least 10 minutes or double the developing time. Return all "wet readings" to the fixer tank after the patient has been treated.
Torn emulsion	Film emulsion is torn off.	Films overlap or touch while drying. They will stick together. In separating the films the emulsion is usually torn off the base in the overlapped areas.	Check that drying films do not touch. If they are stuck together, separate them by applying water.
Scratched films	Radiopaque line on film.	Not carefully placing a second with film rack into a tank already containing one rack. Not discarding racks with broken clips. Fingernails too long.	Be careful not to touch one film rack another film rack when placing them into the tank. Discard any film racks that have sharp edges or broken clips. Keep fingernails trimmed and avoid scratching films with fingernails. Darn gloves when applicable.
Lost films in tank	Missing films/films on bottom of tank.	Films not firmly clipped onto rack.	Check that films are firmly clipped onto the rack before placing them into the developer.

Fluoride artifact	Black mark on radiograph.	Some fluorides, especially stannous fluoride, will produce black marks on radiographs.	Operator should wash hands thoroughly before handling films, or change gloves when applicable.
Reticulation	Image has a wrinkled appearance.	Film developed at an elevated temperature and then placed in a cold water bath; the sudden change in temperature causes the swollen emulsion to shrink rapidly and gives the image a wrinkled appearance.	Avoid a sharp contrast in temperature between processing solutions and the water bath.
Air bubbles	White spots on radiograph.	If air bubbles are trapped on the film, the chemicals cannot affect the emulsion in that area.	Film hanger should be gently agitated when placed into the solutions.
Static marks	Multiple black linear streaks (or spots) seen most often on cold, dry days.	Intraoral film packets forcefully opened in the darkroom. Extraoral film not carefully slid out of the box. Extraoral film not carefully loaded and unloaded into and out of the cassette. Walking over carpeting and not grounding yourself before unwrapping the film.	Carefully remove film from packet or extraoral film box. Carefully load and unload extraoral film in cassette. Operators should ground themselves and should avoid friction that will produce static electricity.

Automatic Processing

Daylight loaders: Light leak	Film fog, a ruined film, or unusual artifacts.	Removing one's hands from the baffles before the film has entered the processor.	Operator must keep hands inside the daylight loader until the film has been completely taken up by the automatic processor.

Continued

COMMON PROCESSING ERRORS—Cont'd

Common Processing Error	Appearance	Cause	Remedy
Dirty rollers	Radiolucent bands or white chalky smudges appear on finished film.	Rollers are not cleaned properly.	Rollers should be cleaned periodically by soaking them according to the manufacturer's recommendations. A piece of extraoral film should be run through the processor every workday to clean the rollers.
Overlapped films	Image of overlapped film on finished film.	Films are fed into the processor too quickly.	The operator should not feed the film into the processor immediately after placing the previous film. The operator should wait at least 10 seconds before putting another film into the processor.

New York University College of Dentistry Radiology Department.

COMMON EXPOSURE ERRORS (See also Chapter 10)

Common Exposure Error	Appearance	Cause	Remedy
Collimator cutoff (cone cutting)	A curved or straight radiopaque border representing an unexposed area on the film.	The x-ray beam is not centered on the film packet.	The central ray of the x-ray beam should be aligned with the center of the film packet. Utilization of a localizing ring with a film-holding device can decrease or eliminate the incidence of collimator cutoff. Make sure the patient does not move after the PID is placed for an exposure.
Film reversal ("herringbone effect")	A light film with the geometric pattern from the lead foil backing embossed on it.	The film packet is placed backward in the mouth.	Always note the front and the back of the film packet. Place the white side (front) of the film toward the lingual (palatal) aspect of the tooth.
Improper film placement	The entire desired area (tooth or teeth) does not appear on the film.	The patient does not bite down completely on the bite piece of the film holder (inadequate closure). The center of the film packet is not aligned with the center of the appropriate tooth (depending on the specific projection being exposed).	Make sure the patient bites completely on the bite piece with both opposing maxillary and mandibular teeth. Align the center of the film packet with the center of the area (tooth or teeth) being radiographed. Place the film securely in the slot of the film holder (1/8 inch of the film

Continued

COMMON EXPOSURE ERRORS—Cont'd

Common Exposure Error	Appearance	Cause	Remedy
		Failing to place the film to the base of the slot in the film holder (the incisal edge or occlusal surface is cut off).	should project above or below the incisal edge or occlusal surface of the teeth).
Horizontal overlapping	The interproximal areas of the teeth appear to be overlapped when they are not actually overlapped in the patient's mouth.	The central ray is not directed perpendicular to the film in the horizontal plane.	Direct the central ray through the contact areas in the horizontal plane.
		The film is not placed parallel to the tooth or teeth in the horizontal plane.	Place the film parallel to the tooth or teeth in the horizontal plane.
Crescent marks	Black marks (artifacts) appear on the film.	Excessive bending of the film packet that results in a cracked emulsion.	Do not bend or over-manipulate the film while placing it in the film holder or in the patient's mouth.
Underexposed film (light image)	Light (thin) in appearance.	Inadequate exposure due to increased FFD or insufficient kVp, mA, or exposure time.	Check all the settings (kVP, mA, time) on the control panel before exposing the film. Keep the PID as close to the patient's face as possible.
			Maintain pressure on the exposure button until the indicator light goes off and the sound signal ends.
Overexposed film (dense image)	Dark (dense) in appearance.	Excessive exposure due to decreased FFD or excessive kVp, mA, or exposure time.	Check all the settings (kVP, mA, time) on the control panel before exposing the film.

Double exposure	Two images appear on one film.	Using the same film packet for more than one exposure.	Separate the exposed films from the unexposed films.
Blurred images	Wavy or fuzzy image.	Patient, film, or tubehead (PID) movement during exposure.	Adjust the tubehead/arm to prevent vibration and drifting. Always keep an eye on the patient, especially when exiting the operatory. Ask the patient "not to move" before exiting the operatory.
Failure to remove dental appliances and facial jewelry	Radiopaque (metal) images are superimposed on the film.	Failure to ask the patient to remove any metallic objects from the mouth or facial area that may be in the way of the primary beam.	For intraoral radiographs, remove any obstructive intraoral appliances, eyeglasses, and facial jewelry before exposure. For panoramic/extraoral radiographs, remove any obstructive intraoral appliances; facial, intra/extra-oral and neck jewelry; hair accessories; and hearing aids before exposure.
Elongation	Lengthening of the image on the film.	Inadequate vertical angulation. Improper occlusal plane orientation because of patient positioning. Poor film placement.	Increase the vertical angulation. The occlusal plane should be parallel to the floor. The film should be placed parallel to the tooth in the paralleling technique and as close to the tooth as possible (forming an angle with the tooth) when utilizing the bisecting angle technique.

Continued

COMMON EXPOSURE ERRORS—Cont'd

Common Exposure Error	Appearance	Cause	Remedy
Foreshortening	Shortening of the image on the film.	Excessive vertical angulation. Improper occlusal plane orientation because of patient positioning. Poor film placement.	Decrease the vertical angulation. The occlusal plane should be parallel to the floor. The film should be placed parallel to the tooth in the paralleling technique and as close to the tooth as possible (forming an angle with the tooth) when utilizing the bisecting angle technique.
Bitewing Radiographs			
Horizontal overlapping	The interproximal areas of the teeth appear to be overlapped when they are not actually overlapped in the patient's mouth.	The central ray is not directed perpendicular to the film in the horizontal plane. The film is not placed parallel to the tooth or teeth in the horizontal plane.	The beam should be aligned in the horizontal plane so that it is at right angles to the tooth and film packet. The film should be placed parallel to the tooth or teeth in the horizontal plane.
Collimator cutoff (cone cutting)	A curved radiopaque border representing an unexposed area on the film.	The operator loses sight of the bitewing tab when the patient's mouth is closed.	The bite tab could be kept visible by asking the patient to smile.

| Improper film placement | The entire desired area (tooth or teeth) does not appear on the film. | Usually occurs with bitewings either when the patient is allowed to bite the film into position after the operator has let go of the tab or the patient does not bite in centric relation, allowing the film to float free and be repositioned by the tongue. | The operator can keep a finger on the tab while positioning the PID and directing the central ray at the tab.
A localizing ring can be used to help center the x-ray beam.
The operator should not let go of the film tab until the patient is biting on it completely in centric occlusion. |

New York University College of Dentistry Radiology Department.

COMMON ERRORS IN PANORAMIC RADIOGRAPHY (See also Chapter 12)

Common Error/Cause	Resultant Image	Panoramic Remedy
Patient positioned too far forward	Upper and lower teeth are blurred and narrow; spinal column is superimposed on ramus; premolars are overlapped.	Patient's teeth or edentulous ridges must be in proper anterior-posterior position on the bite block.
Patient positioned too far back	Upper and lower teeth are blurred and widened; increased ghosting of the mandible also appears.	Patient's teeth or edentulous ridges must be in proper anterior-posterior position on he bite block.
Patient's head tilted up; forehead too far back; chin is too far forward	Upper incisors out of focus; the radiopaque hard palate is superimposed over the apices of the upper teeth; condyles are off the film.	The reference lines on the patient's face, the Frankfort plane or the ala-tragus line, should be aligned parallel to the floor.
Patient's head tilted down; chin is back; forehead is forward	Lower incisors are blurred; the radiopaque image of the hyoid bone is superimposed on the anterior part of the mandible; the superior portions of the condyles may be cut off the film; premolars are overlapped.	The reference lines on the patient's face, the Frankfort plane or the ala-tragus line, should be aligned parallel to the floor.
Patient moved during exposure	The part of the film being exposed at the time of movement appears blurred.	Talk to patients prior to and if possible during exposure to remind them not to move.
Patient failed to place tongue on the roof of the mouth	An airspace is created that produces a radiolucent band below the palate; black shadow is produced on the radiograph.	Remind patients to keep the tongue against the roof of the mouth during exposure.
Patient does not sit or stand erect (patient is slouching)	The spinal column causes a triangular radiopacity to be superimposed on the anterior teeth.	Keep patient's spine erect during positioning.

Failure to remove metal objects such as dentures, jewelry, hair accessories, hearing aids, and eyeglasses from the face, head, neck and mouth	Radiopaque ghosting will appear on the opposite side of the film and may obscure desired structures.	Remove all metallic objects from the face, head, neck and mouth regions before exposure.
Lead apron placed above the level of the clavicles	A large radiopacity will appear on the film.	Keep the lead apron low on the patient (below the level of the clavicles); never use a thyroid collar.
Film cassette slowing down because of patient contact	Black vertical band will appear due to localized overexposure. Exposing the patient with radiation	Position the patient carefully; make sure the film will not contact the patient before (especially patients with large frames).
Static electricity	Electrostatic artifact; black linear streaks resembling bare tree branches without leaves.	Be careful not to pull film quickly and forcefully out of box or rubbing film on film screens during film loading, especially on cold/dry days. The operators should ground themselves and avoid friction that will produce static electricity.

New York University College of Dentistry Radiology Department.

abrasion – The wearing away of tooth structure by mechanical means (e.g., toothbrush).

absorption – A process in which the intensity of a beam of radiation is reduced as a result of the interactions involved in passing through matter.

acquired immunodeficiency syndrome (AIDS) – The group of disease entities caused by the human immunodeficiency virus (HIV).

actual focal area – The true representation of the area of the anode of an x-ray tube that the electrons actually strike.

acute (short-term) effects – The effects of radiation that manifest themselves within minutes, days, or weeks after exposure.

administrative radiograph – A radiograph taken for other than diagnostic purposes, such as a radiograph taken for verification of third-party payment.

advanced caries – Caries that has penetrated through the dentin and is about to reach the pulp chamber.

ALARA – The acronym for "as low as reasonably achievable." In dental radiology, this concept reasonably refers to the cost and convenience to the patient.

ala-tragus line – An imaginary line between the ala of the nose and the tragus of the ear that is kept parallel to the floor for maxillary periapical and bitewing films.

alpha particle – A positively charged particle emitted from an atomic nucleus.

alternating current (AC) – Current that flows in one direction and then in the opposite direction in the circuit.

alveolar bone – The bone of the mandible and maxilla that supports and surrounds the roots of the teeth.

alveolar crest – The most coronal portion of the alveolar bone found between the teeth.

amelogenesis imperfecta – The hereditary developmental defect of enamel seen in both the primary and secondary dentition.

American Academy of Oral and Maxillofacial Radiology (AAOMR) – An organization established to promote and advance the art and science of radiology in dentistry and to provide a forum for communication among and professional advancement of its members.

American National Standards Institute (ANSI) – Institute that designates film speed (sensitivity) by using the letters A through F (A for the slowest film and F for the fastest).

ampere (A) – The unit of measurement of the amount of current flowing in an electric circuit. The unit milliampere (mA) is one-thousandth of an ampere and is the important unit of current measurement pertaining to an x-ray tube.

analog – Relating to a mechanism in which data are represented by continuously variable physical quantities.

angstrom unit (Å) – A unit of measurement equal to one-millionth of a centimeter; x-ray wavelengths are expressed in angstrom units.

angulation – The direction of the primary x-ray beam in relation to the tooth and film.

anode – The positively charged side of the dental x-ray tube. It contains the tungsten target at which the electrons are aimed and from which x-rays are emitted.

anodontia – The developmental absence of teeth. It can be complete or partial.

ANSI – See "American National Standards Institute."

anterior nasal spine – The radiopacity seen in the midline of the maxilla at the inferior termination of the nasal septum.

anterior palatine foramen – The opening in the midline of the palate just posterior to the central incisors through which vessels and nerves emerge.

anteroposterior projection – An extraoral radiograph of the skull seen in the coronal plane.

antibiotic prophylaxis – The antimicrobial drugs prescribed before dental treatment for patients whose medical conditions can be affected by a bacteremia resulting from dental treatment.

antiseptic – A substance that inhibits the growth of bacteria.

arch – The formation of teeth seen in the axial plane.

arthrography – Modality for radiographic evaluation of a bone joint after injection of a radiopaque contrast medium.

atom – The basic unit of matter, composed of a positively charged nucleus around which negatively charged electrons revolve.

atomic number – The number of protons in the nucleus of an atom. The symbol is Z, and it is written as the subscript, for example, $_3$Li.

attenuation – Absorbing or weakening of an x-ray beam because of passage through a material.

attrition – The wearing away of teeth by occlusal forces.

autoclaving – The sterilizing of instruments by steam.

automatic processing – The processing of radiographs by machine, eliminating the need for human interaction to move the films from solution baths.

autotransformer – A transformer that has only one coil and a series of taps that allow it to increase or reduce voltage.

axial plane – The plane in the head that is parallel to the floor.

background radiation – The ever-present ionizing radiation in the environment. Its sources include cosmic rays, radioactive materials, industrial waste, and nuclear fallout.

barrier – A radiation-absorbing material such as lead, concrete, or plaster used to protect an area from radiation. The term also refers to protection used against microorganisms, such as use of gloves, masks, glasses, and surface coverings.

barrier envelope – A plastic bag that the x-ray film packet is placed in to prevent contamination by saliva.

becquerel (Bq) – The Système International (SI) unit of radioactivity produced by the disintegration of unstable elements. It replaces the curie.

bedridden – A term used to describe a patient who cannot leave his or her bed; such patients cannot travel to a dental office to receive treatment.

benign – A term applied to tumors that may be harmful but not life-threatening.

beta particles – Electrons emitted from the nuclei of radioactive atoms.

bilateral lesion – A lesion that is on both sides of the oral cavity. Most bilateral findings are normal anatomic landmarks.

binding energy – The energy (expressed in electron volts) that binds the orbiting electrons around the nucleus of an atom.

bisecting-angle technique – A technique for intraoral periapical radiography in which the film packet is positioned as close to tooth and bone as possible and the central x-ray is directed vertically perpendicular at an imaginary line that bisects the angle formed by the long axis of the tooth and the film packet.

bite block – A device used to support and position dental film in the patient's mouth.

bitewing radiographs – Intraoral films that show only the crown portions of opposing teeth in the biting position.

blurred image – An image showing decreased detail and definition as a result of patient, film, and x-ray source movement.

bone marrow – The soft inner portion of bone.

bone window – The density range in computed tomography in which bone images are seen without superimposition of soft tissue.

bremsstrahlung – Literally "braking radiation," the release of a photon of energy by a bombarding electron slowed and bent off course by an atom.

buccal caries – Demineralization of the hard tissue structure present on the outside surface of the tooth that is difficult to detect radiographically.

buccal-object rule – In localization, if an object on a second radiograph moves in the opposite direction of the horizontal tube shift, then the object is buccally positioned.

buccinator shadow – The radiopaque area seen mostly in the maxillary premolar area that represents the soft tissue density of the cheek.

calcification – Hardening of a structure caused by calcium deposition.

calcium tungstate – The fluorescent material used to coat intensifying screens, emitting a blue light.

calculus – The radiopaque calcification concretion that adheres to the roots of teeth.

cancellous bone – Bone that is composed mainly of marrow.

caries – Demineralization of the hard tooth structure with subsequent destruction. Appears radiolucent on radiographs.

cassette – A wrapping or container for x-ray film that is light-tight yet permits penetration of x-rays. Cassettes may be plastic, cardboard, or metal.

cathode – The negatively charged side of the dental x-ray tube. It contains the tungsten filament and the molybdenum focusing cup.

cathode ray – The stream of electrons in the x-ray tube traveling from filament to target.

cell recovery – The process by which cells heal themselves from the effects of radiation.

cementoenamel junction – That place on the tooth where the enamel ends and the dentin begins.

cementum – The calcified tissue that surrounds the root and helps to support the tooth.

center of rotation – In tomography, the point about which the source of radiation rotates.

Centers for Disease Control and Prevention (CDC) – The U.S. governmental agency based in Atlanta, Georgia, that is responsible for tracking and responding to outbreaks of infectious disease.

central ray– That x-ray located in the center of the x-ray beam as it leaves the tube head.

cephalometric radiography – The modality for measuring the skull by means of radiography.

cephalostat – The head-holding device used in cephalometric radiography.

cervical burnout – The shadow seen interproximally on radiographs that is caused by the concavity in the root surface at that area. It may resemble caries.

chair position – The position of the chair and its head rests and back rests during radiographic procedures.

characteristic radiation – X-rays produced when orbiting electrons in an atom fall from outer shells to inner shells after an orbiting electron is knocked out of one of the inner shells by bombarding electrons.

charged coupling device (CCD) – A type of electronic sensor used in direct digital radiography.

chromosomes – One of a definite number of rodlike bodies, containing genes, found in the nucleus of a cell. At the time of cell division, they duplicate, divide, and distribute evenly in the resulting cells.

chronic effects – See "long-term effects."

clear film – A film that after processing shows no image.

cleft palate – The developmental condition in which embryonic fusion of the palate fails to occur.

coherent scatter – An interaction of x-rays with matter in which the path of the x-ray is deviated without a loss of energy.

coin test – A test carried out in the darkroom to test the effectiveness of the safelighting.

collimation – The process of restricting the size and shape of the x-ray beam.

collimator – A device that limits the size and shape of the x-ray beam.

complementary metal oxide semiconductor (CMOS) – A type of electronic sensor used in digital radiography.

composite – Synthetic restoration primarily used in anterior regions.

Compton interaction – An interaction between x-rays and matter whereby the x-ray photon is deflected from its path after dislodging a loosely bound electron from an atom.

computed tomography (CT) – Tomographic process in which x-ray scanning produces digital data that measure the extent of the energy transmission through an object. This information is stored and transformed by a computer into a density scale that is used to generate an image.

concavity – A depression.

concha – The radiopaque outgrowth of tissue from the lateral walls of the nasal cavity.

concrescence– The condition in which two or more teeth are joined by their cementum.

condensing osteitis – A condition characterized by the formation of dense bone around the apex of a tooth in response to low-grade pulpal necrosis.

cone – The pointed position-indicating device on the dental x-ray machine through which the x-rays travel after leaving the tube.

cone cutting (collimator cutoff) – The error produced by not centering the x-ray beam on the film, producing unexposed areas on the film.

confidentiality – The state of being free from unauthorized disclosure. For example, material in a dental chart is confidential information.

congenital – A condition that is present at birth.

contrast – The difference in densities among adjacent areas on the radiograph.

coronal plane – An orientation plane that divides the head into front and back portions.

coronoid process – The radiopaque part of the mandible that is seen in the distal inferior portions of maxillary molar periapical radiographs.

cortical bone – The dense outer layer of the mandible and maxilla.

cosmic ray – Radiation that has its origin outside of the Earth's atmosphere (e.g., radiation from the sun).

coulombs/kg – The unit for expressing x-ray exposure in the SI system.

CRESO – Certified Radiation Equipment Safety Officer.

critical organ – An organ that if damaged by radiation will seriously affect a patient's quality of life.

cross-contamination – The spreading of microorganisms from one instrument or patient to another.

crown-root ratio – The relationship between the length of tooth that is embedded in bone and the part that is not.

CT number – A number indicating the density of a tissue on a CT scan.

cupping – The change of shape seen radiographically in the crest of the interseptal bone.

curie (Ci) – The unit of measurement of the number of nuclear disintegrations of a radioactive element. The curie was superseded by the becquerel in 1985.

cut – A tomographic plane.

cycle (of electric current) – The sine wave plot of the change in polarity of an alternating current circuit in which the current travels first in the positive direction and then in the negative direction.

cyst – A pathologic radiolucent lesion in which a bone cavity is lined by epithelium.

dark image – A dense or black image.

darkroom – A room with controlled lighting where x-ray film is handled and processed.

darkroom maintenance – Steps taken to ensure quality assurance in the darkroom.

daylight loader – The device attached to an automatic processor that allows the operator to develop film in ambient light.

deciduous – From the primary dentition.

definition (detail) – The degree of clarity on a radiograph.

dens invaginatus – A developmental disturbance whereby the enamel organ invaginates into the pulp of the tooth.

dense image – A dark or black image.

density (film) – The degree of blackness on a radiograph.

density (object) – The relative mass of an object through which an x-ray beam passes, making it appear radiopaque or radiolucent.

dent program (dental exposure normalization technique) – An exposure reduction and quality assurance program for radiologic health agencies developed by the Federal Center for Devices and Radiological Health.

dental papilla – Appears at the root apex as the newly erupted tooth progresses into the oral cavity.

dentigerous cyst – A cyst that develops from the enamel organ of a tooth. It may contain the tooth or be adjacent to it.

dentin – Comprises the major part of the tooth structure and is seen in both the crown and the root portions of the tooth. Dentin is radiopaque on radiographs.

dentoalveolar abscess – An abscess in bone resulting from a necrotic pulp.

detail – See "definition."

detector – See "sensor."

developer – The solution used in the processing of exposed x-ray film that precipitates silver from the silver bromide crystals of the film emulsion that have been energized by x-rays.

developer cutoff – The blank area on processed radiographs that results from an insufficient level of solution in the darkroom developer tank.

diaphragm – The doughnut-shaped, lead-collimating device found in the dental x-ray machine that limits the beam size.

differential diagnosis – The process that the diagnostician goes through with the use of radiographs, clinical examination, and patient history to formulate a diagnosis.

digital image – An image formed by a computer after the conversion of analog penetration data to digital expression.

digitize – Convert to numbers.

dilaceration – A developmental disturbance that results in an abnormally curved root.

dimensional accuracy – The accurate dimensional relationship of one part of a tooth to another.

dimensional distortion – The distortion seen in the bisecting-angle technique in which parts of the object farther from the film are foreshortened in relation to parts of the object that are closer to the film (e.g., the buccal roots of maxillary molars versus palatal root).

direct current (DC) – Electric current that flows in one direction and does not reverse itself.

direct digital radiography – Digital modality that involves use of a sensor wired directly to the computer, with the sensor being either a charged coupling device or a complementary metal oxide semiconductor.

direct effects of radiation – Radiation effects that are the results of the x-radiation striking the affected cell.

direct supervision – Referring to the physical presence of the dentist during a staff member's performance of duties.

disability – A physical or mental condition that limits or impairs a person's life activities.

disclosure – The process of informing the patient about the risks and benefits of a procedure.

disinfection – The process of destroying disease-causing microorganisms by physical or chemical means.

distodens – A supernumerary tooth seen distal to the third molar.

distortion – A change in the size or shape of an object seen on a radiograph.

divergent beam – The primary beam of x-radiation that spreads as it leaves the tube.

dose – The amount of radiation energy absorbed per unit mass of tissue at a particular site.

dose equivalent – A concept that allows for the fact that not all radiations are identical in biologic effects. The dose equivalent is expressed in rems or sieverts.

dose rate – The dose in rads or grays absorbed per unit of time.

dose-response curve – The plot of the effect of radiation as a function of the dose given.

double exposure – An error in which the same film packet is used twice, producing superimposed images.

double film packet – A dental film packet in which there are two pieces of film.

drying – A step in the processing of radiographs where any residual water is removed.

duplicating film – A reversal film used to replicate original images.

duty cycle – The number of seconds in a minute that a dental x-ray machine can be operated without overheating.

duty rating – The number of consecutive seconds in a minute that a dental x-ray machine can be operated without overheating.

effective focal area – The apparent size and shape of the focal spot when viewed from a position in the primary beam.

electric current – The flow of electricity through a circuit.

electromagnetic radiation spectrum – The spectrum of energy-bearing waves whose properties are determined by wavelength. X-rays are invisible electromagnetic radiations.

electron – A negatively charged particle, which is a constituent of every neutral atom.

electron cloud – The electrons at the cathode surrounding the tungsten filament.

electrostatic artifact – Black linear streaks on the radiograph caused by static electricity.

elongation – The distortion on a radiograph that results in lengthening of the image.

emulsion – The silver halide suspension in gelatin that is coated on the x-ray film base.

enamel – The radiopaque covering of the crown of the tooth.

enamel pearl – A small, rounded, hyperplastic area of enamel seen on the roots of the teeth.

enlargement – An increase in size of the image.

eruption – The emergence of teeth into the oral cavity.

exposure – A measure of the ionization in air produced by x-ray or gamma radiation.

exposure routine – The order in which films are taken.

exposure time – The amount of time, expressed in seconds or impulses, that x-rays are generated.

extension paralleling technique – A technique for intraoral radiography that uses a 16-in focal-film distance, film packet placement parallel to the long axis of the teeth, and a central ray direction perpendicular to both object and film.

external oblique ridge – A radiopaque line seen in mandibular posterior periapical radiographs.

external resorption – The idiopathic condition seen radiographically where the tissue from the periodontal ligament causes resorption of the dentin.

extraction socket – The radiolucent area on a radiograph that has not filled with bone after an extraction in the area.

extraoral films – Radiographs that are taken with the film outside the patient's mouth.

fallout – A form of background radiation produced by a nuclear explosion.

federal regulations – A set of regulations promulgated by the U.S. government governing the manufacture and performance of dental x-ray machines.

filament – The tungsten wire found at the cathode in the x-ray tube that when heated boils off electrons.

filling overhang – Poorly contoured filling that allows accumulation of debris.

film – A transparent sheet of cellulose acetate or a similar material that is coated on both sides with an emulsion sensitive to radiation and light.

film badge – A recording device worn to record one's exposure to ionizing radiation.

film base – The cellulose acetate sheet on which the emulsion is coated.

film contrast – The difference in the degrees of density.

film hanger – The device that carries the film through the processing procedure.

film-holding device – The device used to hold film in place for intraoral radiography.

film mount – A cardboard or plastic holder for finished radiographs.

film plane – The plane (axial, sagittal, or coronal) in which the film is held for radiographic exposure.

film position – The description of the relationship between the film and the teeth to be radiographed.

film reversal – The improper placement of the film packet in the patient's mouth that results in an underexposed film with geometric images (herringbone pattern), caused by the useful beam striking the lead foil backing before the film.

film roller – That part of an automatic processor that moves the film along from one step to another.

film speed (sensitivity) – An expression of how much radiation for a given period of time (mAs) is necessary to produce an image on film.

film viewing – The positioning of the finished radiographs on an illuminating device for reading and interpretation.

filter – An aluminum disk placed in the path of the useful beam that absorbs the softer, less penetrating radiations.

filtration – The removal of long (soft), nonpenetrating x-ray photons from the x-ray beam.

fixation – The localization of an object in three planes.

fixer – The solution used in the processing of exposed x-ray film that removes the unaffected silver bromide crystals from the emulsion and preserves the image.

flexible cassette – A cassette that can be wound around a drum for panoramic radiography.

floor of maxillary sinus – The radiopaque horizontal line seen above the apices of the maxillary premolars and molars on periapical films.

floor of nasal cavity – The horizontal radiopaque line seen on maxillary incisor and canine periapical films.

fluorescence – The property of emitting visible light when struck by radiation.

focal-film distance (FFD) – The distance from the focal spot (target) at the anode of the dental x-ray tube to the film. It is usually expressed in inches (e.g., an 8-in FFD).

focal spot – See "target."

focal trough – That plane of an object that is seen clearly on a tomogram.

fog – A detrimental density imparted to a radiographic image by the film base and chemical action on unexposed silver grains. Fog is increased by inadvertent exposure to white light.

foramen – A normal radiolucent opening in bone.

foreshortening – The distortion on a radiograph that results in shortening of the image.

fossa – A depression in bone.

fracture – The breaking of a part, usually resulting in a radiolucency.

Frankfort plane – The imaginary line connecting the floor of the orbit and the external auditory meatus.

free radical – An uncharged molecule that exists with a single unpaired electron in its outer shell.

frequency – The number of oscillations that an energy wave makes per second.

full-mouth survey – A series of intraoral radiographs that gives diagnostic information for all teeth and desired bony areas. It is usually composed of periapical and bitewing films.

furcation – The area between the roots of a multirooted tooth.

fusion – The developmental disturbance in which two teeth are joined, resulting in a large crown and two root canals.

gag reflex – The retching, coughing, or vomiting caused by contact of the film packet, holding device, or operator's fingers with the patient's palate or other intraoral tissues.

gamma rays – Electromagnetic radiation of short wavelengths that emanate from radioactive materials.

gelatin – The material coating the cellulose acetate base of film in which the halide crystals are suspended.

gemination – The developmental disturbance of teeth whereby a tooth has one root canal but two crowns.

gene – The basic unit of inheritance, located in the chromosome, which determines hereditary characteristics.

general supervision – Referring to the fact that the dentist need not be directly present during a licensed staff member's performance of duties.

genetic effects – The changes produced in an individual's genes and chromosomes; usually refers to those changes in reproductive cells.

genial tubercle – The radiopacity seen apical to the teeth on mandibular central incisor periapical radiographs.

ghost image – An artifact seen in panoramic radiography on which the image of the opposite side is superimposed on the side being radiographed.

gray (Gy) – The Système International (SI) unit for absorbed dose. One gray equals 100 rads.

gray level – The density seen on a digital image.

grid – A device used to prevent object scatter from affecting the film.

group D film – An ANSI rating for intermediate-speed film.

group E film – An ANSI rating for fast film.

group F film – An ANSI rating for the fastest film available.

H & D curve – The H & D (Hunter and Driffield) curve is a plot that shows the relationship between film exposure and its resultant density.

half-value layer – The thickness of a specific material that attenuates the x-ray beam intensity to one half. It is an expression of beam quality.

half-wave rectified – The blocking of the reversal of current across the dental x-ray tube.

halide – Compound of metal with the halogen element bromine, chlorine, or iodine.

hard copy – The printout of a digital image.

headrest position – Proper position of the patient's head for radiographic exposure.

Health Insurance Portability and Accountability Act (HIPAA) – Enacted in April 2000 to ensure patient confidentiality in healthcare delivery.

hearing-impaired – Physical disability that affects a person's ability to hear efficiently.

hemostat – An instrument that can serve as an intraoral film holder.

hepatitis – Infectious disease caused by the hepatitis virus. Dental personnel should be immunized (vaccinated) for the hepatitis B virus (HBV).

horizontal angulation – The aiming of the x-ray beam in the horizontal plane.

horizontal bone loss – Interproximal periodontal bone loss in the horizontal plane.

Hounsfield unit – A unit used in computed tomographic scanning to express the density of a specific area of the image.

human immunodeficiency virus (HIV) – The virus that compromises the immune system, leading to acquired immunodeficiency syndrome (AIDS).

hypercementosis – A condition that results in formation of excess cementum on the root of a tooth.

hyperostotic line – Clearly defined borders of slow-growing benign lesions.

illuminator – See "viewbox."

image – A picture or representation of an object.

image acquisition – Acquisition of a computerized image in computed tomographic scanning and digital radiography.

image layer – See "focal trough."

image manipulation – The changing or modification of a digital image.

image receptor – The component of an imaging system that the x-ray photons strike.

imaginary bisecting line – The line that bisects the angle formed by the long axis of the tooth and the film packet.

imaging plate – Reusable plastic storage phosphor sensor that is not wired to the computer but uses a laser scanner to produce an image.

imaging system – The film, "digital sensor," or film-screen combination that the x-rays strike to produce the visible image.

immunization – Protection of an individual from a communicable disease achieved by giving the patient a modified or weakened form of the causative microorganism.

impaction – The condition of a tooth not erupting by its expected time.

implant fixture – The radiopaque metallic device that is placed in a maxilla or mandible.

impulse – The radiation generated during a half cycle of alternating current.

incipient caries – Caries that radiographically is only in the enamel.

incisive foramen – See "nasopalatine foramen."

indirect digital radiography – A kind of digital radiography in which the finished radiograph is scanned to produce a digital image.

indirect effects – Cell damage caused when the cells hit directly by radiation produce toxins that affect cells not in the radiation beam.

infection – Contamination caused by disease-producing microorganisms.

infectious waste – Waste that is contaminated with blood, saliva, or other body fluids.

inferior alveolar canal – The radiolucent band seen on mandibular molar and premolar radiographs.

informed consent – The permission granted or implied by the patient to allow treatment to be rendered after a full explanation of the treatment has been made.

infrabony pocket – The area created and seen on radiographs as the result of crestal bone loss.

intensifying screen – A coating of fluorescent material on a suitable base that intensifies the radiation, thus permitting a decrease in exposure time.

intensity – The product of the quantity and the quality of the x-ray beam per unit of area per time of exposure.

interaction – The result of radiation reacting with any form of matter.

internal alveolar canal – Seen as a radiolucent band below the apices of the posterior teeth.

internal oblique ridge (mylohyoid ridge) – The radiopaque line that is seen running anteriorly on radiographs from the ascending ramus to the genial tubercles of the mandible.

internal resorption – The process in which pulpal cells resorb the walls of the pulp chamber or canal to form a communication to the periodontal ligament.

interpretation – An explanation of radiographic findings.

interproximal caries – Caries on the mesial or distal surfaces of teeth that are best viewed on bitewing radiographs.

intraoffice peer review – Mechanism for maintaining superior levels of chairside technique within a dental office.

inverse square law – An expression of the relationship between the exposure time and focal-film distance. This law states that the intensity of radiation is inversely proportional to the square of the distance between a point source and the irradiated surface.

ion – An electrically charged (+ or −) particle of matter.

ionization – The process by which an electrically stable or neutral atom or molecule gains or loses electrons and thereby acquires a positive or negative charge.

ionizing radiation – The property of radiation that produces ions when interacting with matter.

isotope – An atom whose nucleus has the same number of protons but a different number of neutrons.

kilovolt (kV) – A unit of measurement equal to 1000 V.

kilovolt peak (kVp) – A unit of measurement used in dental radiology to express the kilovoltage setting on the control panel. It implies that not all the x-rays generated are of the penetrating power called for; rather, the numerical setting is the peak.

labial mounting – A means of mounting and viewing processed radiographs so that the observer's point of view is looking into the patient's mouth with the patient's right side on the viewer's left.

lamina dura – A radiopaque line of cortical bone that surrounds the periodontal ligament.

laminogram (tomogram) – A radiograph of a three-dimensional object that shows a predetermined plane clearly while blurring out all other superimposed structures.

latent image – The term used to describe the x-ray film after it has been exposed. The film contains the latent image that will be made visible by film processing.

latent period – The delay between exposure of an organism to radiation and manifestation of change produced by that radiation.

lateral fossa – A depression in the labial plate in the maxillary lateral incisor region. It appears as a radiolucency between the maxillary lateral incisor and canine.

lateral oblique projection of the mandible – Projection used for surveying one side of the mandible.

lateral skull projection – An extraoral radiograph that shows the entire skull in the sagittal plane.

lead apron – The flexible lead or lead-equivalent drape placed over the patient's torso to shield from secondary radiation.

lead foil backing – One of the components of the intraoral x-ray packet that prevents backscatter.

lead-lined boxes – Shielded boxes for unprotected film that over time may contaminate the film with an oxidized leaded white powder.

liability – The responsibility for a deed or decision.

licensure – The permission granted by a governmental body that allows one to work in his or her profession.

light leak – The area where unwanted white light is entering a darkroom.

light-tight – A term used in radiography to indicate that there is no white light in the room.

line pairs per millimeter – A measure of contrast discrimination (gray levels) in an image.

lingual caries – Demineralization of the hard tooth structure on the lingual surface of a tooth.

lingual foramen – A radiolucent opening in the lingual surface of the mandibular anterior bony structure.

lingual mounting – A means of mounting and viewing processed radiographs so that the observer's point of view is looking at the teeth from within the patient's mouth with the patient's right side on the viewer's right.

litigious – Tending to bring legal action.

localization – Locating radiographic structures, particularly in the buccolingual plane.

localized exposure – The measurement of radiation to the area of the body that is in the path of the direct beam of radiation.

localizing ring – That part of an intraoral film-holding device that aligns the x-ray beam with the film or sensor.

long axis – The imaginary line that divides the tooth vertically in two halves.

long cone – Used to refer to position-indicating devices on x-ray machines where focal-film distance is 16 in or greater.

long-scale contrast – Film contrast in which the gray tone is predominant.

long-term effects – Effects of radiation that appear years or decades after exposure to radiation.

magnetic field – The field used in MRI that changes the alignment and orientation of the protons in the patient's body.

magnetic resonance imaging (MRI) – An imaging modality that uses magnetic fields and radio frequencies to view pathologic lesions in soft tissues of the body.

magnification – The proportional enlargement of a radiographic image.

malignancy – A type of tumor that can be locally destructive or metastasize and can result in a fatality.

malposed – A tooth that is out of line with the dental arch.

mandibular canal – See "inferior alveolar canal."

manual processing – The process of developing radiographs where the film hangers are manually placed in the solutions.

marking grid – The device used to superimpose either radiopaque or radiolucent lines in 1-mm vertical and horizontal increments.

mass number – The number of nucleons (protons and neutrons) in the nucleus of an atom.

maxillary sinus – The radiolucent area seen apical to the maxillary posterior teeth.

maxillary tuberosity – The distal portion of the maxillary alveolar ridge.

maximum permissible dose (MPD) – The amount of yearly whole-body radiation to which an occupationally exposed person can be exposed without any harm.

median palatal suture – The radiolucent line seen running vertically between the roots of the maxillary central incisors.

medullary space – A radiolucent area seen in bone representing the bone marrow.

mental foramen – The round radiolucent area seen near the apices of the mandibular premolars.

mental ridge – The V-shaped radiopacity seen in mandibular anterior radiographs.

mesiodens – A supernumerary tooth found in the midline.

metabolic lesion – A radiographic finding caused by a generalized pathologic condition.

microorganism – An organism, such as bacteria, of microscopic or ultramicroscopic size.

midsagittal plane – The imaginary line that divides the skull in equal parts in the sagittal plane.

milliampere (mA) – One thousandth of an ampere.

milliroentgen (mR) – One thousandth of a roentgen.

mixed lesion – A radiographic lesion that has both radiolucent and radiopaque components.

molecule – The smallest particle of a substance that retains the properties of the substance.

monitor – Computer image screen used in digital radiography.

monitoring device – The instrument that measures radiation exposure.

mount – The cardboard or plastic sheet used to hold and view a finished radiograph.

mutation – The chemical effect of a change in a gene or a chromosomal aberration.

mylohyoid ridge – See "internal oblique ridge."

nasal cavity – The bilateral radiolucent areas seen superior to the maxillary central incisors.

nasal septum – The opaque vertical line separating the right and left nasal cavities.

nasopalatine foramen – The oval radiolucent landmark located between the roots of the maxillary central incisors.

negligence – Failure to exercise the care that a prudent person would usually exercise in the same situation.

neutron – A particle that has no charge but has mass. It is found in the nucleus of an atom.

nucleus – The positively charged, relatively heavy inner core of an atom.

nutrient canals – Pathways for blood vessels and nerves that appear as radiolucent vertical lines in alveolar bone.

object – The structure being radiographed, such as tooth or bone.

object-film distance – The distance between the object and the x-ray film.

occlusal caries – Caries that are found on the biting surfaces of teeth and are usually not seen well on radiographs.

occlusal film – A large piece of intraoral film placed on the occlusal surfaces of either upper or lower teeth and used to portray objects in the third dimension.

occlusal plane – The imaginary plane formed by the occlusal contact of upper and lower teeth.

occlusal projection – A radiographic projection of the mandible or maxilla that shows either a larger object area or a right-angle (axial) relationship of the objects.

Occupational Safety and Health Administration (OSHA) – The federal agency that oversees health and safety in the workplace.

open contact – When the interproximal surfaces of teeth or restorations do not touch.

operator concern – Radiation concerns that lie with the operator.

optical scanning – The process in indirect digital imaging whereby a finished radiograph is scanned and then digitized and the information is sent to the computer.

orbit – A prescribed path or ring in which electrons travel around the nucleus of an atom.

output – The amount of radiation produced by the x-ray machine (measured in roentgens per second).

overdeveloped – The condition of a radiograph being too dark because of the film's having been left in the developer bath too long.

overexposed – The condition of a film's being dark or dense owing to excessive exposure (overpenetration) resulting from decreased film-focal distance or excessive kilovolt peak, milliamperage, or exposure time.

overlapping – The state of the interproximal surfaces of adjoining teeth being superimposed on each other because of improper horizontal angulation.

overretention – The state of the deciduous teeth not being shed at the expected time.

packet – A wrapping or container for intraoral x-ray film that is light-tight and permits penetration of x-rays. Packets are usually made of paper or cardboard.

panoramic film – An extraoral radiograph that shows both the mandible and the maxilla in their entirety on a single film.

Panorex – The commercial name for one of the earliest panoramic units.

pantomogram – A panoramic radiograph produced by curved surface tomography.

paperless office – A dental office where all records, including radiographs and photographs, are produced and stored in digital form on a computer.

parallel – Moving or lying in the same plane, equidistant, and never intersecting.

paralleling technique – A technique for intraoral periapical radiography in which the film packet is positioned parallel to the long axis of the tooth and the central ray is directed perpendicular to both tooth and film packet.

pathogen – A disease-causing microorganism.

patient concern – Radiation concerns that lie with the patient.

patient movement – The artifact introduced into a radiograph when a patient moves during an exposure.

penetration – The ability of x-rays to pass through an object and reach the film.

penumbra – The vague or blurred area that surrounds the edge of the radiographic image.

periapical abscess – A type of periapical pathologic process whereby an abscess forms at the apex of a tooth.

periapical cemental dysplasia – A three-stage asymptomatic lesion seen on periapical radiographs.

periapical condensing osteitis – The apical bony response to low-level infection.

periapical cyst – A cyst formed at the apex of a tooth.

periapical film – Intraoral film that is used to image the complete tooth and the surrounding structures.

periapical granuloma – A granuloma formed at the apex of a tooth.

periapical lesion – Radiolucent or radiopaque lesion appearing at the apex of the tooth.

periapical pathologic condition – The infectious condition that arises at the apex of a tooth as the sequela of pulpal necrosis.

periapical radiograph – An intraoral film that shows the entire tooth and surrounding bony structures.

periodontal abscess – A soft tissue abscess of the gingiva that is seen as a radiolucency interproximally on radiographs.

periodontal disease – Disease of the supportive structures of the teeth.

periodontal ligament – Radiolucent area around the root of the tooth between the cementum and the lamina dura.

permissible dose – The amount of radiation that one can receive without suffering any clinical effects.

perpendicular – Intersecting or meeting at a 90-degree angle.

phosphor – A substance that when struck by radiation will emit light.

photoelectron effect – An interaction of an x-ray photon with an atom in which an inner shell electron is released and the total energy of the photon is absorbed.

photon – A discrete unit of energy.

photostimulable phosphor plate – An electronic sensor used in indirect digital radiography that is read by a laser beam scanner.

physical disability – A condition that limits the patient's ability to perform certain movements.

pixel – A discrete point of information.

pocket dosimeters – Small ionization chambers that the operator wears to measure radiation occupational exposure.

point of entry – Anatomic location on the patient's face at which the central x-ray is aimed so that the x-rays strike the center of the film in the patient's mouth.

point of rotation – A point in a tomographic unit around which the sensor and source of energy rotate.

position-indicating device (PID) – That part of the x-ray machine (cone, rectangle, or cylinder) that aligns the useful beam to the object and film.

posteroanterior projection – The companion projection to the lateral skull used to survey the skull in the anteroposterior plane, which provides a means of localizing changes in a mediolateral direction.

pregnancy – The condition in which a woman is carrying a fetus in her womb.

primary dentition – The first (deciduous) set of teeth.

primary radiation – X-rays coming directly from the target of the x-ray tube.

primordial cyst – A cyst seen in the jaws that forms instead of a tooth.

progeny – The descendants of an individual.

proton – A positively charged particle that has mass. It is found in the nucleus of an atom.

pulp calcification – The condition in which the pulp canals and chamber are completely filled with dentin.

pulp canal and chamber – The space within the crown and root of the tissue where the soft tissue of the pulp is found.

pulp denticle (calcification) – A calcification formed in either the pulp chamber or the pulp canal.

quality assurance (QA) – A series of tests and procedures to ensure that all components of the radiographic system are functioning at an acceptable level of quality so as to ensure the best radiograph for the radiation exposure.

quality factor – An expression of the different types of effects that radiation produces in human tissue (for x-rays, $Q = 1$).

radiation – The emission and propagation of energy in the form of waves or particles.

radiation absorbed dose (rad) – A unit of absorbed radiation equal to 100 ergs per gram. In dental radiology, 1 rad is equal to approximately 1 roentgen.

radiation caries – The type of caries caused by a decrease and changes in saliva secondary to radiation therapy of the head and neck.

radiation exposure – The process of being struck by radiation, either primary or secondary.

radiation history – The record of a patient's exposure to radiation for diagnostic and therapeutic needs.

radiation inspection – The monitoring of x-ray equipment and procedures by some governmental body or CRESO.

radiation risk – The likelihood of ill effects from radiation.

radioactive process – The process whereby certain unstable elements undergo spontaneous degeneration and produce high-energy waves called *gamma* and *particulate radiations*.

radio frequency – The frequency in the electromagnetic spectrum at which radio waves are found.

radiograph – The visual image produced by chemically processing the effects of x-rays on film.

radiolucent – Refers to areas on the radiograph that appear dark.

radiolucent lesion – A pathologic lesion that is dark on radiographs.

radionuclide – A radioactive substance.

radiopaque – Refers to areas on the radiograph that appear light.

radiopaque lesion – A pathologic lesion that is light on radiographs.

radiopaque medium – A liquid that is injected into body vessels or spaces whose outline is radiopaque on the radiograph.

radioresistant cell – A cell that is relatively unaffected by radiation.

radiosensitive cell – A cell that is sensitive to radiation.

rapid processing – The processing of radiographs by either elevated solution temperature or concentration, which markedly shortens the time needed to produce an image.

rare earth elements – A group of metallic elements that contain oxides classified as rare earths. Such elements are used in intensifying screens to produce light.

receptor – The material (film, film screen, or digital sensor) that is affected by the x-ray beam and from which the visible image is formed.

receptor holder – The device that holds and positions the receptor (e.g., film) in the patient's mouth.

recessed target – The design of a dental x-ray machine in which the tube is positioned at the back of the tube head that allows for a 16-in focal-film distance and a short position-indicating device (PID).

recessed tube – An x-ray tube that is placed in the rear part of the tube head, with the rest of the components placed on both sides of the beam. This design extends the focal distance without increasing the length of the position-indicating device.

records – The written or electronic description and images of treatment given to a patient.

rectangular collimation – Limiting the shape of an x-ray beam to a rectangle instead of the conventional circle.

rectification – Blocking of the flow of current in one direction in an alternating current circuit.

reference film – An ideally processed film, which is kept on the darkroom viewbox, to which densities can be compared to check processing solutions.

reformatting – In computed tomography, changing the plane of orientation in which the image is portrayed.

replenisher – A concentrated form of either the developer or fixer solutions that is used to maintain concentrations of the solutions.

residual cyst – A cyst that was not removed with the extraction of the tooth and continues to grow.

residual granuloma – A granuloma that was not removed with the extraction of the tooth and continues to grow.

resolution – The discernible separation of closely adjacent image details.

resonance – The transition from one energy level to another.

respondent superior – The legal doctrine that states that liability, both professionally and legally, rests with the dentist and not the hygienist or dental assistant.

retake – The repeating of a nondiagnostic exposure.

reticulation – An unsatisfactory image caused by a sudden change in temperature from one processing bath to another.

reverse bitewing – A variation of a bitewing whereby the film is placed in the buccal sulcus and the central rays directed at the film from the other side of the jaw as in a lateral oblique projection.

ridge – A radiopaque line representing extra bone seen on radiographs.

right-angle technique (projection) – See "paralleling technique."

risk estimate – The comparing of the presence of a finding between irradiated and nonirradiated populations.

risk management – Office procedures and policies that reduce the likelihood of litigation.

roentgen (R) – The basic unit for measuring x-ray (ionizing radiation) exposure in air. It is the amount of radiation needed to produce one electrostatic charge in 1 cm^3 of air. The milliroentgen (mR) is one thousandth of a roentgen.

roentgen equivalent man (rem) – The expression of dose equivalent; the dose of radiation that produces the same biologic effects in humans as are produced by 1 roentgen of x-radiation. For x-rays the rem equals the rad.

root resorption – The destruction of the root structure by some process.

root sack – The radiolucent ball seen at the apices of developing teeth.

RVG – One of the earliest dental digital units to be put on the market.

safelight – Illumination used in the darkroom that does not affect the film emulsion.

sagittal plane of head – A vertical longitudinal plane that divides the head into right and left sections.

scanner – A device that senses the grayscales of a radiograph and records it in the digital form for a printout or computer storage.

scatter radiation – Radiation that during its passage through a substance has been deviated in direction. It also may have been modified by an increase in wave-length. It is one form of secondary radiation.

secondary dentin – Dentin produced by the pulp in response to an irritation or aging.

secondary radiation – Radiation that comes from any matter being struck by primary radiation. Secondary x-rays are less penetrating than primary x-rays.

selection criteria – Those factors that dictate whether radiographs are necessary and useful in a specific clinical situation.

self- or half-wave–rectified – The blocking of the reversal of a current (rectification) that the dental x-ray tube is designed to produce.

sensor – An electronic detector plate that is placed in the patient's mouth to record the penetrating x-ray photons in digital radiography.

septa – Radiopaque lines seen dividing bony spaces.

shell – See "orbit."

shielding – Preventing or reducing the passage of radiation.

short cone – A position-indicating device on dental x-ray machines for which focal-film distance is 8 in.

short-scale contrast – A reduced range of grays on a radiograph (i.e., high contrast).

sialography – A modality for radiographic visualization of salivary glands following the injection of a contrast medium into the salivary ducts.

sialolith – A salivary calcification (stone).

sievert (Sv) – The Système International (SI) unit for the dose equivalent. One sievert equals 100 rem.

sight development – An unacceptable film-processing technique in which the time the film stays in the developer is determined by periodically looking at the developing image under safelight conditions.

signal intensity – The strength of the radiofrequency wave that comes from the patient back to the detector in magnetic resonance imaging.

silver bromides (halide) – The x-ray–sensitive crystals used in the film emulsion.

sinus – A radiolucent cavity in bone.

slit beam – An extremely narrow, rectangular x-ray beam used in pantomography.

soft tissue window – A density range seen in computed tomographic scans that portrays mainly soft tissue.

soft x-rays – X-rays of longer wavelengths and low penetration.

software – A computer program.

somatic effects – Effects of radiation on all cells except the reproductive cells.

standard of care – The quality of care that is provided by dental practitioners in a similar location under the same or similar conditions.

statute of limitations – The period of time in which a patient can bring suit against a dentist or dental health professional.

step-down transformer – A transformer designed to decrease the voltage.

step-up transformer – A transformer designed to increase the voltage.

step wedge – The device used to measure the penetration of a dental x-ray beam.

sterilization – The process used to destroy all pathogens, including highly resistant bacteria and spores.

stop bath – The solution (water in x-ray processing) in which films are placed after the developer.

storage phosphor – A type of indirect digital radiography that uses photostimulable phosphor plate technology.

submandibular fossa – The broad radiolucent band seen apical to the mandibular molars that represents a medial bone depression.

submentovertex – An extraoral projection whereby jaws are seen from an inferior view.

Système International (SI) units – The units of radiation measurement that standardize measurement to the metric system.

target – That part of the anode that the high-speed electrons strike and that produces x-rays and heat. In dental x-ray tubes, the target usually is made of tungsten.

taurodontia – A developmental defect of teeth in which the crowns have longitudinally enlarged pulp chambers with short roots.

temporomandibular joint – The joint formed by the articulation of the mandibular condyle and the temporal bone of the maxilla.

tesla (T) – The unit of measurement for the strength of the magnetic field in an MRI unit.

thermionic emission effect – Production of free electrons by the passing of an electric current through a tungsten filament with resultant heating of the filament.

thermometer – The device found in the developer solution used to measure the temperature of the solution.

thermostatic valve – A device used to control the temperature of the incoming water in the developing tanks.

thin image – A light image, lacking in density.

threshold erythema dose (TED) – The minimal dose of radiation to the skin that will produce a reddening of the skin on the most sensitive patient's skin.

thyroid collar – The lead drape put around the patient's neck to shield the thyroid gland during intraoral radiographic procedures.

timer – The parameter on the x-ray unit control panel that regulates the exposure time.

time-temperature technique – A technique used to process x-ray films in which the time the film stays in the developer is calibrated to the temperature of the solution within a stated acceptable range.

tissue sensitivity – That scale of sensitivity of various tissues in the body to radiation. Some tissues (e.g., epithelium) are very radiosensitive, whereas others (e.g., bone) are relatively radioresistant.

tomogram – A radiograph of a three-dimensional object that shows a predetermined plane with blurring of all other superimposed structures.

tomography – A radiographic modality that allows imaging in one plane of an object while blurring or eliminating images from structures in other planes.

topographic projection – A type of occlusal radiographic technique that shows a large area, although the image may be distorted.

torn emulsion – Film-processing error that occurs when the emulsion is removed from the acetate base in a finished radiograph.

total body exposure – The radiation dosage that reflects the effects on the whole body of the person exposed.

trabecula – Radiopaque line separating marrow spaces in bone.

trabecular pattern – The expression of the radiographic appearance of alveolar bone.

transcranial projection – An extraoral projection used to visualize the temporomandibular joint.

transformer – An electric device that can either increase (step up) or decrease (step down) voltage.

transposed – Tooth development in another position in the dental arch.

triangulation – A description of the shape of interproximal bone loss.

trismus – The state of being unable to open one's mouth.

tube head drift – Drift of the x-ray tube head from its set position.

tube head leakage – Leakage of x-rays from an area in the tube head other than the port.

tube shift – A technique used to localize objects in the buccolingual plane by shifting the tube for a comparative radiograph.

tuberosity – A normal anatomic bony protrusion.

ultrasound – Mechanical radiant energy above the audible range used in diagnostic imaging.

umbra – The sharp area that surrounds the edge of the radiographic image.

underdevelopment – A thin (light) film that is the result of weak solutions or incorrect developing time.

underexposed – The condition of a film's being light or thin as a result of insufficient exposure time, inadequate kVp or mA, or excessive FFD.

unilateral lesion – A lesion seen only on one side of a patient.

universal precautions – An infection control protocol that is followed for all patients regardless of history and clinical findings.

useful beam – The part of the primary radiation that passes through the diaphragm aperture and filter and exits through the position-indicating device.

vaccination – The introduction of vaccine (i.e., a weakened, dead, or genetically altered form of a microorganism) for the purpose of inducing immunity.

vertical angulation – The angle made between the x-ray beam and a line parallel to the floor.

vertical bitewing – Bitewing projection in which the film is placed in the patient's mouth with the long dimension running vertically.

vertical bone loss – Interproximal bone loss in periodontal disease in the vertical plane.

viewbox – An illuminated device used to view radiographs.

visually impaired – A person who has lost all or part of the ability to see.

vitality testing – The technique that uses either thermal or electrical stimulation to determine whether a tooth is vital or nonvital.

voltage – The difference in potential in an electric circuit. It is this difference that causes the current to flow.

water bath – The second and fourth solution (water) in the processing of dental radiographs.

Waters' view – The type of posteroanterior extraoral projection that enlarges the middle third of the skull to prevent superimposition, usually used for viewing the maxillary sinus.

wavelength – The distance from the crest of one wave to the crest of the next wave. In radiology, wavelength is a measure of energy.

wet reading – Interpretation of a radiograph approximately 3 minutes after its initial fixation.

wheelchair access – The design of an office that permits unrestricted access and placement of all patients.

x-rays – Penetrating electromagnetic radiations having wavelengths shorter than those of visible light and that are produced by bombarding a metal target with high-speed electrons.

zygoma – The radiopaque bone seen apical to the maxillary molars.

zygomatic process – The cranial bone that runs from the maxilla distally to the temporal bone.

INDEX

Note: Page numbers followed by "*b*" indicate boxes; "*f*" indicate figures.